"The best and most up-to-date resource for men who want to understand and enjoy their sexuality."

—Richard C. Reznichek, M.D., Assistant Clinical Professor
of Surgery/Urology, UCLA

"This is an excellent self-help book and information source for men of all ages. It is a guide to breaking out of the old, restrictive model of male sexuality. It is a treatise for becoming a richer and more humane person."

—*Contemporary Psychology*

"The best practical guide I've seen for anyone—male or female, young or old, coupled or single—who wants better relationships and better sex."

—Sandra L. Caron, Ph.D., Associate Professor of Family Relations/
Human Sexuality, University of Maine

"Bernie Zilbergeld has done it again. He has written another comprehensive and up-to-date book with a great combination of theoretical and practical knowledge. I recommend it highly for men seeking good information on sexual matters."

—Ira D. Sharlip, M.D., Pan Pacific Urology, San Francisco
Secretary, Society for the Study of Impotence, Inc.

"For years, I have prescribed to *The New Male Sexuality* for my patients with sexual dysfunction and their partners, with fabulous feedback. Recently our understanding of erectile dysfunction and its treatment has evolved dramatically. Bernie Zilbergeld takes a great book and incorporates this new knowledge into an up-to-date guide that provides useful information for every man and woman, which will be relevant and beneficial well into the twenty-first century."

—Ken Goldberg, M.D., founder and director of the Male Health Institute
and author of *When the Man You Love Won't Take Care of His Health*

"This book will be an aid for helping men and women get along better sexually and more sensitively. It dispels many harmful myths, it is a peaceful, and informed approach to very delicate subject matter. No man who wants to understand himself and his partner should be without this book."

—John Gottman, Ph.D., Professor, University of Washington, and author
of *Seven Principles for Making Marriage Work*

"This book sets a new standard in popular books on male sexuality. Dr. Zilbergeld brings a lifetime of experience to bear on the subject, and has provided men of all ages a well-balanced, and completely up-to-date perspective on the topic. It is must-reading for anyone with questions or concerns about the subject."

—Raymond C. Rosen, Ph.D., author of *Sexuality in Modern Life* and
Patterns of Sexual Arousal

THE · NEW
MALE
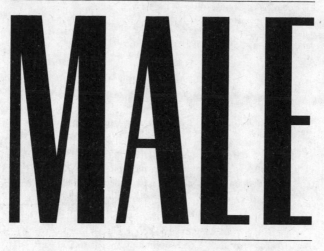

SEXUALITY

—REVISED EDITION—

Bernie Zilbergeld, Ph.D.

BANTAM BOOKS
New York Toronto London Sydney Auckland

THE NEW MALE SEXUALITY—REVISED EDITION
A Bantam Book
PUBLISHING HISTORY
Bantam hardcover edition published July 1992
Bantam paperback edition published June 1993
Bantam revised trade paperback edition / July 1999

Library of Congress Cataloging-in-Publication Data
Zilbergeld, Bernie.
The new male sexuality / Bernie Zilbergeld.—Rev. ed.
p.   cm.
Includes bibliographical references.
ISBN 0-553-38042-7
1. Sex instruction for men.   2. Sex role.   3. Masculinity.
I. Title.
HQ36.Z55   1999   99-12946
613.9'6'081—dc21   CIP

Published simultaneously in the United States and Canada

Bantam Books are published by Bantam Books, a division of Random House,
Inc. Its trademark, consisting of the words "Bantam Books" and the portrayal
of a rooster, is Registered in U.S. Patent and Trademark Office and in other
countries. Marca Registrada. Bantam Books, 1540 Broadway, New York, New
York 10036.

PRINTED IN THE UNITED STATES OF AMERICA

20 19 18 17 16 15 14

For Ian, with love

and the hope that the boys and girls of your generation
will grow up to enjoy a safer, saner, more loving,
and more fulfilling sexuality

Contents

RESOLVING PROBLEMS

Introduction

This book is for any man or woman who wants to know more about the sexual development, thoughts, feelings, behavior, and potential of men. It's for those in relationships and those not, those currently having sex with a partner and those who aren't. It's for those who want information, those who want advice and exercises on how to make sex better, and those who want help in resolving sexual problems.

For men interested in love and sex—and I assume that means virtually all of us—these are challenging yet exciting times. They're challenging because masculinity itself seems to be under attack. We are told over and over that we are overly aggressive, unexpressive, and insensitive brutes who think with our genitals and don't have any idea of what real life is about. For those who don't fit this description, well, they're just passive wimps who have neither balls nor a clue as to what real life is about. After all, what do you expect of a man?

Challenging because all the other rules of relating and sex have gone the way of the dinosaur. I was reminded of this by a fifty-two-year-old client who was dating again after the death of his wife. He was "shaken to the roots," as he put it, by the behavior of a woman he had had three dates with. She took the lead in every way. She was the one who asked for the first date, initiated the first kiss, invited him to spend the night, and orchestrated every move of their sexual activity.

In bed she acted like I thought only men were supposed to act. Touch me here, lick me there, let me put this condom on you, let's move over here, turn around, take me this way, now let's switch to that way. I have never in my whole life done so many different things and been in so many positions. I had two fantastic orgasms and have nothing to complain about. But my question is, what am I, as the man, supposed to be doing?

It's not that all women are behaving more aggressively. Many are not, but in a way that only makes things more confusing. As a forty-four-year-old client put it:

The one sure thing I know about life right now is that it's bewildering. It's not clear what it means to be a man or a woman, how to have a relationship, or even how to act in bed. I see lots of people trying to get clear by reading John Gray's books, but I don't think that helps. Things are in flux; there are no answers. While I know that's the truth, I wish it were otherwise. It's so much hassle the way it is.

Challenging, too, because men and women alike are experiencing grave difficulties in making relationships work. Half or more of marriages end in divorce, and I don't know anyone who would argue that singles and live-ins are any happier. An old-fashioned guy might say, "So what's that have to do with sex?" The answer, as more and more men are understanding, is practically everything. Good sex usually takes place within the context of a good relationship. And despite propaganda to the contrary, men are heavily dependent on their relationships with women. If these relationships are not going well, that in itself is a problem.

But life and this book are about more than challenges and problems. There are also many opportunities and sources of excitement for today's man.

NEW SOLUTIONS FOR MEN'S SEXUAL PROBLEMS

The last ten years have been a period of intense creativity and progress in the study of male sexuality. The new solutions that have had the most media presence have been the pharmaceutical ones, especially Viagra.

Viagra is not the first pharmaceutical sexual aid. Far from it. But this blue pill caught the public imagination like no other drug. In the three months after its introduction on April 10, 1998, three million prescriptions were filled, making it the most popular drug ever introduced in America. Men who wouldn't have dreamed of injecting a drug into their penises to induce erection were clearly more than happy to pop a pill.

Viagra is changing not only the state of some men's erections but also how we think of sex. The penis, which was always conceded to have a mind of its own, is being brought under voluntary control. For better or worse, being too old, too tired, too anxious, or too upset no longer need keep a man from getting erect. This in itself is not sufficient, of course, to guarantee good sex, but there's no question that Viagra has been a godsend to many men who had thought their sex lives were over.

Although the media, having discovered the term *impotence,* can't seem to repeat it often enough (as in "the impotence pill Viagra"), the effects of Viagra extend far beyond men who might be considered impotent. For example, some men are using it to overcome their "stage fright" the first time or two with a new partner. And listen to this man's account of his weekend escapades:

I think I'm starting to show the effects of age even though I'm not yet forty. Tania and I have had this ritual since the beginning of going away every few months for a weekend of sex. But in the last year or two I found that by the last day, my mind is willing, as they say, but the flesh is weak. It's not the end of the world. I can always use my fingers or tongue on her, but there are times I'd really like to be inside her again. Viagra does the trick. No matter how many times we've already fucked, it always gets me another hard-on.

As I write these pages, clinical trials are starting on the use of Viagra in women. What a brave new world seems in the offing, with Viagra-aroused men coupling with Viagra-enhanced women.

New solutions have also emerged for the other perennial sex problem for men: staying power. Since the 1950s there have been sexual exercises that a man could use with his partner to learn better ejaculatory control. While these exercises are effective, they require time and effort. In the first edition of this book I said only a few cautious words about a then recent development, the use of small doses of antidepressant drugs to help men last longer. Although these drugs seemed effective with some of my clients, there hadn't been much research and I didn't want to raise unrealistic expectations. But in the intervening years it has been demonstrated that they do indeed work, either on their own or as part of a sex therapy program.

Nondrug sex therapy has also become far more sophisticated and effective since it was introduced by Masters and Johnson in the early 1970s. Over the past twenty-five years, a wide range of new therapeutic methods has been incorporated—including various cognitive therapy interventions, eye movement desensitization and reprocessing (EMDR), meditation, neurolinguistic programming, and relaxation training—to deal with fears, traumas, and relationship difficulties. Where appropriate, traditional and newer tools of sex therapy are used in combination with Viagra and other chemical helpers.

In short—as you'll see in the pages that follow—there's hope for almost every man and every couple with a sexual problem.

BETTER UNDERSTANDING OF RELATIONSHIPS

Sex therapy has also been powerfully enhanced by our better understanding of relationships, and it is one of the primary goals of this revised edition to show what it takes to have the kind of relationship that supports and encourages satisfying sex. It has become abundantly clear that—very short flings with strangers or near strangers aside—good sex depends on having a decent relationship. Although men aren't always happy to hear this, you simply cannot have good sex in the long run when partners don't know each other, don't spend a lot of fun time together, and don't regularly show their care and concern for each other. When sex therapy fails, the most common reason by far is not a lack of therapeutic technology or therapist skill, but rather a strained relationship. Even Viagra has failed to make a difference in some cases; yes, it produced erections, but it didn't make the partners want to make love, or automatically create good sex.

In this new edition, I draw on the brilliant work of John Gottman, of the University of Washington, who has been studying couples for twenty-five years. Gottman has given us what we never before had: real data about how happy couples interact and how their behavior differs from that of discontented couples. As a result, I am now able to pass along not only my own observations from twenty-eight years of working with couples in therapy but specific guidelines that have been scientifically verified (to the extent possible given the infinite variability of human behavior).

By incorporating such new understandings, we sex doctors are helping more people than ever before. When I called one male client a few months after his therapy ended, he kept repeating, "It's nothing short of a miracle." His wife gave the specifics:

We are absolutely delighted. After the chemo for his prostate cancer, we thought we'd never have sex again. When we tried to do anything sexual, there was so much tension and anxiety on both our parts; the whole experience was agonizing. But the shots have been very helpful with his erections [this was several years before Viagra], and the main thing is we're making love in a way we never did before. We talk more, we're more open, we get downright silly at times, and we have far more fun, not only in sex but all the time. It's truly wonderful.

MEN ARE MORE OPEN

I have seen encouraging signs of change in men in the last few years, and this is another reason that sex therapy can be more effective. Many men whose fathers never expressed a feeling, made a bed or a sandwich, or even considered getting medical or psychological help for problems are doing precisely those things. Many men are questioning their priorities and values. I have known men to turn down much-desired promotions at work so that their children could remain in the same school or their wives could continue in their jobs.

Men seem much more receptive than even ten years ago to the relating skills I teach in my therapy and have included in this book. They may be uncomfortable and awkward at first, and they become reluctant at times, but they have come to understand that, no matter how "girly" this stuff seemed when they were younger, they need to listen, talk, share, and open up with their loved ones. And younger men, those born after 1960, as a group seem very much open to their own feelings and those of others, and to what were once called "feminine" values and characteristics.

It's exciting to me as a therapist that most of the men I work with these days don't have to be talked into trying to be more communicative and sensitive. They are already sold on the idea. What they need is the practical how-to of doing these things, and that is what I try to supply.

In this regard, one specific tool that's been beneficial to many men is scripts—examples of how to talk to your partner about various issues, some sexual, some not. We men simply have not had enough examples in our own upbringing and in the media of how to express our desires and go after what we want while at the same time being sensitive to the other person's needs and not trampling on her rights.

A NEW MODEL OF SEX

We men now have opportunities to enjoy a sexuality superior to anything we've had before. The traditional model of sex, the one most of us were trained in, focuses on male performance. The man has to make the right moves, has to get and keep an erection for as long as necessary—however long that might be—and now that women are entitled to sexual satisfaction, he also has to provide an ecstatic experience for his partner. This model puts enormous pressure on the man to perform and leads to unnecessary anxiety and fakery of all sorts (pretending to be interested when he isn't, pretending to have knowledge he doesn't, and even pretending to have orgasms; women aren't the only ones who do this).

For men, the traditional model of sex amounts to playing against a stacked deck. The results have been widespread anxiety among men about performing, lots of joyless sex, and even a fairly large group of men who've given up sex altogether; it was just more than they felt they could deal with. For years my caseload has been full of couples in which it's the woman saying she wants more sex and the man rejecting her advances, a topic I address in the chapter on problems of sexual desire and frequency.

Maybe we men need to start stacking the deck on our side. Throughout the book I offer the elements of a new model of sex, one that emphasizes pleasure, closeness, and self- and partner enhancement rather than performance and scoring. This model broadens the acts we usually think of as sexual and also how we go about them. Good sex doesn't have to stop at the traditional foreplay-intercourse routine. There are whole menus of choices that can give pleasure and fit the relationship and situation precisely. This model has a lot to offer both men and women because it allows us to more closely integrate sex with the rest of our lives and values, to be free of performance pressures and anxiety, to be more honest with ourselves and each other, and to feel better about what we're doing.

In recent years we have learned a great deal about how society influences young girls as they grow up and how this helps to account for the behavior and problems of adult women. A great deal of understanding and sympathy has been generated for girls and women, and I believe we have all become wiser and more compassionate as a result.

But not much has been said about what society does to boys and men. Males are still assumed, by themselves and by women, to have a better deal. They are the privileged ones, with all sorts of perks and power that women usually don't have, and they make more money and have more options in many areas.

I suggest that it's not easy being a woman or a man and that our training and treatment of men has been as misdirected and harmful as our training and treatment of women. The pressures and problems are somewhat different, but both sexes get battered in the process. My goal is to help both men and women come to a more compassionate understanding of what it's like to be a man, in bed and out.

THE SELF-HELP PROGRAMS

Although this is a self-help book—that is, it contains suggestions and exercises for making changes in your life—some people also need competent professional help from a therapist or physician. This applies particularly to those in relationships mired in hostility and those who may have a physical basis for their sexual difficulties. Even in such cases, this book may resolve the problem or give some assistance. In fact, I've been pleased over the years by how many doctors and therapists have made it assigned reading.

The suggestions and exercises are based on more than twenty-five years of experience working with men individually and in groups, with couples, and with women individually. While most of this work was in my private psychotherapy practice, I also draw on nine years of experience at a large sex clinic at the University of California, San Francisco, and in conducting scores of workshops on sexual enhancement. All of the suggestions and exercises in the book have been tested time and again by me and other therapists, and only those that have proven themselves are included here.

The instructions are detailed and comprehensive. I try to give sufficient information so you'll know exactly what to do and what to be aware of, and what problems may arise and how to deal with them.

But be warned: Reading alone rarely changes behavior or resolves problems. You need to follow the suggestions and do the relevant exercises if you want to make changes. I realize that those who have an urgent problem may want to zoom right in on the self-help chapters, but that is a mistake. You would do better to read the book straight through before turning to specific exercises.

A NOTE ON MY USE OF WORDS

In some sense there is no such entity as "men" or "male sexuality." There are only individual men and only the sexuality of individual men. But at times we need to generalize. In this book I make frequent use of qualifiers such as *many, some, often,* and so on, but to do that in every sentence becomes boring. I ask for your understanding. Just because I say "Men do . . ." or "Men say . . ." I don't mean to imply that every single man in the world does or says that thing. The same applies to generalizations about women.

When I talk about the other person, the one you're relating to or having sex with, I use a number of terms synonymously: *partner, lover, spouse, wife,* and *mate.* Just because I use *wife* or *spouse* does not mean I think you are or should be married to her.

My examples and language reflect my own heterosexuality and that of the vast majority of men I have worked with. But much of the material and all of the techniques apply equally to bisexual and homosexual men. Gay readers, however, will have to translate some of my words into language more appropriate to their own situations.

TAKING GREATER CONTROL OF OUR LIVES

Although men often give the impression of being in control of their lives—that's the impression they are supposed to convey—and although women often believe this impression and envy it, I have been surprised over the years by how many men feel exactly the opposite. In bed and out, they feel buffeted like leaves in a strong wind. They often aren't getting what they want. They often feel powerless to affect the course of their work, their relationships, and even what happens in sex. One cause of sadness for me in the last three decades is that the great debates about taking charge of one's life have been conducted almost entirely by and for women. They are the ones who've been working to redefine traditional concepts of gender and sexuality. I'm sad not about what women are doing—I think it's great—but about the fact that more men haven't been doing the same. It goes against our grain. We're too busy performing to think about such issues, we don't want to be seen as whiners and complainers, and we don't want to admit to problems we don't have ready answers for.

Nonetheless, we men have a lot to gain from taking greater control over our lives. We don't have to be at the mercy of our genitals or hormones or the traditional sex roles we were brought up on. We don't have to forgo the incredible joys and benefits of truly loving relationships. We don't have to put up with boring, joyless, or dysfunctional sex. We can develop personal styles, relationships, and sexual patterns that more closely fit our own values, preferences, and interests, that more closely fit our human selves. For those who are willing to make the effort, that's what this book is about.

The Making of Anxious Performers

I hear girls had it rougher, but you couldn't prove it by me. Growing up was the pits. Incredible pressures all the time, everywhere. Had to do well in school, had to do well in sports, had to maintain my manly image and couldn't walk away from a fight, and later had to do well with girls and pretend I knew all about sex and was getting it regularly. I often wished the whole world would just go away and leave me alone. I don't know what I would have done, but it couldn't have been any worse.—*Man, 36*

It took me half a century to realize that I'd been living a half life, that I had buried important feelings and parts of myself. I was a shit father and husband. Not abusive or anything like that, but I wasn't even home most of the time. Aside from money and fixing things around the house, I didn't contribute anything. Only when my grandson arrived did I make a shift. With him, I am a whole person. I can love him, cuddle him, listen to him, and really talk to him. Sounds funny, listening and talking to a four-year-old, but it's true. His expression of emotion has allowed me to unblock my own feelings. I'm sad that my wife died before I could be a real partner to her. I'm sad that I didn't give more to my own children and that I missed out on so much.—*Man, 54*

MEN IN OUR culture walk a thin line. Like their fathers and grandfathers, they must be sure their behavior conforms to what is considered manly. It takes very little—maybe as little as one failure or one sign of weakness—to lose one's place in the charmed circle of men and to be called "lady," "woman," or "pussy"—all signifying a non-man or less than a man. But if a man isn't a man, what then is he? The answer most men seem to believe is: nothing at all.

The concern of being considered a non-man keeps men in a state of almost perpetual vigilance and anxiety. It also makes for a certain inflexibility. If the results of changing one's behavior can be so dire as a loss of identity, one doesn't take change lightly. There is nothing new about this situation for men; it has existed in Western societies for hundreds of years. What is new is that the traditional definition of masculinity has come under scrutiny and attack and that the messages men get have become quite confused. Men are still supposed to exhibit all the manly virtues, but now they should also be sensitive and emotionally expressive, attributes that used to be considered feminine. Being a man has become more difficult than ever before.

What follows is, in my mind, not a pretty story. It shows how we transform male babies into adult beings who are somewhat less than human, who are cut off from huge portions of themselves, the parts that have to do with caring, nurturing, and expressing, who must wear a suit of armor almost all day and night, and who in a very real sense are only pale reflections of who they might be. At least in the old days, they were heavily rewarded for succeeding at being who society wanted them to be. But in recent times, men have come under unrelenting criticism for being who they are trained to be and for not being who they were discouraged from being. The cry is heard on media talk shows, in countless books and articles, in therapy offices, and in bedrooms and kitchens throughout the land: "Why aren't men more interested in relationships, why aren't they softer, why don't they express feelings, why aren't they more interested in household chores and child care?" The questions are of course not really questions, but accusations.

But why should men be this way? Where did they learn to focus on relationships, to express emotion, to be interested in children? The answer is: nowhere at all.

MAKING THE MAN

By the age of three or so, boys and girls are aware that they are not just children—they are boy children or girl children, and these distinctions are extremely important. Later learning is always filtered through the lens of gender. Even such neutral-seeming activities as cooking, soccer, and math are influenced by these lenses. Very early on, the child has a notion that soccer and math are things boys are interested in, while cooking is for girls. These notions are easily modifiable at early ages—a boy whose father takes pride in his culinary skills may well conclude that cooking is for males—but the point remains that everything is seen in terms of gender.

What a culture teaches its boys and girls is dependent on its images of men and women, what it wants these youngsters to grow up to be. Although in recent years we have been reevaluating what we want from men and women, the traditional definitions still exert a very strong pull. A number of researchers have found that a small number of characteristics comprise most of what we expect from our men: strength and self-reliance, success, no sissy stuff (in other words, don't be like women), and sexual interest and prowess. Here's a description from a Harold Robbins novel: "This was a strong man. . . . The earth moved before him when he walked, men loved and feared him, women trembled at the power in his loins, people sought his favors." That may seem a bit outdated, but here's how a recent Sidney Sheldon novel describes the hero: "He was like a force of nature, taking over everything in his path." In a 1989 novel titled *Sophisticated Lady*, we read of the hero (who had, of course, a "tall, powerfully built body"): "Just standing there, he radiated a quiet kind of strength and authority." He's the modern version: less raucous, more sophisticated, but still strong, successful, independent.

Of course there are contrary images: weak men, passive men, and general bunglers like Dagwood Bumstead. But we know they aren't what's wanted, that their bungling is precisely what makes them funny. Real men don't behave like this.

Little boys and little girls are certainly not the same—boys, for example, are on the average more active and aggressive—but they are more similar than adult men and women. Boys, like girls, are playful, warm, open, expressive, loving, vulnerable, and all the other things that make children so attractive. But when we look at adult men, we may wonder what happened to all these wonderful qualities. As adults, men display them to a far lesser degree, if at all. A lot of their best stuff has been trained out of them. In addition, some of their worst and most dangerous tendencies—toward aggressiveness and even violence—have been overdeveloped.

Although I emphasize the role of learning or socialization in the discussion that follows, I do not mean to imply there are no biological differences between the sexes. There certainly are. Nature had different purposes in mind for males and females and programmed them accordingly. Nonetheless, the training given to boys and girls is strikingly different and has an important influence. While we may not be able totally to undo a genetic disposition, we can shape it to some extent. It is probably true, for instance, that males are genetically more aggressive than females, but how frequently and in what ways aggressiveness is manifested are significantly influenced by societal messages boys and men get about it.

Little boys present a huge problem for all societies, because the societies don't want men to be like these boys. The question is how to make these open, expressive boys who wear their vulnerabilities and fears on their sleeves into strong, decisive performers who will be able to do whatever the society deems manly. We may think it's cute for a young boy to say, trembling, "I'm scared a monster is gonna get me," but we don't want a twenty- or thirty-year-old to act that way. Instead, we want him to deny his fear ("Monsters don't scare *me*!") and announce he's going to kick some monster ass.

Training in masculinity begins as soon as the child is born and continues for the rest of his life. By the age of six or seven, important lessons have already taken hold. An image of this process comes from a scene in a recent novel about a shooting at an elementary school. There was the usual mass confusion, shots, and a dead body being carried out; in short, a trauma. How did the kids react? A "little girl burst into tears. A chubby boy, five or six, cried. The boy next to him was older, maybe eight. Staring straight ahead and biting his lip, straining for macho." Between the ages of five and eight, he has learned lessons about being male. He will not cry, maybe never again. Nor will he show fear or dependency or tenderness, and he may not even be able to ask for directions when he's lost. He will lose his ability not only to show feelings, but also to experience and know them. He won't understand why his girlfriend or wife just wants to cuddle, to hear his fears and express hers, simply to talk.

You can see the results of men's training everywhere, and such examples serve to reinforce the training for all men who observe. One football-highlights TV show I saw in the fall of 1990 focused on New York Giants coach Bill Parcells, who coached his team that Sunday despite suffering from painful kidney stones. (The very fact of working while in great pain itself conveys a powerful message regarding what a man is.) As Parcells talked to reporters after the game, his discomfort was obvious. A reporter yelled out, "How do you feel, Bill?" Since it was apparent how he felt, all that was required was that he give a few words to his pain. But his response was this: "I'm going into the hospital tomorrow morning and I'll probably be there a day or two." Feelings? What's that? The message that men watching the show will take away is as clear as the pain that Parcells felt but couldn't put into words.

An important ingredient of the socialization of boys is the message "Don't be like a girl." Since females of all ages are the softer ones—the people who express feelings, who cry, who are more people-oriented—not being like them is an effective way to suppress the softer side of males. Girls and women are allowed far greater leeway. *Tomboy* has nowhere near the derogatory punch of *girl* or *sissy*. Girls can participate in boys' games, play with boys' toys, wear boys' clothes. But can you imagine what others will call a boy after the age of four or five who wears a dress or plays house or with dolls?

The primary focus of males and females is very different. Connection to others is the name of the game for females of all ages, even in their play. Dolls (the typical plaything of girls) are more conducive to intimacy training than the toy trucks and weapons boys get. You can cuddle a doll, comfort it, feed it, talk to it, sleep with it. But what can you do with a fire truck that has anything to do with relationships?

Ask little girls about their best friends, and this is what you get: "Janie is my best friend because we talk and share secrets." Research shows that girls spend much more time than boys in one-to-one interaction with their friends, in what one researcher called "chumships." Boys go in a different direction. They learn that the primary thing in life is doing or performing in the world out there, not in the family in here. When little boys are asked about their best friends, their answers usually are about activities: "Robert is my best friend because we play baseball and do lots of other things." Much more so than girls, boys spend time in large groups, often playing games.

These separate emphases set the stage for huge problems in adult relationships. Both men and women say they want love and intimacy, but they mean different things by these terms. Women favor what has been called face-to-face intimacy: They want to talk. Men prefer side-by-side intimacy: They want to do.

In almost all societies, femininity is given by having the right genitals. Masculinity or manhood is not. It is conditional. Having the right genitals is necessary but not sufficient. As Norman Mailer put it: "Nobody was born a man; you earned your manhood provided you were good enough, bold enough." In his book *Manhood in the Making,* anthropologist David Gilmore notes a recurring notion "that real manhood is different from simple anatomical maleness, that it is not a natural condition that comes about spontaneously through biological maturation but rather is a precarious or artificial state that boys must win against powerful odds." It is assumed that girls will grow up to be women simply by getting older, but boys need something special to become men. Thus, most societies have had special rituals, usually difficult and painful, sometimes life-threatening, that boys had to go through before they themselves and the rest of the group considered them to be worthy of the name of men. The good thing about these rituals was that once one had navigated his way through them, one's manhood could never again be questioned.

Western societies long ago got rid of these rituals. But in the process, something valuable was lost and men were left in a perpetual state of anxiety. Now one's manhood is always on the line. One deviant act is all it takes for your manhood to be questioned. Maybe you really aren't good enough or bold enough; maybe you don't have what it took. This is why men walk the thin line I mentioned earlier.

Early on the boy gets the idea that he can't be like the person who means the most to him, his mother. No longer is it acceptable to bask in her warmth and nurturance, except occasionally, and no longer is it possible to think that he, as she did, will someday give birth to babies. She's a woman, and he can't be like her or any other woman. In effect, he's wrenched away from the closest relationship he's had and may ever have. In most primitive societies, boys were also wrenched away from Mom, but they were entrusted to the care of one or more men who guided their development. In our society, there is no such arrangement.

There is only Dad, or whoever is playing that role for the boy. It is from him that the boy will learn his most important lessons about masculinity. Unfortunately, that relationship is rarely nurturing or positive in our society. Fathers are often not physically present and when they are, often are not emotionally present. Physical affection, emotional sharing, expression of approval and love—these are the human experiences that very few boys get from their dads. It is a tragedy of the greatest magnitude for men not to have been respected, nurtured, loved, and guided by their fathers.

Martial arts expert Richard Heckler recalls what happened when he was a child and his sailor father returned from a year-long cruise:

> I felt proud of him, proud that he was my father, proud that after not seeing him for a year and not even sure what he looked like, I still had a father. He came up to me and extended his hand in his stiff, formal way. "Hello son. Have you been taking care of your mother and sister while I was away?" I was nine years old and I wanted him to hold me and have him say that he loved me. But he didn't then or ever.

What boys do get from their dads, if anything at all, is reinforcement of macho tendencies and the necessity for performance and achievement. Therapist Terrance O'Connor relates this story:

I was struggling in my first year of high school. My father had just given me holy hell for the scores I had received on a standardized test. I felt terrible. In my room, I went over the results again and again. . . . Suddenly I realized that the numbers were raw scores. They needed to be converted. I was astonished. In percentiles, my scores were in the nineties. Vastly relieved, I rushed out to show my father. "Then why in hell don't you get better grades?" he yelled. It was a dagger in my heart. Never a word of love. Never a word of praise.

This is not to blame our fathers, who were only doing what was done to them. Nonetheless, the wounds opened by this lack of care run deep and are rarely healed. If you want to see grown men cry, give them a safe setting and get them talking about their fathers. That's all it takes.

Because the boy is wrenched away from his first real intimate relationship, does not get to experience one with his father, and is taught a body of attitudes, beliefs, and behaviors that are not conducive to intimacy, he will arrive at adulthood quite unprepared for the requirements of a mature relationship. The point is simple and frightening: The socialization of males provides very little that is of value in the formation and maintenance of intimate relationships.

Since so much of male training is in opposition to female qualities, males come to believe that these qualities, and therefore femaleness as a whole, are strange and inferior. The result is the development of a habit of not taking women seriously. Although a man may dearly love a woman and want very much to be considerate, fair, and respectful, he has years of training pulling in the other direction. Women are icky, weird, and disgusting; they're weak and dependent rather than strong and independent, as he's supposed to be; they're overly emotional and not logical; they're at the mercy of their hormones; and, well, they just don't see things the way men do. Since the boy had to break away from his mother and feminine ways to establish his masculinity, there's also a fear of once again coming under the domination of a woman. To be in this situation is too much like childhood, when he was a non-man. The last thing any man wants is to be "pussy-whipped" or "henpecked" because that's a clear indication that he's not man enough to keep "the little woman" under control. This, too, often leads men, no matter how much they love their partners, to be not quite able to treat them as full human beings with equal rights. This inability to take women seriously can cause much friction in adult relationships and negatively affects sex itself, as we will see later.

Since strength and self-reliance are the primary goals we have for our males, they are trained to mistrust and dislike the more vulnerable and expressive side of themselves. Boys are rewarded for "toughing it out," "hanging tough," not crying, not being weak. By the time my son Ian was four, he was using the words *tough* and *strong* in an admiring way. By the time he was five, *wimp* and *sissy* had entered his vocabulary as negative terms for males. Sometimes when he was angry at me, he would explode, "You're just a wimp."

Part of being tough is not getting or needing the loving touching that all babies get. Parents stop touching their boys early on; it seems somehow feminine or treating him like a baby or sissy. Girls, on the other hand, continue to be touched and hugged. We end up with women who understand touch as a basic human need and like to touch and be touched as a way of reinforcing contact and demonstrating affection; men, in contrast, lose sight of their need for touching except as a part of roughhousing or sex.

Boys learn that competition is an aid in proving oneself. If you're as good as or better than other males, then at least you're some kind of man. Most of us experienced no choice: We had to demonstrate our masculinity no matter how ill equipped and ill prepared we felt. In his essay "Being a Boy," Julius Lester captures the agony so many of us felt. Comparing himself to girls, he says:

> There was the life, I thought! No constant pressure to prove oneself. No necessity always to be competing. While I humiliated myself on football and baseball fields, the girls stood on the sidelines laughing at me, because they didn't have to do anything except be girls. The rising of each sun brought me to the starting line of yet another day's Olympic decathlon, with no hope of ever winning even a bronze medal.

Competitiveness turned out to be one of the uglier manifestations of male upbringing. First, few of us could win and therefore feel good about ourselves. After all, how many boys can excel at baseball, basketball, and football? And what are the others supposed to do? Countless men have stories to tell about how humiliated they felt as boys when they weren't successful on the athletic field, couldn't even do well enough to be chosen when teams were selected. They felt bad not only because they didn't get to play, but because their very personhood or manhood was questioned.

Second, competition is antithetical to intimacy. As psychologist Ayala Pines points out, in competition the question is "Who's on top?" or "Who's in front?" In intimacy the question is "How close are we or do we want to be?" Closeness is tied to openness, how much we can share of ourselves. But it's difficult to be open if you have a competitive mental set, for the fear is that what is revealed can be used to the other person's advantage.

Because of the emphasis on strength and self-reliance, men have trouble admitting to unresolved personal problems. It's not that problems don't come up, but you handle them, solve them, master them without help and without complaint. That's a large part of what being tough and independent—of being a man—means.

Like so many of the other ideas that men learn, this one puts them in a bind. What is a man supposed to be when he's confused, when he's frightened, when he needs help? Almost by definition, if he acknowledges his confusion or fear and asks for help, there's something wrong with him. He's not as tough as he ought to be. If, on the other hand, he doesn't acknowledge what's bothering him and get help, he may literally make himself sick and do worse at the task he's working on. On a mundane level, this belief results in the ridiculous behavior of men driving around endlessly in their cars because to stop and ask for directions would suggest they need help, which they do.

Not being able to talk about problems works against intimacy. As linguist Deborah Tannen points out, women use such "troubles talk" as a way of getting support and maintaining connection. But men aren't used to expressing their own problems or having to deal with anyone else's, so while troubles talk can be a wonderful way to maintain closeness between two women, it often doesn't work very well between a man and a woman.

Another consequence of being unable to express problems is that men often don't get what they need. They are slow to admit to illness and other physical problems, and they are even slower to admit to emotional distress. And the idea of needing to go to an expert for help in dealing with personal or relationship problems is anathema to many of them. Men are changing in this respect—more men, for example, are coming to therapists' offices—but the change is slow, and men are still nowhere near as willing as women to admit to personal problems.

It's not easy for boys and men. It's not easy to give up the warm, tender side of themselves. It's not easy to squelch feelings of dependency, love, fear, and anxiety. It's not always easy to be posturing, pretending to be more knowledgeable, more self-reliant, more confident, and more fierce than you really are. There are many times when a man feels fearful or defeated and wants nothing more than to be held and comforted, just as his mother held and comforted him long ago. But he can't get it. He can't admit his feelings, and he can't ask to be held. And that is very sad. Like some men, he may choose to drown his feelings in alcohol or sex; at least in sex he will get some body contact and a distraction from his feelings. But neither the alcohol nor the sex is the same as real physical and emotional comforting. Too bad he can't get what he really needs and wants.

It's not easy to always have to perform and succeed, whether on the athletic field, in the boardroom, or in the bedroom. Although the whole process has been romanticized, the fact is that boys and men often make themselves sick and crazy in getting ready to perform. It's not unusual for athletes to throw up in the locker room before competition (romanticize that if you can) and to get themselves into a murderous rage that under any other circumstances would rightfully be considered psychotic. This process, by the way, is often called "getting it up." It's not easy for a man to go into a sexual situation believing that everything rides on how well he performs (especially with a part of himself that he can't control), but what else is he to do?

Being a male is like living in a suit of armor, ready for battle to prove himself. The armor may offer protection (although it's not clear against what), but it's horribly confining and not much fun. In fact, fun is exactly what it's not. Maybe this is why so many men take to alcohol and other ways of deadening themselves. And it may help explain men's fascination with sports.

In sports many of the usual prohibitions on males are lifted. A man can be as emotional and expressive about his favorite team and players as he wants. He can cheer them on with unabashed enthusiasm and what might even pass for love. He can be ecstatic and jump up and down when they win, and he can feel despair and weep when they lose. Playfulness and creativity are allowed. He can dress up in ridiculous hats and shirts, make up posters and poems and songs, and just be plain silly. There's even a lot of physical contact: back- and butt-slapping, touching of shoulders and arms, and hugging. And cursing a bad call, a decision, or a mistake is a way of expressing anger without much risk. Sports is one of the few places where men can safely drop the facade of Mr. Uptight-and-in-Control and just play.

LEARNING ABOUT SEX

Through no fault of my own I reached adolescence. While the pressure to prove myself on the athletic field lessened, the overall situation got worse—

because now I had to prove myself with girls. Just how I was supposed to
go about doing this was beyond me.... Nonetheless, duty called, and with
my ninth-grade gym-class jockstrap flapping between my legs, off I went.
—*Julius Lester*

Between the ages of eleven and fourteen, children enter puberty. The brain
signals the pituitary gland to increase its production of growth hormones
and, in males, of testosterone. One of the first outward signs of puberty is
a spurt of the rate of physical growth, unmatched since the first few years
of life. During the next few years, in boys the penis and scrotum enlarge to
adult size, facial and pubic hair appear, and sperm and semen are manu-
factured. By the age of thirteen or so, boys (and girls as well) are capable of
sexual reproduction. And they feel different than before, trying to get accustomed to their new bodies, trying to make sense of new sensations they
experience, trying to deal with the hormonal gush. Testosterone in boys
and estrogen in girls make a crucial difference, causing the boys and girls
to seek each other out, but also propelling them along separate paths that
are already well developed.

Before they start having sex with partners or even themselves, boys
know that sexual interest and prowess are crucial to being a man. The
message permeates our culture. Here's how the hero of a romance novel
thinks of himself: "He was, after all, a very physical man with a highly active sex drive. He enjoyed women, all kinds of women." All kinds: short
ones, tall ones, young ones, old ones, fat ones, thin ones, smart ones, dumb
ones. He likes to get it on and presumably isn't too particular about partners. After all, you can't be a hero if you don't have a whopping sex drive.

It's interesting that in the liberated '90s we still have a double standard
for males and females regarding sex. Boys will be boys, after all, and how
can you be against a boy's sowing his wild oats? We tend to admire males
who get around. But although women are no longer expected to be virgins, God help any of them who has had sex with too many men, however
many that might be.

Since sexuality is such a crucial component of masculinity, males feel
pressured to act interested in sex whether or not they really are. They have
to join in the jokes and banter. "Getting any, Fred?" "Oh yeah, more than I
know what to do with." And they have to face the derision of their peers if
they're still—God forbid—virgins at the advanced age of eighteen or
twenty-three. This is a great setup for faking, lying, and feeling inadequate.

Perhaps no one has captured the angst of boys' sexual learning better
than Bill Cosby in an article he wrote about his first sexual nonexperience.

Believing that other boys are doing what he isn't, Cosby asks his girlfriend if she'll have sex with him. She agrees to do so next Saturday, at which point Cosby realizes he has a problem: He doesn't know what sex is or what to do.

I'm trying to ask people questions about how they get some p-u-s-s-y. And I don't want guys to know that I don't know nothin' about gettin' no p-u-s-s-y. But how do you find out how to do it without blowin' the fact that you don't know how to do it? So I come up to a guy and I say, Say man, have you ever had any p-u-s-s-y? And the guy says, Yeah. And I say, Well, man, what's your favorite way of gettin' it? He says, Well, you know, just the regular way. And I say, Well, do you do it like I do it? And the cat says, How's that? And I say, Well, hey, I heard that there was different ways of doin' it, man. He says, Well, there's a lotta ways of doin' it, you know, but I think that . . . you know, the regular way. . . . I say, Yeah, good ol' regular way of gettin' that p-u-s-s-y.

As he continues his ruminations on the way to the girl's house, Cosby shows how well he has learned that a man should be able to do it all on his own.

So now, I'm walkin', and I'm trying to figure out how to do it. And when I get there, the most embarrassing thing is gonna be when I have to take my pants down. See, right away, then, I'm buck naked in front of this girl. Now, what happens then? Do you . . . do you just . . . I don't even know what to do . . . I'm gonna just stand there and she's gonna say, You don't know how to do it. And I'm gonna say, Yes I do, but I forgot. I never thought of her showing me, because I'm a man and I don't want her to show me—I don't want nobody to show me, but I wish somebody would kinda slip me a note.

The sex that adolescent boys learn about is totally penis-centered. The focus is narrow-mindedly on what can be done with their frequent erections. But this penis orientation has to do with more than just immediate pleasure and release. Boys are aware, even if only vaguely, that having and using erections has something to do with masculinity. Popular literature abounds with statements linking the two, phrases about a woman grasping or feeling his "throbbing manhood" or reaching for the "essence of his masculinity." And it goes even further: She reached for *him*, or she grasped *him* gently, the *him* in both cases referring to his penis. From a recent novel: "Her hands left my neck and scrambled at my fly. More fumbling, eyes closed. Then she located me." What she located, of course, was his penis. This creates an incredible confusion between personhood or identity and one's sexual organ. No wonder men get so perturbed when their penis isn't the "right" size or doesn't operate according to spec. No penis, no person.

The sex that boys learn about is also largely impersonal. Although this message may serve one of nature's goals (for men to spread their seed as widely as possible regardless of love or commitment) and therefore be programmed into men, there is no shortage of cultural messages to reinforce the idea. For example, one of the characters in Irving Wallace's *Guest of Honor* is the secretary of state. He's approached by the resident's adviser for a favor requested by the First Lady. "I'd do her any favor, if she'd do one for me. I'd love to fuck her." And then: "Not that I care for her that much. I just have a hunch she'd be fun between the sheets."

The message is clear: For men, sex doesn't have to be connected to anything except lust, and it doesn't matter much toward whom it's directed. A boy may have fantasies about girls in his classes, his friends' mothers, neighbors, girls or women in the street, movie and TV stars, and anyone else. The female in his fantasies is simply a tool to gain release. And then to do it again, and again, and again. Next time it will probably be a different female. And he certainly doesn't have to like the girl to want to have sex with her. This is clearly demonstrated in an old practice where teenage boys have sex with unpopular girls they despise and wouldn't be seen with in daylight. It's enough if she'll give the boy sex. At this early age, we can see the start of the male split between love and sex. Sex is a thing unto itself for adolescent boys, cut off from the rest of life and centered on their desire for physical release and the need to prove themselves.

Girls go in a different direction. Perhaps because their genitals are internal, less obvious and less obtrusive than boys', their attention isn't constantly drawn downward. Probably of greater importance is that nature had a different task in mind for women than for men: to find a mate to help to care for and raise the children they produced. Although in recent years girls have started masturbating earlier and more frequently than in the past, the percentage of girls who do masturbate is far smaller than the percentage of boys. And the girls who do masturbate don't do it as much as boys of the same age.

Teenage girls aren't as focused on physical sex as boys. "Getting off" in itself isn't nearly as important to them. Girls' sexuality is channeled or filtered through personal connection. They want to have sex with Prince Charming or Mr. Right in the context of a relationship. The idea of a group of girls getting together to have sex with Joe Dork just because he's willing to put out is almost unthinkable. More so than men's, women's first sexual experience with a partner is likely to be with someone they love. And women are far less likely than men to seek sex for its own sake. It's not surprising that when Lonnie Barbach and Linda Levine asked women what qualities make for a good sexual experience, relationship factors were mentioned most often: "Women talked about the security, comfort, and sharing that took place in the emotional relationship as being necessary prerequisites for good sex."

Here we see a male-female difference that persists into adult life. For women, sex is intertwined with personal connection. For men, sex is more a thing in itself, an act to be engaged in with or without love, with or without commitment, with or without connection. Although in surveys men agree with women that the best sex occurs in loving relationships, much more so than women they'll take it any way they can get it.

That the sex boys learn about is performance-oriented goes without saying. What else could it be for a person who has already had over a decade of training in becoming a performance machine?

It's Two Feet Long, Hard as Steel, and Will Knock Your Socks Off: The Fantasy Model of Sex

I learned so much crap about sex as a kid that it took most of the rest of my life to unlearn it and come up with something better. It's still hard to believe how much hassle I caused myself and what a poor lover I was in my early years. I wish I could apologize to every woman I was with before I shaped up.—*Man, 49*

WHEN I STARTED working with men with sex problems nearly thirty years ago, I was immediately struck by the absolutely fantastic beliefs they held. They seemed to believe, for example, that they needed a penis as big and hard as a telephone pole to satisfy a woman, that male and female orgasm were absolutely necessary, that intercourse was the only real sexual act, that good sex had to be spontaneous, without planning or talking, and that it was a crime against humanity if a man had any questions, doubts, or problems in sex. As I reflected on these beliefs, I was shocked to realize that I shared many of them myself, and so did most men who weren't clients, and many women as well.

Where, I wondered, did we get these messages? They weren't taught in most sex courses or in sex books by professionals. I was making the mistake, of course, of assuming that most knowledge about sex comes in formal ways, from courses and books. But before boys and girls get to sex courses and books, they already have had years of learning about the subject.

Whether we know it or not, whether it's intended or not, sex education goes on all the time, from the day we're born until the day we die, with an especially heavy dose coming during puberty. Long before we are exposed to the realities of sex, our heads are filled with all sorts of nonsense. Every time we tell or listen to a sexual joke, watch a movie that depicts sexuality explicitly or implicitly, read a novel or see a television program that involves sex or adult relationships—at all these times and many others, either we learn something about sex or, more likely, something we already believe is reinforced and strengthened.

The messages get through because of our basic insecurity about sex and our sensitivity to any information about it. Whether we are trying to learn anything or whether we are aware of having learned anything is irrelevant. Most men, I suspect, would deny that they are affected by all the positive references in jokes and novels to large penises and the denigrating references to small ones. I suggest, however, that these references do indeed have a cumulative effect and help explain why so many men feel their own penises are inadequate. Many of the things that we believe are natural, real, or "the way it is" are in fact absorbed in this way but, because of our insistence to the contrary, are resistant to change or even examination.

Because all the media portray essentially the same sexual messages, it's virtually certain that all men and women will learn the same model of sex, although, to be sure, the messages are filtered through the different gender training males and females have undergone. What is picked up from one source is reinforced by the others. Even if you never read a book or saw a movie, you'd still learn the model. It pervades our culture. Our friends learned it (and you probably learned a lot from them), our parents learned it, and so did everyone else.

The sexual messages conveyed in our culture are the stuff of fantasy, of overheated imaginations run wild, and that's why I call them collectively the fantasy model of sex. It is a model of total unreality about how bodies look and function, how people relate, and how they have sex. The main actors in this model are not actually people but sexual organs, especially the penis. These penises are not like anything real but instead are, according to historian Steven Marcus, "magical instruments of infinite powers." The men these penises are attached to are not exactly average, either. They are always well-built and muscular, even if they're over sixty and even if they do nothing but shuffle papers all day. They are usually tall, with "strong, intelligent" faces; they "radiate power"; most are extremely successful at work; and sexual energy oozes from every pore.

The women in fantasyland are incredible, with beautiful faces, sensuous lips and hips, lustrous hair, slim bodies, full breasts always pointing outward and upward, and long, shapely legs you wouldn't believe. It might be thought that the combination of slimness and big breasts would create a problem of balance, but fear not—none of the women ever tips over. And these women are mainly young, meaning in their twenties or early thirties. The few older women we encounter, except for those who are someone's mother, look half their age and could pass for college sophomores. For instance: "She was a month away from her fortieth birthday and looked thirty, even on a bad morning."

Regardless of age, these women have some interesting features. Barbara, in John Gardner's *Secret Houses*, is, well, kind of perfect: "As she leaned over him, he noticed that her hair, like her breasts, stayed in perfect order." It wouldn't do to have any hairs or breasts flopping about. Her breasts are worth another few words. They "remained the same whichever way she turned. They did not even seem to flatten when she was on her back, as some girls' did." Ain't life wonderful?

Another interesting feature of women in fantasyland is that they are seriously into sex. They go around with dripping panties, are ready for action at a moment's notice, and can express their desires as some men have always done: "That's right, honey, eat me, hurt me, talk dirty to me, and fuck me. That's all I want." Unless they're virgins, foreplay is not something they need much of. Orgasms, dozens of them, come quickly and easily to them.

Some women complain that this emphasis on perfect female forms is a male conspiracy, but the women created by female writers—for example, most of those who write romance novels—also tend to be young and physically perfect. The fantasy model is equally hard on men and women. The male bodies, organs, and performances are just as far out of reach for the ordinary man as the female bodies and performances are for the average woman.

Here's a little passage from a Harold Robbins novel that sums up a lot of the action of the fantasy model. Try to keep in mind that this book is not only not pornographic by any of the usual definitions, but for decades has been available at many drugstores and supermarkets. Robbins is one of the best-selling authors of fiction in the world, and he along with other popular writers such as Henry Miller, Norman Mailer, Mario Puzo, Sidney Sheldon, Erica Jong, Judith Krantz, and Jackie Collins—all of whose books have sold millions of copies and all of whom share some rather interesting ideas about sex—may be a far more influential sex educator than Masters and Johnson and Dr. Ruth.

The man in the story is a wealthy businessman and the woman is his wife's dressmaker, whom he has just met. He got aroused and asked her how much. She indicated she wanted to open a small shop, and he said, "You've got it." With that for introduction and foreplay, we begin:

> Gently her fingers opened his union suit and he sprang out at her like an angry lion from its cage. Carefully she . . . took him in both hands, one behind the other as if she were grasping a baseball bat. She stared at it in wonder. . . .
>
> [After placing his hands under her armpits and lifting her in the air] he began to lower her on him. Her legs came up, circling his waist, as he began to enter her. Her breath caught in her throat. It was as if a giant of white hot steel were penetrating her. She began to moan as it opened her and climbed higher into her body, past her womb, past her stomach, under her heart, up into her throat. She was panting now, like a bitch in heat. . . .
>
> [He then lifts her off him and throws her onto the bed.] Then he was posed over her. . . . His hands reached and grasped each of her heavy breasts as if he wanted to tear them from her body. She moaned in pain and writhed, her pelvis suddenly arching and thrusting toward him. Then he entered her again.
>
> "My God," she cried, "my God!" She began to climax almost before he was fully inside her. Then she couldn't stop them, one coming rapidly after the other as he slammed into her with the force of the giant body press she had seen working in his factory. She became confused, the man and the machine they were one and the same and the strength was something she had never known before. And finally, when orgasm after orgasm had racked her body into a searing sheet of flame and she could bear no more, she cried out at him: "Take your pleasure . . . Quick, before I die!"
>
> A roar came from deep inside his throat. . . . She felt the hot on-rushing gusher of his semen turning her insides into hot, flowing lava. She discovered herself climaxing again.

You may be wondering what's wrong with this kind of material. Isn't it more exciting and more fun to view, read about, and fantasize about perfectly built people and flawless performances than about real people? I admit it can be great fun to get away from the shortcomings and hassles of real life and imagine only perfection. That's one of the main purposes of fantasy. But there is a problem. Because we don't have any realistic models or standards in sex, little idea of what is customary or even possible in the real world, we tend to measure ourselves against these fantasies. We often don't remember that what we're comparing ourselves to is for the most part unattainable by human beings. We usually aren't even aware that we're comparing ourselves to anything. We just know that we feel bad because our equipment and performances aren't what we wish they were.

In a society that doesn't give us realistic models of sexuality, where else would people go for standards? It's rare, for example, to read of or see an average-looking couple having sex, so we end up feeling inadequate about our own and our partners' bodies. It's rare to read about or see a couple having the kind of sex that is possible in the real world, so we feel bad about our less-than-cataclysmic experiences. It's rare to read of or see a couple discussing a sexual problem, so we learn that sex problems don't or shouldn't exist, and we fail to learn how to deal with them when they do occur.

We compare ourselves to what we've learned, and almost everyone feels that they've come out on the short end. No matter what kind of equipment you have, no matter what partner, no matter what you do, no matter what the results—none of it equals what you heard and read about. Good sex is always somewhere else with someone else.

The myths generate huge amounts of anxiety and bad feelings about ourselves and our partners. They help create sex problems and make resolving them difficult, they bring misery to relationships and individuals, and, in general, they make good sex hard to come by.

Virtually all of the men and women I've talked to over the years who say they have good relationships and good sex report that they had to unlearn or give up a number of harmful notions and replace them with ideas that were more realistic and constructive. The purpose of this chapter is to give you an opportunity to look at some of the main destructive myths men hold about connecting and sex.

MYTH 1: WE'RE LIBERATED FOLKS WHO ARE VERY COMFORTABLE WITH SEX

Beginning with the sexual revolution of the 1960s and '70s, the idea has spread that we have overthrown and overcome the prudishness and inhibitions of our Victorian ancestors. Sexual pleasure is our birthright, and we don't much care what our religions or churches or parents say about it. We're going to do what we want with whom we want, and we're going to enjoy it. In other words, we are fairly calm about and accepting of sex. This view is now held by many people, especially men.

This belief is reinforced by media portrayals of erotica. Everyone in movies and books seems so comfortable with sex. No woman is concerned with her weight or the state of her breasts, thighs, or hips, or about her ability to lubricate and be orgasmic. No man is concerned about the size and hardness of his penis or his sexual endurance. No one questions his ability to provide a mind-blowing experience for himself and his partner. Everyone is comfortable with everything: vaginal, oral, and anal sex, sex with and without drugs, sex in public places, sex with several partners at the same time, and sex without protection against pregnancy and disease. In fact, people in fantasyland are usually so comfortable that it doesn't make any difference whether the partners even know each other.

While I'm not saying that greater comfort with impersonal sex is a desirable goal, it certainly would be nice if we were more comfortable with our bodies, our sexual organs, and sexuality in general than we are now. But it seems quite clear that we have not quite reached nirvana yet. I have yet to meet a man or woman who I think is totally comfortable with sex, and that of course includes myself. We all seem to have hang-ups of one kind or another.

How else could it be in a society where parents are still very uncomfortable with their children's playing doctor with the boy or girl next door and with, God forbid, their children's masturbatory behavior? How else could it be in a society where even supposedly liberated parents still protect children from movies that show more or less explicit sexuality? We allow our children to see violence in all its ugly faces—the average fifteen-year-old has seen more bombings, shootings, and knifings on television than most soldiers see in actual combat—but we draw the line at erotic pleasure. What messages do you think get across? Kids aren't stupid. They get the point: There's something wrong with sex. As the children grow up, they also learn that sex is pleasurable. But if you scratch the surface you often find the earlier belief, that there's something wrong with sex.

If we're so accepting of sex, why is there so little decent sex education in this country? How come so few of us can talk about it with our partners? How come so many of us feel so bad and guilty about our own self-stimulation? And how come so many of us have trouble consistently and effectively using protection against disease and unwanted pregnancy?

In her book *Erotic Wars*, Lillian Rubin notes that although sex is now openly discussed and displayed, it's a different matter in our private lives.

"There, sex still is relegated to a shadow existence, and silence is the rule. There, the old taboos still hold: sex is a private affair, something we don't talk about, not with friends, often not even with lovers or mates."

Believing that we are so liberated about sex leads to arrogance and narrow-mindedness. It makes it difficult to examine our own knowledge and attitudes, to see and appreciate our own ignorance and discomfort. And this makes it hard to change our behavior.

MYTH 2: A REAL MAN ISN'T INTO SISSY STUFF LIKE FEELINGS AND COMMUNICATING

In the last chapter we saw that men don't have much practice discerning their feelings or talking about them. Women want to talk, men want to do.

Because men have trouble directly expressing feelings except for sexual ones, they tend to get sneaky. In one scene in the movie *Three Men and a Baby*, Tom Selleck asks his woman friend to spend the night, and the subject of feelings comes up. She says, "I thought sentiment made you uncomfortable." His reply: "I can handle it, as long as it's disguised as sex."

A man in a research study spoke for a lot of men when he said, "What it really comes down to is that I guess I'm not very comfortable with expressing my emotions—I don't think that many men are—but I am pretty comfortable with sex, so I just sort of let sex speak for me." A woman in the same study [commented]: "Sex is his one and only way to be intimate. But how close can you get to someone who only communicates with his cock?"

Talking is important in sex. One reason it's important is so that you can protect yourself. Sex has always been a risky activity, and these days the ante has been upped considerably. At the very least, you need to be able to say, "Wait a sec, I've got to put this rubber on."

Of course, in fantasyland there is nothing to talk about. There are no STDs, and it goes without saying that no man in fantasyland has sexual questions, doubts, or problems. It's all perfect and wonderful, just like in a fairy tale, which is exactly what it is.

The absence of sex problems in the media, especially in men, is unfortunate because it plays into the larger fiction discussed in Chapter 1, that men don't have personal problems of any kind. Because having personal problems means a man doesn't have it all together, men are much less willing than women to acknowledge such difficulties and get help for them. The whole thing gets magnified dramatically when it comes to sex. This makes it extremely difficult for a man to discuss with a new partner or even a long-term mate that he's concerned about his desire, arousal, erections, or early ejaculations. The usual case when a couple comes for sex therapy is that even if the problem is primarily the man's, he's there only because the woman dragged him in. He doesn't want to acknowledge the problem; he'd prefer that the whole matter just go away. Needless to say, this only makes the therapy more difficult and the chances of a successful outcome less likely.

The reality is that men have as many personal problems as women, including problems with sex. But because it's so fraught with meaning if a man has a difficulty, he's in an incredible bind. Not being able to acknowledge it means he can't try to resolve it on his own or with his partner. She knows there's a problem but can't get him to acknowledge it, which puts her in a bind as well. It doesn't take long before the partners are distant and the relationship deteriorates. This is sad, because in the majority of these cases the problem could have been easily dealt with, if only it could have been confronted.

Obviously, this myth works against being able to talk about sex. This is unfortunate, because we know that talking about sex leads to better sex. People who have good sex say that you need to be able to speak your preferences and desires (that is, your feelings), to ask for changes, and so on. This is one of the main keys to sexual happiness.

The ability to talk is also important in another way. In many relationships there's less sex than the man wants precisely because his partner feels the absence of connection. He doesn't listen to her or talk to her, so she feels estranged and isn't receptive when he comes on to her.

MYTH 3: ALL TOUCHING IS SEXUAL OR SHOULD LEAD TO SEX

Boys and girls learn different things about touching, and men and women use touch in different ways. Women tend to see touching as a goal in itself; that is, they hug in order to hug, not in order to get someplace else. For men, touching is more often a means to an end; hugging is a part of the foreplay to sex.

As a result, misunderstandings and conflicts over touch are common.

SHE: Why can't we just touch sometimes without having to go on to sex?

HE: But touching turns me on, and I want sex. What's wrong with that?

Touching soothes us, makes us feel loved and supported, makes us feel good. Readers in their late and middle years may recall how wonderful it felt when they were hospitalized (which in general didn't feel good at all) and got a nightly back rub from a nurse. As one who had several such experiences, I remember thinking that those back rubs did more for me than most of the medicines I was receiving. Unfortunately, nurses' back rubs have gone the way of the horse and buggy, and many patients feel worse as a result.

The idea that touching is sexual is so deeply ingrained that many men don't consider having physical contact unless it is part of or going to lead to sex. Women complain about not getting as much touching as they want, but they aren't the only ones being deprived. Men need touching, if only they knew it, and cheat themselves as well. If sex isn't possible—because of illness, a sexual problem, or something else—touching becomes even more important as a source of support and bonding. But many men don't see this and distance themselves physically from their partners in times of trouble.

There are many times when all we need is a hug or to be held. It's ridiculous to go through a whole sexual act to get that. And we go through other acts as well to get touched. Many women point out a hidden purpose for the wrestling that men often engage in with their children. As one puts it clearly: "He can't ask for a touch or a hug, not from me or the boys. So he wrestles with them and with me. Seems like a lot of sweat and effort just to get a hug. Must be terrible to be a man."

This myth robs us of the joys of "just" touching, confuses us as to what we want, and puts pressure on us to be sexual whenever we touch or are touched.

MYTH 4: A MAN IS ALWAYS INTERESTED IN AND ALWAYS READY FOR SEX

As I indicated in the last chapter, sexual interest and activity are part of the model of manhood we learn. A real man is someone who's always interested in sex and ready for it. Here's an example from a novel about a man's needs: "Ike Vesper had had his fill of girlie magazines. Ten weeks without a woman was nine weeks and six days too long." Poor guy! And from another novel:

> Now all Alexis wanted was to be inside a woman. Nothing gave him more pleasure than fucking women, in every way. He had all three of them, going from one to the other in every position imaginable. Juju begged to be sodomized and the two women prepared her, for Alexis's sheer size would have ripped her apart had she not been helped. Before he left the bed he had filled each of them with his sperm.

Having to be ever eager for sex makes it difficult for a man to refuse a sexual invitation. If someone within five miles is interested in sex, far be it from him to say no. Not being able to say no leads to trouble, because there's nothing more likely to result in a sex problem than having sex when you're not interested.

A young man came to see me years ago about an erection problem. He was telling me about his latest failure, a woman he had been with a few nights before. I asked him to think back if he really wanted to have sex with her. He thought about it awhile and then admitted he didn't. I asked what he would have preferred. He said his muscles were sore from moving furniture that day and a back rub would have been really nice. So I asked why he didn't ask her for one. He looked at me as if I was crazy and blurted out: "How could I have asked her for a back rub? It was our first date. I hardly knew her!"

Since that story was published in my book *Male Sexuality*, a number of men I've seen have said that reading it made them think about themselves. They realized there were times when they wanted physical affection (usually having to do with getting comfort) but had problems getting it without having sex.

One man related to me what happened when he lost his job:

> I felt utterly crushed. I'd been riding on top of the world for several years, pulling in more bucks than I imagined possible. I felt so proud about giving my family that great new house and all the other goodies. And now we were going to lose it all. I felt like nothing. I realized later that what I needed was for my wife to take me in her arms and hold and rock me, just like my mother used to do. To let me know she

loved me and that things would be okay. But I didn't know this then. All I could think of was to have a few drinks and go home and make love with her. The sex wasn't bad, it helped, but I know it would have been better had I not had the drinks, but just told her what happened and let her hold me.

The reality is that no one is always interested in any one activity. Of course there are times when a man would rather read or sleep or walk or talk or be comforted than have sex. Too bad it's so hard to admit this.

This myth also puts tremendous pressure on young men to be sexual as early as possible. But why should a boy get into sex if he isn't interested or ready? Some young men won't be ready to have sex with a partner until they're out of college. Too bad they and their friends can't see there's nothing wrong with this.

If you aren't ready to talk to someone about sex and if you aren't ready to ask them for a back rub or a hug, you're definitely not ready to have good sex with them.

MYTH 5: A REAL MAN PERFORMS IN SEX

You've got to have good equipment and you've got to use it right. Sex isn't mainly for enjoyment or to express love or caring or lust; it's mainly to prove that you're a man. This performance orientation explains why men are so much into measurements. If sex is to enjoy and express personal feelings, then you just do and enjoy. But if you're into proving something, then you have to know how you measure up. How big is it, how long did it last, how many orgasms were there? The performance orientation also explains why some men brag about sex to their friends. What's the point of a great performance if no one knows about it?

The quote from Harold Robbins earlier in the chapter is one kind of great performance. Here's another one, from Erica Jong's best-seller *Parachutes and Kisses*:

He heaped the pillows in front of her for her to lean on, and cupping her breasts, he took her from behind, ramming her harder than before. Her cunt throbbed, ached, tingled. She screamed for him to ram her even harder, to smack her, to pound her. . . .

She had never come before in this position—but when she did, it was as if thirty-nine years of comes were released and she howled and growled like an animal—whereupon he was aroused beyond containment and he began to come with a pelvis and cock gone wild, pounding her fiercely, filling her with come.

Whew! I get tired just reading this stuff.

One fascinating fact is that fictional accounts of sex almost invariably depict male *performance* and female *pleasure*. He *acts* (rams, pounds, thrusts, bangs) and she *feels* ("unbearable pleasure," "overwhelming joy," "delirious ecstasy")—the usual male-female dichotomy. Although she sometimes performs (she too can thrust and bang), it's rarely clear what he feels and experiences. It's as if his feelings and pleasure are beside the point.

Now let's look at the main performance specifications.

MYTH 6: SEX IS CENTERED ON A HARD PENIS AND WHAT'S DONE WITH IT

The adolescent male's fixation on his penis remains constant throughout life. When men think of sex, they think of what they can do with, or what can be done to, their erections. That's what it's all about. And not any old penis or erection will do. Men have a set of specifications for what's required.

Size: Penises in fantasyland come in only three sizes: large, extra large, and so big you can't get them through the door. "Massive," "huge," and "enormous" are commonly mentioned in fiction. "She reached inside his pants and freed his huge erection." "He was so big that she could not reach her fingers all around him." Sometimes we get numbers: "She swears that her Italian singer's cock is over ten inches long." In Mario Puzo's *Godfather*, Sonny Corleone's main claim to fame is the possession of the biggest cock in the known universe. Here's the experience of one of his many lovers with it: "Her hand closed around an enormous, blood-gorged pole of muscle. It pulsated in her hand like an animal and almost weeping with grateful ecstasy she pointed it into her own wet, turgid flesh."

Not only are penises huge to begin with, they can get still bigger during intercourse. "She wailed in hot flooding ecstasy. It went on and on, one climax after another, and as Craig's penis lengthened unbelievably, his semen erupting within her, she wailed again, this time in unison with him." With that penis expanding the way it was, it's no wonder everyone was wailing.

Hardness: These organs that might be mistaken for telephone poles are not mere flesh and blood but "hard as steel," "hard as a rock," or a "diamond cutter." One wonders whether we're talking about making war or making love with these tools. There is, of course, no joy in a penis that's sort of hard, semihard, or "only 70 percent" erect.

Activity: These rocklike monstrosities manifest an excess of exuberance, for they are forever leaping, surging, springing, and, in general, behaving in a manner that might be considered dangerous for objects so large and hard. Two examples from novels: "He sprang swollen into her hand" and "She captured his surging phallus." (Sounds like that one almost got away.) Nowhere does one read of a penis that quietly moseyed out for a look at what was going on before springing and crashing into action.

The desired penis functions automatically and predictably, just like a well-oiled machine. It should immediately spring into full readiness whenever its owner decides he will use it. If you're dancing close with someone, your penis should be fully erect, pressing mightily against your pants and making its presence clearly felt. If a woman unzips your fly, your erection ought to spring out at her. If you kiss, well, here's how one novel put it: "The lingering kiss [the first one that day, it should be said] induced an immediate erection." The way some men talk about it, I have the impression they think their penises should stand fully erect if a woman even says hello to them.

Automatic functioning means that the penis should function regardless of any other considerations. Neither rain nor snow nor sleet shall keep the almighty penis from its appointed rounds. No matter if you're sick or well, tired or fresh, preoccupied or fully present, if you like your partner or not, if you're angry or not, if you're anxious or relaxed, or if you've gotten any stimulation or not—your penis should immediately come to full attention and do its manly thing.

Penises in fantasyland are also distinguished by their ability to last. They can literally go all night. The admiring wife in one novel: "With Dax it's like having a machine gun inside you. It never stops shooting and neither does he." In one scene, she and Dax have intercourse and both have orgasms (naturally). Immediately after: "She looked at him in surprise. 'You're still hard,' she exclaimed, a note of wonder coming into her voice. She threw her head back . . . as he thrust himself into her again."

The clear message to men and to women is that a man showing up at a sexual event without a rock-hard penis is as inappropriate as a carpenter showing up for work without his hammer and tape measure. You simply can't leave home without your stiff dick. Almost needless to say, these requirements make men feel inadequate about the size and power of their penises and under a bit of pressure to have and keep erections.

MYTH 7: IF YOUR PENIS ISN'T UP TO SNUFF, WE HAVE A PILL THAT WILL TAKE CARE OF EVERYTHING

This is the newest myth, brought on by the advent of Viagra in the spring of 1998. The news was incredible: All you had to do is take a little pill and *voilà*—a man would have a great, long-lasting erection. Some thought we were on the verge of sexual nirvana.

It is true that Viagra does give many men an erection. If that is all that is wanted and if the pill works for you, it's like magic. But Viagra does not fix most sexual problems, because being erect is hardly all there is to good sex. Viagra does not make you a good lover—or even make you want to make love—and it does not heal relationship problems.

I saw a couple in which the man was eagerly waiting for Viagra to go on sale. His wife didn't say much until it was announced that the pill would be available soon and he said he was calling his doctor for a prescription, whereupon she announced that she would leave him if he brought the pill into the house. He was shocked and asked why. Her response: "Because, as I've been trying to make clear for a very long time, the problem is not that you sometimes can't keep your erection. What's making me crazy is that you aren't with me in bed. Hard or soft, all you're relating to is your penis. I want you to relate to me. Until we've ironed this part out, I don't want anything to do with erection pills."

She was right. Viagra-induced erections would not make him more present and attentive. He accepted her perspective and worked with me on being more present. With that goal achieved, their sex life improved so dramatically that he never did get the prescription filled.

Pills are tools and, like most tools, have their place. But they usually are only part of what is needed, and that's definitely the case with sex.

Another couple had had serious relationship problems for over twenty years. Given the state of war between them, it was not surprising that the man was not getting erections. Nonetheless, in a last-ditch effort to save the marriage, they agreed he should take Viagra. But his wife wasn't interested in sex with him even when he came into the bedroom with a full erection. More surprising to both of them was that he wasn't interested, either. When he thought about it, he realized that when he ran into the bedroom with his erection, he was much more excited about the fact of the erection than the possibility of having sex with his wife. It was evident that after so many years of tension and hostility, the relationship was over. Not all the king's horses and men, not even Viagra, could make a difference.

Let us celebrate Viagra and all the other wonderful tools medical science is providing us, and let us also use them appropriately. That means thinking clearly about what they can and cannot do.

MYTH 8: SEX EQUALS INTERCOURSE

Both men and women learn that the main thing in sex is intercourse, and for most of us the two terms are synonymous. Almost all resources that deal with sex—medical books, textbooks, popular books, and articles, as well as erotic materials—treat sex and intercourse as if they were the same. Kissing, caressing, and manual and oral stimulation of genitals are all fine, but mainly as preliminaries to the ultimate: having the penis in the vagina. The very term we use to describe these other activities—*foreplay*—indicates their lowly status relative to intercourse. They are presumably important only as means to that main event.

This is silly. Since the goal of the vast majority of sexual encounters is *not* conception, there is no good reason why they have to include or end in intercourse, unless that is what the participants desire. There is no "normal" or "natural" way for sex to proceed. There are lots of possibilities, most of which do not include intercourse. These are discussed in the next chapter.

But we men continue to expect and press for intercourse. Although women in general are more likely to enjoy other aspects of sex, many of them also demand intercourse even though they may not be orgasmic with it.

Insisting on intercourse as a necessary part of sex—the only real way to go—creates a number of problems. One is that it reinforces our performance orientation and makes it difficult to enjoy other aspects of what's going on because we're so focused about getting to intercourse. In this way we rob ourselves of pleasure and of fully experiencing the stimulation necessary for an enjoyable sexual response.

Because intercourse requires some kind of erection (not as much as most men think, but still some hardness), making it a mandatory part of sex reinforces our anxiety about erections. And this, not surprisingly, is likely to result in erection problems.

I'm not against erections or intercourse. If it were up to me, you'd have as many and as much as you wanted. But the absolute need to have them causes lots of problems. When the penis doesn't operate as we want it to, many of us get upset and refuse to have sex at all. If we can't do it the "right way," why do it at all? Should we deprive ourselves of all sexual pleasure because we can't do sex one particular way? Does this make any sense?

Say a man is fortunate enough to have a Mercedes, a car he gets a lot of pleasure from. Then his luck changes and he has to sell the car. What would we think if he refused to drive any other car or take public transportation, saying, "If I can't go the right way, I won't go at all"? Wouldn't we consider him silly or even mad? Suppose he finally came to terms with taking buses or driving another car, but his wife refused to go with him because she considered a bus or Toyota "settling for second best"? Wouldn't we see her as a bit rigid in her thinking?

Yet when it comes to sex, people behave in these peculiar ways all the time. Some men who have trouble with erections stop having sex altogether. Others are willing to try sex but give up as soon as it's clear they're not going to get hard. Still others will do other things—for example, stimulate their partners by hand or mouth—but still feel terrible because they didn't have an erection. And some women whose partners are having erection problems do the same: "I don't want to get myself all worked up and be left hanging. To the suggestion that he could satisfy her another way, she replies: "It's not the same. I'd rather do without."

There's nothing wrong with wanting a Mercedes and erections and intercourse. But there's also a lot to be said for flexibility. In fact, it's one of the hallmarks of maturity.

MYTH 9: A MAN SHOULD MAKE THE EARTH MOVE FOR HIS PARTNER, OR AT THE VERY LEAST KNOCK HER SOCKS OFF

It used to be that scoring was all that mattered. Any man who got a lot of sex could consider himself fulfilling the male role in the sex department. But now we are much more focused on the pleasure of our partners. You can't consider yourself a good lover unless you give your partner an earth-shaking experience.

Here are a few examples from novels of what a man should be able to bring about. From Sidney Sheldon's *If Tomorrow Comes:*

Then Jeff rolled on top of her and was inside of her and it began again, more exciting than before, a fountain spilling over with unbearable pleasure, and Tracy thought, *Now I know. For the first time, I know.*

Sometimes it's more than purely physical. In *Nightwalker,* the beautiful Grey has sex with Khan (who, of course, had a "large, rigid penis [that] was formidable"). This was not a one-shot affair: "He took her time after time. When she thought she could bear no more, he took her again." And there was variety: "He was gentle, softly stroking, coaxing, his soft lips teasing, then suddenly he was again demanding, hard, plummeting the very depths of her passion." The outcome: "She was all woman now, spirit truly touched by the earth-shaking revelations her body had revealed. . . . There were no words to describe the intensity of her feelings."

But another popular author found the words: "Alix felt as if she had been thrown into a fire, felt as if her bones were melting. She had never felt such overwhelming pleasure." Once her bones start melting, you know you're doing it right.

If you're in doubt, she'll probably tell you. In a novel by Irving Wallace, a man receives the ultimate accolade from his lover: "You're good, Ezra, very good. You're the best I know. You're spoiling me for all other men." And a woman in another novel: "You're the most man I ever had."

In fantasyland, sex is always the best, the greatest, the most wonderful. The earth always moves. At minimum, you should be able to "give" your woman at least one and preferably several orgasms. It is now rare to view a sexual scene in a movie or read of one in a book that doesn't include at least one per experience. Ever since Masters and Johnson's research showed that some women are capable of multiple orgasms, expectations have soared. "One climax after another" is a common way of putting it in novels. Here's one happy woman: "Deeper, harder, faster, until she cried out again, barely recovered from her first overwhelming orgasm before she was thrust into her second." Any man who can't generate at least a dozen or so orgasms in his partner is hardly worth considering.

There's also concern about the type of orgasm women have. In fantasyland, they are quick and furious. Women have orgasms "instantaneously" or "almost before he was fully inside her," always accompanied by screams and a thrashing of limbs. "With three violent thrusts he brought her to orgasm" is one example, as is "Within seconds they reached orgasm simultaneously."

The equating of sex with orgasm has become so common that many men might react with incredulity to my calling it a myth, asking, "What's the point of sex without a climax?" What's the point indeed? And what's the point of dinner without dessert? Or a football game without a touchdown?

The point is simple. With or without an orgasm, with or without dessert, with or without a touchdown, the sex, dinner, and game go on. There's interesting stuff to be had, if only you can pay attention and not get upset because it doesn't have the ending you want.

I have nothing against orgasms. If it can happen without making everyone miserable, enjoy it. But what's the point of twisting oneself into a pretzel in order to have an orgasm? Many men try to force their own orgasms by thrusting wildly and calling up every fantasy they can think of. Although it surprises many people when I say this, more than a few men I've talked to have faked orgasm. They felt bad about doing this, but they didn't want their partners to know they didn't come. Besides, they had no idea of how to stop the activity without an orgasm.

Men also put pressure on their partners to have quick, loud orgasms so that they, the men, will be able to feel good about themselves. No wonder that faking orgasms on the part of women hasn't gone out of style. Even if she has a real one, she may feel pressured to fake several more, or to make it more dramatic than it really is. What's the point of doing this to one's partner?

There is a point, come to think of it, understandable but still harmful. We men are obsessed with specifications and indicators. Now that women are supposed to enjoy sex—which men take to mean that we are supposed to make it enjoyable for them—how do we know they enjoyed it? We need a clear sign, and orgasm is the clearest sign we can think of.

Yet all of this is foolishness. There can be good sex that doesn't include orgasm for either partner, that has orgasm for only one partner, that has only one orgasm for the woman, that involves less than house-shaking and bed-breaking orgasms.

One result of this myth is added pressure on a man to perform. Not only does he have to get it up and keep it up, he also has to use his tool, and everything else he has, to give his partner a mind-blowing experience. And of course no one ever tells him exactly how he's supposed to accomplish that.

This belief has another unfortunate consequence. It can make it difficult for a man to feel good about a sexual encounter that consists solely of being pleasured by his partner. Sometimes when the woman is not in the mood and the man is, she can engage in intercourse or some other act for his pleasure. As long as she feels good about what she's doing and there's no coercion, I don't see anything wrong with this, just as I don't see anything wrong with a man's stimulating his partner for her satisfaction when he isn't in the mood for something for himself. This practice can be quite helpful in a relationship where one partner wants sex more frequently than the other.

But because of the idea that sex isn't complete unless the woman has orgasmic convulsions, many men put such activities down as "servicing" and say they aren't interested. So the man may deprive himself of the sex he could have had and feels frustrated, annoyed, or angry. The woman is also in a bad place. What she was able and willing to provide isn't good enough, and now she's got an upset partner. Should she just accept that, or should she try to force feelings that aren't there or even fake them? This kind of stuff does not make for happy relationships.

MYTH 10: GOOD SEX IS SPONTANEOUS, WITH NO PLANNING AND NO TALKING

Fantasyland sex is spontaneous. People get turned on to each other and one thing leads to another, as we like to say. Of course, one or both partners may have been thinking about sex beforehand, hoping for it, anticipating it. And the partners may hint, flirt, tease, and seduce. But apparently it's not okay to talk openly and plan together for sex.

A quote from best-selling author Jackie Collins illustrates part of this myth. A man and woman who don't know each other and who have barely exchanged a dozen words start having sex: "There was nothing awkward about their lovemaking. He entered her smoothly and she moved with him as if they had been together many times before. Instinctively she knew his rhythm and he knew hers." Isn't that nice? Nothing was awkward, and each "instinctively" knew the other's rhythm and presumably desires as well. Just like in real life, right? Later, as the man recalls the experience, he thinks this: "No corny lines or bullshit. Just wonderfully uninhibited silent sex." The message is clear: Discussing sex, or even getting to know one another—all this is "corny lines or bullshit." Only silent sex is real and meaningful.

This shows why fantasy sex is so popular. It feeds into the childish fantasies we all carry around, where people instinctively know what the other wants and willingly provide it, where there are no serious problems, where we can have whatever we want and all we want of it.

We have no trouble planning dates and social events. Few people show up at airports, laden with suitcases, asking, "Do you have planes going to any interesting places today?" Rather, they plan their vacations, and no one seems to suffer because of this. And few people have any problems discussing what to do about dinner tonight: "Do you want to eat in or go out? Early or late? Chinese, Mexican, Italian, or what?"

But because we still view sex, even in marriage, as not quite all right, we'd rather sneak our way into it—and call it spontaneity. Planning sex usually involves talking about it, something that makes most of us very uncomfortable. So the less we plan and the less we talk about it, the less real it seems and the less embarrassed we have to get.

We pay heavily for our desire for spontaneity. Because of a lack of planning, we often have less sex than we want. Our spontaneous invitations often get rebuffed because of insufficient time or energy. Because we don't want to plan and talk, we often fail to use necessary protections against disease and conception. Yet another price is that sex often isn't as good as it could be if we were willing to plan for it (by making time, anticipating it, setting the appropriate mood, and so on).

If you want more sex, safer sex, and better sex, you might want to re-think whether spontaneity is really crucial. And while you're thinking, keep in mind that planning does not rule out spontaneity. Couples who have good sex talk about it and plan for it, and also take advantage of spontaneous opportunities.

These and similar myths have made men and women anxious, created problems and dissatisfactions, and made resolution of existing problems more difficult. But we are not stuck with these destructive notions. We can reject them and put in their place more realistic and more constructive ideas. In the process, we can make our sex lives a true reflection of our values, feelings, thoughts, and the best interests of ourselves and our relationships, rather than trying to measure up to ridiculous standards set by others. In the rest of the book, you'll have numerous opportunities to examine and modify beliefs that may be creating problems in your sex life.

SEXUAL REALITY

What Is This Thing Called Sex?

Sex! Everything connected with it. People spend more time thinking, worrying, agonizing over it than all the rest of the woes of man put together. Nothing so drives people—men, women—off the rails. I sometimes think God had begun to doze, was excessively fatigued, hadn't worked it out properly, when he put that part in place.—*William Brinkley*

I used to think I was a hot stud in college and knew everything about sex. Turned out that I knew very little: just get her hot, stick it in, hump away, and come. Took me a while to find out sex is a lot more than that. —*Man, 31*

THE MAIN PROBLEM with the fantasy model of sex is that it holds up standards that are for the most part unattainable by human beings and probably not desirable even if they could be reached. But because people take the model as defining what's normal, as a standard against which to measure their own behavior and feelings, they not only end up feeling inadequate but also miss the obvious. They don't ask if they're getting what they want and if their erotic activity in fact enhances their pleasure, self-esteem, and relationship.

In many ways, the sex people actually have doesn't differ that much from the sex animals have. And that's depressing, to think that what you're doing isn't much different from what a mouse or chicken or monkey does. And in some ways, lower animals have it better. They may not have long-lasting intercourse, but at least they aren't sneaky about their matings and apparently they don't feel guilty about what they do, and I doubt they worry about their performance. In a reproductive sense, it doesn't make much difference, of course—just whatever gets the job done. But humans are capable of so much more.

The model of sex I discuss in this chapter and that will take me most of the rest of the book to illustrate is more distinctly human and more intimate than what we've had before. It's a sexuality in which *people* inter-act and relate, not just genitals; in which deceit and coercion play no part; in which what's between your ears is as important as what's between your legs; in which you can plan for sex and talk about it before, during, or after the actual events; in which you can change directions or stop at any point. The goals of this intimate model of sex are pleasure, closeness, and self- and partner enhancement, not performance or conquest.

This is a freer and better-feeling kind of sex. It's freer because you have more options: You and your partner can select from a huge range of ways to express your sexual feelings and are no longer limited to just the old foreplay-followed-by-intercourse routine. You can even decide not to plan or talk or be intimate; in other words, part of this new sex is the option to have sex in the old way. It's more enjoyable because it's understood that pleasure rather than performance or obligation is the goal; you don't *have* to do anything, and there's permission to be yourself and get what you want and need. You can be loving, playful, silly, lusty, or whatever else you want. You can have affection without sex, sex with or without affection, or none of the above. You're freer to enjoy yourself because of all the choices and because most of the worry is taken away: The emphasis on talking and planning allows you and your partner to protect yourself against un-wanted consequences.

The freedoms gained in the sexual revolution allow us to create a smarter, more enjoyable, more exciting and satisfying, and more humane sexuality. Unless we want to continue paying the price that sex has exacted from the beginning of time (bad feelings, unnecessary anxiety, dysfunc-tions and dissatisfactions, unwanted conception, debilitating and even fa-tal diseases), maybe it's time to try something different.

GOOD SEX

Although good sex is often defined in terms of specific behaviors and spe-cific body parts, feelings are paramount. And this is as true for men as for women. Even though men tend to think and talk in terms of activities— "I'd like to fuck [make love to] her"; "I'd like her to give me head"—it seems clear that what's really wanted is the feelings these actions will pro-duce. They will make him feel sexy, excited, satisfied, manly, powerful, and so on.

Good sex is not about using any particular organ, following any par-ticular script, or doing any particular act. Rather, it has to do with the emotions generated by whatever you and your partner do. The best definition I've heard derives from an idea of San Francisco sex therapist Carol Ellison and goes like this: You're having good sex if you feel good about yourself, good about your partner, and good about what you're doing. If later, after you've had time for reflection, you still feel good about yourself, your partner, and what you did, you know you've had good sex. As such, it need not include intercourse or any other specific act or sequence of acts, need not include orgasm, and can take anywhere from a few seconds to several hours.

Certain things, however, are excluded—any kind of coercion, for example. If coercion is used, whether physical or psychological, at least one partner is not going to feel good during and after the activity. The same is true for deception. I would make a similar point for impulsive sex that goes against one's interests and values. If you don't want conception to occur, yet take no measures to protect against it, you're going to worry and feel bad afterward. I wouldn't call that good sex.

Let's take an example from another area, driving. If you believe the ads on TV, a good drive consists of quickly shifting through the gears and getting your car to do 150 miles an hour. Given the condition of today's roads and traffic, it's a mystery where you could do this—on most roads these days you're happy if you can get up to 20 mph—but it's clear that lots of people buy the fantasy, always looking for a place to "open it up."

Even assuming you could safely drive at 150 mph, it would still represent only one kind of good drive. Suppose you took a leisurely drive through the country, looking at the sights and smelling the scents. Couldn't that be a good drive? Or suppose you took a drive with a friend and had a stimulating conversation. Wouldn't that constitute a good drive? And wouldn't it also be a good drive if during it you worked out a problem in your head, had an interesting fantasy, or enjoyed listening to the radio? And what about the unlikely circumstance where there was little traffic and good weather and you simply got to your destination without hassle— might that not be a good drive as well? Isn't it also possible to have a good trip by letting someone else do the driving, by carpooling, or by taking a bus? You could also consider using a bicycle rather than a motorized vehicle. Couldn't that be a good drive as well as good exercise?

Just as there are lots of ways to have a good drive and lots of kinds of good meals and good experiences, there are lots of ways to have good sex.

Before getting to sexual options, let's take a closer look at what they're alternatives to, the traditional sexual script.

THE PRIMACY OF INTERCOURSE

As I mentioned when discussing sexual myths, almost everyone seems to believe that intercourse is what sex is mainly about. Even people who consider themselves liberated and are comfortable with many different sexual acts feel cheated if intercourse isn't part of the routine. This goes for women as well as men.

Although there's no doubt that social conditioning plays a role in reinforcing the belief that intercourse is *the* sexual act, common sense requires us to acknowledge that the desire for sexual intercourse is also, perhaps mainly, caused by something else. Intercourse is the only way to reproduce the species, and reproducing the species is nature's main interest. All of us, women and men, are programmed to want intercourse. That much is fact, and it is folly to ignore or deny it.

Culture follows nature, at least in the most important areas. While political and religious authorities often are uncomfortable with anything sexual, no reproduction means the whole enterprise will soon go out of business. So while many authorities through history have been unable to stomach the idea of masturbation, homosexuality, or oral or anal sex, they always make provision for heterosexual intercourse under certain circumstances.

Most people, of course, do not think they want intercourse because they are following nature's programming or in order to produce more of the faithful or more soldiers or customers. Their desires are always experienced in more personal terms. One woman said this about intercourse:

> It's not as exciting as oral sex or a vibrator, it's certainly not orgasmic, but I feel incomplete without it. It's just something I have to have.

A man put it differently:

> I love when she goes down on me. My orgasms in her mouth are unbelievable. I even love a quick hand job. But there's something special about intercourse. A sense of having her, possessing her, that I only get when my penis is in her vagina and I come inside of her.

Because of feelings like this, and also because of the sexual conditioning we're given, the standard sexual script is simple: foreplay (which may include oral or manual stimulation of genitals, and the main purpose of which is usually thought to be getting the woman ready for what is to follow) and then intercourse.

And it seems so natural, which of course it is, and makes so much sense. After all, he has a pole, she has a hole, so it seems only right that the pole should go in the hole. This can also be seen in apparently more sophisticated ways, having to do with the merging of the yin and the yang, the union of bodies and maybe souls. There's also the silly fact that humans tend to make possibilities into imperatives. Since a man can get hard, he ought to get hard. Since we can stick poles in holes, we ought to; otherwise there's something wrong.

Although from an evolutionary standpoint there is good reason for us to desire intercourse, there is a lot wrong with intercourse as an imperative, having to have it and seeing everything else as second best. The problems with intercourse as the main course can be grouped into six categories:

1. Since intercourse demands some kind of erection (not as hard as most men think, but still some hardness), it puts tremendous pressure on a man to get erect. The pressure would be less if the man could just will himself erect, as many men wish they could. But the penis is not subject to this kind of control.

Bad feelings result if the man doesn't get and stay erect. He feels inadequate and less of a man, a very heavy burden indeed. And the woman often feels that his "failure" is a comment about her: She's not sexy or skillful enough to get him hard. What is the point of all this self-inflicted misery?

2. Women are also put in a difficult situation. Thanks to Sigmund Freud and thousands of writers of pornography, it was assumed that both men and women would climax in intercourse. But the majority of women require direct clitoral stimulation and do not climax solely by means of intercourse. Thanks to the women's movement of the 1960s and '70s and the advent of sex therapy in the 1970s, this fact got lots of exposure, and women were given permission and encouragement to get the kinds of stimulation they needed. Many men and women, however, continue to believe that women should somehow climax during intercourse, and both sexes feel bad when that doesn't happen.

3. Intercourse as generally done takes more time and effort than some other sex acts, and also, as already noted, puts more pressure on both partners. This means that there is less sex than might be the case if other sexual activities were given equal significance.

4. It's also a fact that many sex problems occur mainly or only during intercourse. Many men who ejaculate very quickly in intercourse, for instance, can enjoy manual or oral stimulation for much longer.

5. The emphasis on erections and intercourse fails to take into account our aging population, people with various kinds of illnesses and disabilities, and couples in which the woman is in the last stages of pregnancy or has recently given birth. Many people in these groups have difficulties with erections or intercourse and don't fit the traditional sexual script very well. What are they supposed to do about sex?

6. Intercourse is also the most dangerous sexual act. One huge risk is pregnancy itself. I realize, of course, that Mother Nature would have a tough time with that one. She did not foresee a time when reproducing the species would be the least of our problems. Conception is the goal only a tiny proportion of the times men and women get together sexually. Disease is another problem. Although most STDs can be transmitted through oral-genital contact, the main risk by far is vaginal or anal intercourse. Why are we so intent on emphasizing a sexual act that can be so risky?

Given the stage we've reached in our historical development, given that pleasure and relationship enhancement are what we want from sex rather than reproduction, to some extent it's fair to say that we have to go against Mother Nature's design. But not by much. After all, while giving primacy to intercourse, she also built us to feel great pleasure with masturbation, oral sex, and lots of other kinds of stimulation. In addition to genitals, she gave us hands and mouths and tongues and sensitive skin all over. Consider for a moment the fact that no matter how large your penis is, even if it's twelve inches long and eight inches around, that represents only a fraction of your total body area. Why should great feelings and great pleasure be limited to this tiny portion of your anatomy? And women have a clitoris, an organ that has nothing to do with reproduction and whose only function is sexual pleasure. Interestingly, it's in a place that makes it difficult for a penis, thrusting or not, to stimulate it. Maybe Mother Nature thought that other kinds of sex besides intercourse should be part of the plan.

I believe that the fairest interpretation of Mother Nature's plan these days is that it allows humans the freedom to choose how to enjoy sex. We can choose to enjoy it alone or with a partner, and with a partner we can choose from a whole range of options.

The more you accept the idea that there are many ways to give and receive sexual pleasure, the erections, intercourse, and even orgasm are nice but not necessary, the more frequent and better sex you will have. Since you'll be putting fewer demands on your penis, it will be free to do its best, and you'll be able to enjoy a wide variety of sexual activities, including intercourse.

Some people might say, **"Other things can be fun, but it doesn't feel like making love unless we have intercourse."** That's to be expected, because traditionally "making love" has meant intercourse and not other kinds of sexual activity. I suggest, however, that *making love has to do with feelings rather than with specific acts.* People can feel very loved and loving with all sorts of acts, many of them not even sexual. If you can allow this idea to be your guide—that it's the feelings rather than the acts that define making love—I think you'll agree. If your partner lovingly caresses you all over your body or lovingly stimulates your penis with her hand or mouth, why can't that be lovemaking as much as intercourse is?

SEXUAL OPTIONS

I'm not suggesting you never have intercourse with an erection. Whenever you and your partner are agreed that's what you both want, that's what you should have. But you'll have more sex, and probably more fun and satisfaction as well, if you're willing to consider other options like the following:

▲ Flirting with your partner although you both know nothing physical can take place now.

▲ Flirting with another woman although you both know nothing physical will ever take place between you.

"Flirting is OK, but it's not the same as physical sex." Of course it isn't. But that doesn't mean it can't feel sexual and be the source of great pleasure. Why not just enjoy the feelings?

"Flirting is OK as far as it goes, but it doesn't go far enough. I'm afraid I'd get all worked up and get frustrated." Let me assure you that no one has ever been taken to a hospital emergency room because of sexual frustration. Don't worry, you won't explode. Why not allow yourself to enjoy the good feelings and then let them subside? Or, if you know you and your partner will be together later, why not let the flirting start your juices flowing and build the turn-on?

▲ Bathing your partner, or she you, or both of you bathing each other. Take your time and remember that getting clean is not the main purpose.

▲ Giving or receiving a sensuous massage that does not include genital stimulation.

▲ Giving or receiving a sensuous massage that does include genital stimulation.

▲ Giving or receiving a session of toe sucking or finger licking and sucking. This may sound weird if you haven't done it before, but giving it a try won't cost you much.

▲ Kissing and hugging followed by rubbing your bodies and pelvises together while clothed (called "dry humping" when I was growing up). You can do this in elevators, stairwells, up against walls, in parked cars, and so forth.

▲ Dirty dancing, which is dry humping on a dance floor. Want a hint? Each of you puts one leg between your partner's legs, and you take it from there.

▲ Petting, kissing, and fondling breasts and genitals while clothed or partially clothed. Petting and dry humping remind many adults of the sexual activity they engaged in during adolescence, when that's all they could do. Many adults feel deliciously wicked when doing these things now.

▲ Kissing and hugging followed by one of you stimulating the other by hand.

▲ Kissing and hugging followed by one of you stimulating the other orally.

▲ One of you stimulating the other by hand or mouth without any kissing or hugging.

"My partner and I often do oral and manual stimulation as part of foreplay. But it would seem strange for one or both of them to be the main course." The strangeness comes from your idea of what "real" sex is. But that idea can change. Why can't manual or oral stimulation, as well as some other items, be the main course sometimes? You might find you enjoy a more varied menu.

"It seems unequal if I'm getting all the pleasure or if she's getting all the pleasure." But who said that you have to be equally excited or derive equal pleasure? It is often the case, even in intercourse, that one partner is more excited and gets more out of it than the other. What's wrong with your getting most of the goodies sometimes? What's wrong with her getting most of the goodies at other times?

"Your-turn, my-turn kind of sex seems so artificial and unnatural." The traditional model of sex is a reciprocal one: while she's kissing your neck or touching your penis, you're kissing her neck, fondling her breasts, or touching her clitoris, and then you both participate in intercourse. But who says it has to be this way? Suppose she does all the "work" while you just sit or lie back and enjoy? Can't that also be a loving or passionate or caring experience?

The main problem with the reciprocal model is that your attention is always split. One moment you're focusing on the stimulation you're getting, the next moment on the stimulation you're giving. This has its benefits, of course, but because of the split attention, you're never able to focus on your own pleasure for long.

The main advantage of the taking-turns kind of sex is that the receiver can just receive, focusing only on pleasure, without also being concerned about giving anything in return. This allows a total concentration on sensations and feelings that often results in a powerful experience.

▲ You masturbating while your partner holds and touches you.

"Masturbation is something I do myself. I don't see it as something to do with a partner." Of course. A lot of people see masturbation as something they do themselves, not with a partner. That's part of our traditional model. In partner sex, you touch your partner and she touches you, but no one touches himself or herself. But why not? Why can't touching yourself be part of what you do with a partner? Masturbating with some kind of partner participation is just another way of having good sex.

Many men say their most intense orgasms come through masturbation. The reason is simple: No one knows or can know your body as well as you do. I realize that intense orgasms are not the only reason to have sex. There are many other rewards as well. But what's wrong with masturbating with partner involvement and giving yourself an incredible climax?

"The idea sounds fine, but I'm shy about touching myself with her watching." Many men (and women as well) feel shy at first about touching themselves while their partner watches. Fortunately, all it takes is the courage to do it once or twice. The shyness and embarrassment usually evaporate quickly. By the way, most women like watching their partners masturbate; it's a turn-on. As one woman put it: "I enjoy it because I love to see a man doing something loving for himself."

▲ You masturbating while your partner tells you an exciting fantasy, perhaps over the phone.

▲ Your partner masturbating with her hand or a vibrator while you hold and touch her.

▲ Your partner masturbating while you tell her an interesting fantasy, perhaps over the phone.

▲ One of you orally or manually stimulating the other one, who is talking on the phone with someone else. The third party, the one on the other end of the telephone line, does not know what is going on. It can add to the excitement if the third party is someone in authority: a parent, teacher, coach, or employer.

▲ Each of you masturbating while you lie side by side or facing one another (so you can see each other's faces).

▲ During any sexual activity, change what you do with your eyes. If you usually keep them closed, open them. If you usually have them open, close them. Experience the difference.

▲ Your partner uses a finger or two to massage your perineum (the area between the scrotum and the anus) or anus, or inserts a well-lubricated finger into your anus during any other sexual activity. Although as children we were all warned away from the anal area, it is richly endowed with nerve endings and a source of great erotic pleasure to many men (and women).

▲ Your partner stimulating your soft penis with her hand or mouth.

I hope it goes without saying by now that all of the above acts can be enjoyed with or without orgasm. Too many people don't enjoy sex because they're so focused on the Big O that's supposed to happen and then get upset when it doesn't. Orgasms are nice and I'm all for them, but you can have lots of pleasure without them.

Remember, as long as you feel good about yourself, good about your partner, and good about what you're doing or have done, that's good sex.

EXPRESSING DIFFERENT FEELINGS IN SEX

So far we've been talking about options involving different activities. But there is also another kind of option having to do with the main feeling that's expressed in sex. Sexual activity with a partner can be a fine way to express a number of feelings. These days, it seems that the main goal of both women and men in this regard is to connect deeply to another person we care about. And there are times when a couple really makes love. What they do is a reflection of the deep feelings they have for each other, and the result is an openness and bonding that lasts for hours or days, regardless of what they actually did sexually. Individual boundaries may diminish or disappear, and it really feels like a unity or oneness, as if two people have merged. You can't plan for this kind of sex and you can't make it happen. But if you really care about one another and are open to yourself and each other, sometimes it just happens. And when it does, it makes everything right, like the sun suddenly appearing on a dark and rainy day.

But good sex can be far more than an expression of loving feelings. In the old days, women complained that men were rough and quick; apparently the main feelings the men expressed were their own lust and desire for gratification. But men have changed, as have women, and now a frequent complaint is that men are too timid, too careful, too unassertive and unpassionate. My experiences working with men tend to support this idea. Many men are really hanging back in sex.

There's nothing wrong with expressing love and caring through sex; it's a great vehicle for showing these feelings. But there's also nothing wrong with expressing lust in sex, or fun, or other feelings. If sex is a vehicle for only one kind of feeling, you'll be limited in the amount of sex you have—you can be sexual only when, say, you feel loving or only when you feel lustful. Also, expressing only one kind of feeling in sex can lead to boredom.

Many couples differentiate between at least two kinds of sex: making love (gentle, concerned with expressing romance, caring, and love) and fucking (more passionate and expressing only desire).

Too much sensitivity can inhibit passion. Writer Myron Brenton relates the story of Allan, a law student in love with his partner, Marie. He was always soft and gentle, holding himself back in sex for fear of hurting her. While on vacation, he met a seductive, teasing woman who finally managed to get him in bed with her. Not caring much about her, and feeling angry toward her, he thrusted hard and vigorously when they had intercourse. He expected to be criticized for this and was surprised when she said it was terrific. When Allan returned to school, he decided to try this kind of sex with Marie, even though he feared she might not like it. Her reaction was to ask why they hadn't always made love like this.

Passion and love are far from all the emotions that can be expressed. Good sex can also be playful, fun, and even silly. For the most part we're talking about differences in perspective and feeling rather than different activities. You may do the same things while making love, being playful, or fucking. But you do them with a different attitude and spirit. A long-married woman told me that one of the aspects of sex with her husband that she most appreciates is the silliness:

> After all, the whole thing—the positions and all—is pretty ridiculous to begin with. It sometimes reminds me of being a child and engaging in explorations of my own and friend's bodies. I feel so secure with my husband that I can let that little girl's silly side come out. It's great fun.

Some couples sometimes revert to baby talk during sex; some enjoy teasing and being teased.

One of the most memorable experiences I had wouldn't even fit most people's definition of sex. My girlfriend and I were in bed one afternoon. Just as she was guiding my penis into her, she came out with phrases she had gotten from a book of pornography she had looked at earlier that day: "Stick that huge, hard cock into my hot and juicy pussy. I want to feel all twelve inches of you, filling me up, fucking and thrusting as hard as you want, spilling gobs of seed into me." We both broke up into gales of laughter, and I fell off of her. We laughed and laughed for what seemed like hours. Every time we tried to talk, we started laughing again. There was no intercourse, no other sexual activity, and no orgasm for either of us. But it was an incredibly wonderful experience that I recall vividly and lovingly over twenty years later.

Sex can also be a great tension reliever. We have all sorts of nostrums for reducing stress—everything from physical exercise to meditation to various drugs—but sex is one of nature's best ways to feel relaxed. I know a man who usually gets tense before he has to give a public talk. He's tried beta-blockers and other pills, relaxation tapes, and other remedies, but the one that works the best, with no side effects, is an orgasm produced by his partner's hand or mouth. How does she feel about it? "Absolutely fine. I'm happy to be able to do this for him. And he reciprocates when I need it, usually when I have trouble falling asleep." Of course, this won't work if your anxiety is about sex itself. But for stress related to work and other matters, it's often quite useful.

Although some people have trouble with this one, I also believe it's fine to express anger through sex—provided, of course, that this doesn't happen all the time, that it's okay with both partners, and that the anger doesn't turn to violence. Physiologically, anger and sexual arousal are quite similar. Both excite the nervous system. While it's true that some people can't even think about sex when they're angry, let alone do something about it, others find that anger—regardless of its source—can serve to heighten the sexual experience. Recall that anger at his new partner was partly what caused Allan, the law student mentioned on page 47, to let go and find a new way of being sexual. This isn't unusual. Some couples report that their best sex occurs in the midst of an argument.

Anger is a strong emotion and should be treated with caution. Nonetheless, anger is a fact of life, and it can be used to enhance one's sex life.

The most important thing about expressing different feelings is that the partners have to agree on what they're doing. It can lead to confusion, frustration, and other negative feelings if one partner is fucking while the other is trying to make love, or if one wants a stress reliever or sleeping potion while the other has something else in mind. Clear communication is a must.

I hope you'll go over the ideas in this chapter and share them, or at least the ideas that appeal to you, with your partner. While I certainly haven't covered all the possibilities, I hope I've made you aware that sex isn't any one thing and isn't confined to any one script or routine. With skin all over our bodies, with hands, mouths, breasts, penises (hard or soft), clitorides, vaginas (wet or dry), and anuses, and with incredibly powerful and creative minds to work with and lots of different emotions that we can experience, we have lots and lots of possibilities.

Of course, there's no rule that you have to like all the options. Some may not appeal to you, and some may not appeal to your partner. But I hope that at least a few of them will sound attractive enough to both of you to warrant a bit of experimentation. You'll have more sex and better sex if you're open to a number of possibilities.

CHAPTER FOUR

What Is This Thing Called a Penis?

You would think I'd know better. I mean, I'm well educated and have read a lot about sex. But I still believe that I'd be more attractive to women and a better lover if my penis was an inch or two longer and an inch wider. —*Man, 28*

My big wish is that my cock were exactly like my hand. If I told it to stand up, it would stand up. If I told it to lie down, it would lie down. Why can't I have the same control over my penis that I have over all my other appendages?—*Man, 50*

IN THIS CHAPTER I discuss the issues about penises that have been of most interest to the men I've worked with. I've been surprised to discover over the years how ignorant many men are about this organ that means so much to them. Some basic knowledge can be helpful. I won't bore you with irrelevant details, but I will discuss what penises are, what can reasonably be expected from them, and what happens to them as they age.

Let's start with how we think and feel about our penises.

TOWARD A FRIENDLIER AND MORE REALISTIC VIEW OF OUR PENISES

To say the least, we men have mixed feelings. Our penises are very important to us. They are the main distinguishing characteristic between us and women, and they are a source of great pleasure. But there's often a sense of unease or discontent with our organs. We fear that they may not be up to snuff in terms of size, power, and predictability. This does not feel right or good. We fear that, sooner or later, they are going to disappoint and embarrass us.

Some men are on friendly terms with their penises. They like them for the pleasure they provide and see them as a kind of friend, sometimes even giving them pet names. Other men, however, are in a state of near war with their cocks. They speak cajolingly, angrily, or threateningly to them: "Come on, please, you can do it, yes you can"; "You better come through for me, you son of a bitch"; "I'll break your neck if you don't get hard." This kind of self-talk is often caused by the penis's failure to do what its owner wants, or fear of such a failure. Whatever the reason, it is not conducive to friendly relations.

Being on better terms with our penises is made difficult by the common terms we have for them—*cock, prick, rod, tool, ramrod, hard-on, dick.* These words sound harsh and do not contribute to a sense of warmth, gentleness, or friendliness. They fit right in, of course, with the view of penises in fantasyland, always throbbing, thrashing, banging, ramming, thrusting. You'd think a penis was a weapon of war rather than an instrument of pleasure and love.

This depiction is neither realistic nor useful. We need something more accurate and helpful. Consider that the penis is very soft. Even when fully erect, the skin is velvety and smooth. Consider also that the penis spends the vast majority of its time in a flaccid state, just lying there all crinkled up and cuddled against the body. Even the fabled adolescent penis spends most of its time just resting.

In addition, we should take into account the age-old idea that penises have minds of their own. A man usually comes to this conclusion when he feels aroused and ready for sex but his penis isn't cooperating. A useful way of looking at this situation is to ask, "Why won't it cooperate?" or, better still, "What does it need that it isn't getting?" I used to ask men with erection problems to take the role of their penis and write a letter or essay giving its point of view. The results were quite revealing. Often the penis complained mightily about not getting what it needed (a relaxed owner, a booze-free environment, proper stimulation, and so on) and resented the demands being made on it. An example:

> You never pay attention to me unless you want something, and then you want it exactly when you want it, and get angry and threaten me unless I comply. Half the situations you get into scare the hell out of you and that scares me. I'm not at my best when I'm scared. I want

you to know that unless you pay more attention and give me what I need, like more appealing and less frightening situations, you're getting zilch. And that's that!

It may sound strange to hear that penises have needs and can get frightened. But real penises are far more vulnerable and frail than the robotlike machines in the fantasy model. They do have needs. Just as athletes have long known that their muscles and systems work better under certain conditions than others (having to do with rest, nutrition, exercise, temperature, and so on), we now know that penises and sexual systems do the same. In Chapter 6 I'll talk more about what you and your penis need.

It will pay you to start thinking of your penis as the human organ it is. The more you can regard your penis in a gentler and more humane way, the more you take care of it, the better relationship you'll have with it and the more it will behave as you want. And when your penis doesn't do what you want, it pays to listen carefully. It's trying to tell you something.

PENIS ENVY

Sigmund Freud, the founder of psychoanalysis, had a theory that girls and women were dissatisfied with their own genitals and envied men their penises. They wanted them, too. I have yet to meet a woman who wanted to have her own penis (except on camping trips), although many would like to borrow one from time to time. As a woman friend once put it: "Why would I want a thing like that hanging between my legs? I'd be afraid I'd sit on it."

I think, however, that Freud was partly right about penis envy. It exists, but only in males. Almost every male seems to envy someone else's penis. He wants one that's longer, wider, harder, with more staying power, and he assumes that some other man or lots of other men have one just like that.

One reason we are so unhappy with our penises is the superhuman expectations we have learned. Having repeatedly read and heard about gargantuan, hard-as-steel ramrods, our own real penises don't seem like much. How can anything real seem adequate compared to the telephone poles we read about?

And most heterosexual men have never seen another erect penis, or at least not a typical one. The ones we are likely to have seen, in pornographic movies and magazines, are not representative. The producers of these films conduct broad searches for the biggest phalluses in existence.

Given the absence of reasonable standards, there is good reason for us to wonder about the adequacy of our own organs.

HOW LARGE IS ENOUGH?

Like all other physical characteristics, penises do differ in size and shape. As indicated in Figures 1 and 2 on pages 54 and 55, some are longer, some shorter; some are broader or wider, some narrower; some curve or bend to the right, some to the left, some not at all; some point upward when erect, some downward, some straight out. Although penises differ in size, there is less variation among hard penises than among soft ones because a smaller soft penis will increase more in size during erection than a larger soft penis. Nonetheless, there is still some variation, and there's nothing that can be done about that.

Men almost invariably assume that a bigger penis is better and is what women prefer. Women think much less about penis size than do men. The vast majority of women I've talked to could not recall a conversation about sex with women friends where penis size was even mentioned. When I questioned these women about size preference, they gave surprising answers. There are, to be sure, a few who said they like very large penises, which give them a "filled-up" feeling in intercourse. But the vast majority of women I've talked to do not desire large penises. Here's what a thirty-seven-year-old woman had to say: "The penises in my fantasies are always very large and thick, but in real life a large penis can be hard to take. I'm much more orgasmic with an average-size penis; a large one is distracting. The old adage 'It's not the meat but the motion' most definitely applies."

I've also talked to a number of men with very large penises. You'd think they'd be quite content, because they're the ones who measure up to the fantasies of most men. Surprisingly, many of these men are anything but happy. Most of them say they wish they had smaller organs. They complain about women gasping—not in ecstasy, but in horror—when they first lay eyes on their outsized organs. Some women have refused to have intercourse with them at all, and many have refused to do oral sex on them, fearing they would choke. And some of these men said they often have to be careful when having sex lest they do hurt their partners. Sometimes living up to a fantasy isn't all it's cracked up to be.

Most women I've talked to prefer average-size penises, and that's nice, because that's what most men have. But what about smaller-than-average

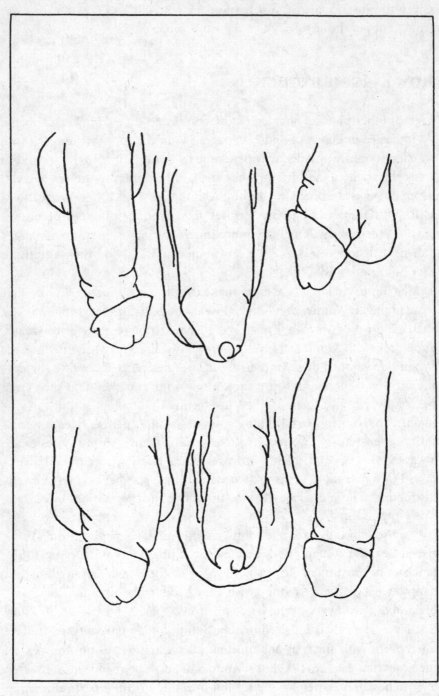

Figure 1: Flaccid penises

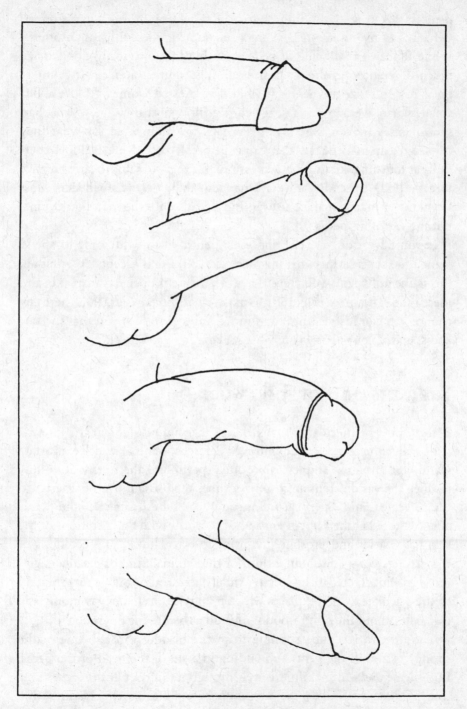

Figure 2: Erect penises

penises? It's true that some men's erections are shorter than average (which is to five to six inches long) and some are less thick than others. While it may be difficult to believe, such variations really don't make much difference. As already indicated, most women aren't half as interested in penis size as men. But when I've pressed women to talk about smaller-than-average penises, several said the guys they knew who had such penises were terrific lovers. Perhaps to compensate for what they considered an inadequacy (their small penises), these men developed their skills at touching, kissing, and caressing. But this does not mean you have to get a Ph.D. in sex if your penis happens to be on the small side. Most women said that a small penis was fine, because "it's the man that counts, not the size of his penis."

If you have trouble accepting your penis, you might want to spend some time considering what it would take to make it acceptable. After all, this is the only penis you'll ever have. There are no penis transplants and there is no safe and effective way to make what you have larger. Is there any chance you can just accept it and move on? I guarantee you that the size and shape of your penis is not what makes for a good lover.

THE PARTS AND HOW THEY WORK

Before going further with the penis, let's take a quick look at the internal sex organs: the testes, epididymis, vas deferens, seminal vesicles, prostate gland, and urethra. The testes produce sperm and the hormone testosterone. The vas deferens are two firm tubes that extend from the testes to the prostate gland. Sperm travel through the tubes from the epididymis and are stored at their upper ends until they mix with the secretions of the seminal vesicles and prostate just prior to ejaculation. The secretions of the prostate comprise about a third of the seminal fluid or ejaculate, giving it its whitish color. The sperm actually account for only a tiny fraction of the ejaculate, which explains why a man who has had a vasectomy still ejaculates about the same amount of fluid as before the operation.

The urethra is a tube running from the bladder through one of the spongy tissues in the penis and ending in a slit in the head of the penis. Both urine and seminal fluid travel through it, but not at the same time. The prostate surrounds the urethra where it leaves the bladder, and prostate problems such as inflammation or enlargement can cause urinary difficulties.

The external male genitalia consist of the penis and the scrotum, the

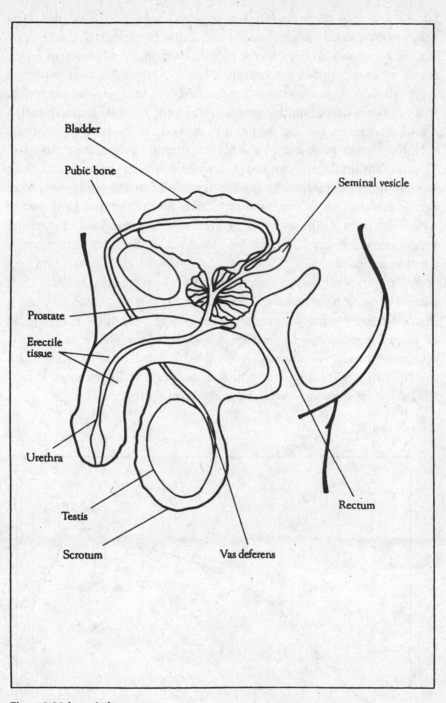

Bladder

Pubic bone

Seminal vesicle

Prostate

Erectile tissue

Urethra

Rectum

Testis

Scrotum

Vas deferens

Figure 3: Male genital anatomy

latter containing the testes. Despite what many people think, the penis contains no striated muscle tissue, the kind that can be enlarged with exercise. There is also no bone in the penis, giving the lie to the term *boner*, which many of us used as teenagers. Most of the penis is filled with two large cylinders of spongy tissue surrounded by a tough fibrous covering. In a healthy male, the spongy tissues become engorged with blood during sexual excitement, causing the penis to expand. As the spongy tissues fill with blood, they push against the fibrous sheath, making the penis hard. This is quite similar to what happens when you fill a tire with air. As air fills the tube (comparable to the spongy tissues in the penis), it pushes against the tire, which limits the expansion. So the tire gets hard, just as your penis does. As the spongy areas in the penis expand with blood and press against the sheath, the flow of blood out of the penis, through very small veins, is reduced.

In terms of sensitivity to stimulation, most men find the heads of their penises to be the most sensitive. This is not to say that the rest of the penis is insensitive, merely that for the most pleasure, the head of the penis should be included in whatever stimulation is done. Many men also like their scrotums stimulated—touched, rubbed, held, licked, or squeezed (though not too firmly)—during sex. Another area of sensitivity for many men is the perineum, the area between the scrotum and the rectum.

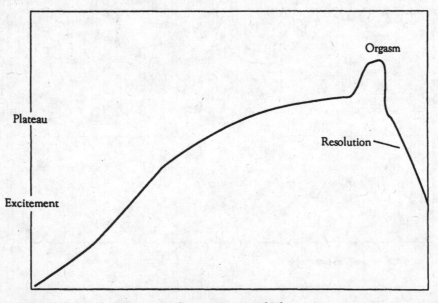

Figure 4: Male sexual response according to Masters and Johnson

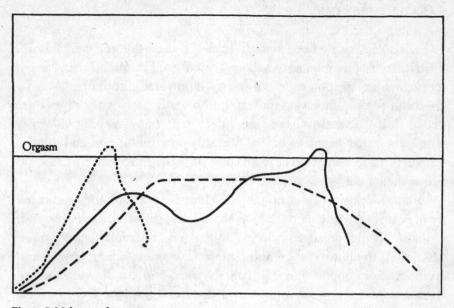

Orgasm

Figure 5: Male sexual responses

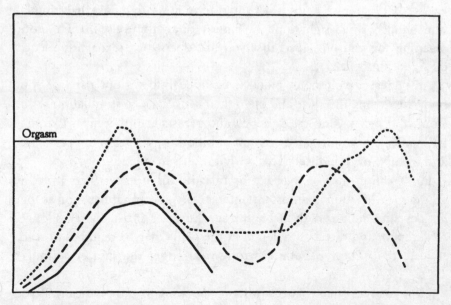

Orgasm

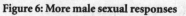

Figure 6: More male sexual responses

SEXUAL RESPONSE

In their pioneering work *Human Sexual Response,* Masters and Johnson described the physiological changes a man goes through during sex in terms of a sexual response cycle arbitrarily divided into four phases: excitement, plateau, orgasm, and resolution. This part of their work has been widely popularized and accepted, but many men's (and many women's) sexual responses do not fit neatly into the Masters and Johnson scheme, and some people have asked what was wrong with them for not fitting the model.

I think Kinsey was more on target: "There is nothing more characteristic of sexual response than the fact that it is not the same in any two individuals." There is no right or normal way to have a sexual experience. Your response is the result of a complex interaction among many variables, including, for example, your age, your physical and emotional state, how turned on you are, what your partner does, and how you feel about her. Lots of types of response cycles are possible, as shown in Figures 5 and 6.

The main physical changes that occur during a sexual experience are the result of vasocongestion, the accumulation of blood in various parts of the body. Muscular tension increases and other changes occur. With orgasm, the muscular tension is released or discharged and blood flow resumes its normal or nonsexual pattern, but these phenomena happen even without orgasm, though more slowly.

A sexual response begins when you receive some kind of sexual stimulation: a touch, smell, sight, thought, fantasy, or anything else that has erotic meaning for you. Provided that you are open to a sexual experience, changes commence.

An increased volume of blood is pumped into various parts of your body, increasing their size and often their sensitivity to stimulation. Aside from your penis, your lips, earlobes, and breasts are other areas that may be so affected. An increased amount of blood is pumped into your penis, and the outflow is reduced. This is what results in erection.

Full erection may or may not occur early in an experience. In many young men, erection is almost instantaneous; they get hard as soon as they get any stimulation. With increasing age, however, it usually takes longer to get hard, and direct stimulation of the penis may be required to reach full erection. There is nothing wrong with either the shorter or longer route.

How you feel directly affects what's happening to you physically. If you get bored, distracted, or anxious, or aren't getting optimal physical stimulation, you may lose some or all of your erection and experience other changes that reflect your lowered level of excitement. Usually this is not something to get concerned about. You can probably return to a higher level of arousal and regain your erection when you reinstate the conditions and activities that got you there in the first place. If you get very nervous, however, you might lose your erection and ejaculate. Many men are surprised by this, but it's not uncommon. Anxiety can cause both loss of erection and ejaculation.

It is normal for erections to wax and wane during lovemaking, especially if it goes on for some time. Many men, for instance, find that although they enjoy giving oral stimulation to their partners, they lose their erections during it. This does not mean these men don't like oral sex. It only means that, while pleasurable, what they're doing isn't the kind of stimulation that keeps their erections going. Erections can go down during other activities as well. The only important thing about the waxing and waning is that you don't get upset if you notice your penis is getting soft. In most cases it can get hard again.

The scrotum and testes undergo some interesting changes during sex. The skin of the scrotal sac thickens and contracts, while the testes increase in size because of the engorgement of blood. The testes are also pulled up within the sac until they press against the wall of the pelvis. This elevation of the testes anticipates ejaculation and is necessary for it to occur.

Ejaculation is a spinal reflex that releases the built-up muscular tension and reverses the flow of blood in the body, draining it away from the penis and other engorged areas. Two distinct steps are involved in ejaculation. First, the prostate, seminal vesicles, and vas deferens contract, pouring their contents into the urethra. The sperm mix with the secretions of the seminal vesicles and the prostate to form the ejaculate. The contractions are the beginning of ejaculation. To you, it feels like "I'm going to come" or "It's coming." Masters and Johnson have called this "ejaculatory inevitability." Since the ejaculatory process is already in motion, ejaculation is inevitable. Nothing can stop it once the point of inevitability has been reached.

During the second step of the ejaculatory process, which follows immediately after the first step, the fluid is propelled through the urethra by contractions of the pelvic muscles. The semen may spurt several inches or even feet beyond the tip of the penis, or it may just ooze out. The force and amount of ejaculate expelled are determined by a number of factors, including your age and the length of time since the last ejaculation.

Ejaculation is a total-body response, not just something that happens in the crotch. Respiration, blood pressure, and heartbeat increase as the man approaches ejaculation, usually peaking at the moment of ejaculation. Involuntary muscle contraction and spasm may occur in various parts of the body, including legs, stomach, arms, and back.

Although many people use ejaculation and orgasm synonymously, I find it is useful to draw a distinction between them. Ejaculation is the physical part, the propulsion of seminal fluid. Orgasm is the peak feeling in sex. This peak feeling usually occurs in men during ejaculation, but not always. Sometimes there is no peak feeling, and sometimes that feeling comes long before ejaculation. Some men don't have a lot of feeling when they ejaculate, and some men have lots of peak feelings, with and without ejaculations. There is no good and bad, right and wrong, about any of this.

What would happen if you got very excited, had an erection, but for one reason or another did not ejaculate? Many men believe that this would lead to the condition commonly called "blue balls" or "lover's nuts": discomfort, pain, and soreness in the testes. This belief is easy to understand. The fantasy model of sex invariably includes orgasm for the male, and the implication seems to be that its absence would be disastrous.

In fact, it is not disastrous. There may be soreness or pain, but this is rare. You might want to think back over your sexual experiences and see if this is true for you. Be sure to include all instances where, whether with masturbation or with a partner, you got very aroused and did not ejaculate. How many times was there pain? Probably very few, although those are the ones we tend to remember. It is not necessary to ejaculate every time you have sex. It's nice when it happens, but there's no reason to try to force it. You and your partner will probably feel better stopping while you are still feeling good. Working at producing an ejaculation has a way of making sex tedious.

After ejaculation, your body starts to return to where it was before the sex began. Blood flows out of your penis and it returns to its nonerect state. The rate at which this happens depends on many factors and varies with each occurrence. Sometimes your erection may go down immediately, while at other times it may stay relatively firm for many minutes after ejaculation. Blood pressure, pulse, and breathing rates gradually return to their prearousal levels. The scrotum and testes descend to their normal position. A thin film of perspiration may appear over much of your body.

When there has been excitement and no orgasm, resolution usually takes longer. The muscular tension and accumulation of blood are released more slowly than when there has been an ejaculation. Because of this, you may feel a bit congested in the pelvis and perhaps a little tense or jittery. If there is pain, a short period of rest will help, or perhaps you'll want to stimulate yourself, or have your partner stimulate you, to ejaculation.

After ejaculation, many men experience feelings of lassitude and deep relaxation. For some this immediately leads to sleep, often to the chagrin of their partners. Women usually prefer a continued connection—holding, cuddling, relaxed talking, and so on—which some call afterplay. Most men I've worked with have found they can become comfortable with these activities if they desire to do so. And sometimes, of course, sleep is just the right thing to do.

WHAT DOES AN ERECTION MEAN?

Many men, and women as well, assume that an erection means the man wants sex. If only life were that simple. Of course an erection may mean the man desires sex, but it also may mean nothing of the kind.

Consider that during rapid eye movement (REM) sleep, the part of sleep in which we dream, males—from one-day-old infants to men ninety and older—usually have erections. This means three to five erections a night, each lasting from a few minutes to an hour. Does this mean all men want to have sex three to five times a night? While they're asleep? We really don't know why these erections occur or what they mean, but studies have been done in which the men were awakened during their dreams and asked what they were dreaming about. Sex isn't one of the main topics.

Consider that males often have erections at times when they will tell you they're not interested in sex. Teenage boys, for example, have erections in class when they're trying to concentrate on the classroom material, when walking down the street not thinking about sex, and on many other occasions. This causes embarrassment and frantic efforts to hide the bulge behind books, packages, and jackets. I played football in high school and invariably had an erection when "The Star-Spangled Banner" was played before each game. I guarantee that sex was the farthest thing from my mind at the moment.

To make things even more complex, consider that erections can be produced by certain kinds of fear (while other kinds of fear can prevent erections). There have been a few reported cases of men being forced at the point of a knife or gun to have intercourse with one or more women. This isn't the kind of rape we usually hear about, but the evidence is clear that the male victims did get erect and were able to have intercourse. Erections are not only produced by positive, loving, or lusty feelings.

An erection means only that your penis is hard. Whether or not you *want* sex has to do with how you feel, how excited you are. Whether or not you *should* have sex has to do with your appraisal of the situation, what your head tells you. You may have an erection and you may be wonderfully turned on, but if your head reminds you that the woman in question is your best friend's or boss's wife, or that you have no protection against disease or unwanted pregnancy, you may want to think carefully about what to do.

WHAT DOES LACK OF ERECTION MEAN?

Just as many people confuse erection with an interest in sex, they also confuse lack of erection with a lack of interest. Women are especially likely to make this error and to personalize it. If you don't have an erection in a sexual situation, your partner may well assume that you're not turned on to her or that she doesn't know what to do to turn you on. It's possible, of course, that she's right. Maybe you're not aroused by her at the moment or ever, or maybe she's not doing what you'd like.

But most of the time lack of erection in a sexual situation means something else entirely. Let's say you are sexually aroused; you want to have sex. But your penis doesn't respond. Although this situation is enormously frustrating to men, and often their partners as well, there is always an answer. There is an obstacle preventing your arousal from translating into an erection. In some cases the barrier is obvious and simple. For example, perhaps you require a certain kind of stimulation to get hard and you're not getting it. Maybe your partner doesn't know that's what you need, maybe she forgot, or maybe she's upset and doesn't want to supply it. Or maybe because you've had so much sex in the last day or so, your penis is simply too tired to get hard again. But usually the obstacle is something else.

Erection requires a whole constellation of things to be right. Your nervous and vascular systems have to be capable of responding properly, and your emotions have to be capable of aiding or at least not impeding the process. Anything, physical or emotional, that gets in the way of sufficient blood getting and staying in the penis can cause problems.

It used to be thought that erection problems were almost always due to psychological factors. But we have learned in recent years that this isn't the case. Many erection problems are caused by disease or drugs by themselves or in combination with emotional factors.

Any disease that interferes with blood getting to the penis, with blood being kept in the penis, or with the nervous system's control over blood flow may cause erection problems. A number of medical conditions are known to affect the nervous system's ability to control blood flow or the ability of blood to get into and stay in the penis. Hormonal imbalances, diabetes, heart disease, multiple sclerosis, spinal cord injuries and back problems, injuries to the pelvis, long-term cigarette smoking, and alcoholism are some of these conditions.

Just because you have hardening of the arteries or any of the other problems mentioned above does not necessarily mean that they are the cause of your erection problems. Such problems may also be caused by anxiety and other emotions. But it is important to determine what's going on.

The penis can also be affected by anything taken into the body—for example, drugs you take for depression, anxiety, high blood pressure, and many other conditions, as well as for recreation. In the Appendix I list a number of common drugs that can adversely affect sexual functioning.

Your ability to get and maintain erections can also be influenced by your emotions and the state of your relationship. Anxiety about whether you'll get or maintain an erection is a common obstacle to getting erections. But other feelings also enter in. Anger, for instance, no matter who it's directed at, can block your ability to get hard. So can the absence of a feeling, the lack of arousal. If you're not turned on, perhaps because you're highly anxious, because your mind is preoccupied with something else, or because you don't like your partner or don't find her attractive, this may be enough to prevent stimulation from translating into erection.

I hope it's clear that not having an erection doesn't necessarily mean you don't want sex. It just means that your penis is less stiff than you'd like.

THE PLEASURES OF THE SOFT PENIS

Penises do not have to be hard to produce pleasure. A soft penis has just as many nerve endings as a hard one and is therefore capable of generating good feelings. Whether it is exactly as enjoyable as an erect penis is difficult to say. Although the number of nerve endings doesn't change, it's possible that the engorgement of the hard penis with blood amplifies the sensations. Some men say it's more pleasurable to be stimulated with an erection, and some say it doesn't make any difference. And it's also possible to have an orgasm with a soft penis.

You already know how much pleasure can be gotten from the stimulation of a soft penis. Think about it for a minute. Have you ever started a sexual experience, alone or with a partner, without an erection? How did it feel as you or your partner stimulated your soft penis? Didn't it feel good? And it probably didn't feel as good as it could because you or you and your partner were focused on making it hard and were therefore anticipating what was to come rather than what was happening at the moment.

There are two reasons for taking more seriously the pleasure that can be yielded by a flaccid penis. One is that doing so takes some pressure off it to get hard. And the fewer demands put on a penis to behave in certain ways, the better it will function. The other reason is that it simply gives you more options. You can enjoy sex without an erection. And your partner will know she can give you pleasure without your having an erection.

It's also possible to have intercourse with a soft penis. But be warned: This works only if both of you are comfortable with the soft penis, if you're not going to get upset if it doesn't get hard, if you're willing to experiment with different positions, and if you can talk about what's happening. It sometimes happens that once you start having intercourse, your penis will get harder. If that happens, it's fine. And it's also fine if it doesn't.

A number of men have been surprised by my earlier statement that orgasm is possible without a full erection. Nonetheless, it's true. Erection and orgasm are separate entities and not dependent on each other. Just as you can have an erection without an orgasm, so, too, you can have orgasm without erection.

THE PENIS THROUGH THE LIFE CYCLE

Like all parts of the body, the penis changes as it ages. The truly young penis—in babies and grade-school boys—is basically a sleeper. True, it gets hard during dreams and at other times, especially when stimulated, but it doesn't do much otherwise except for resting and urinating.

The adolescent penis is another story altogether. It is rambunctious and rowdy; it gets hard frequently and at the most inappropriate times. The problem for many teenage boys is not getting it up but trying to keep it down. The writer Julius Lester recalls just how ubiquitous and embarrassing the adolescent penis can be:

God, how I envied girls. . . . Whatever it was on them, it didn't dangle between their legs like an elephant's trunk. No wonder boys talked about nothing but sex. That thing was always there. Every time we went to the john, there it was, twitching around like a fat little worm on a fishing hook. When we took baths, it floated in the water like a lazy fish and God forbid we should touch it! It sprang to life like lightning leaping from a cloud. . . . I was helpless. It was there, with a life and mind of its own, having no other function than to embarrass me.

The idea that penises are hard as steel comes from the adolescent penis. The adolescent penis seemingly wants to explode to orgasm every few minutes. It comes, and ten minutes later it's hard again and wants to come again. And what orgasms these are. The force is explosive and the pressure is immense; large amounts of semen fly across the room. And if the owner doesn't stimulate himself to orgasm, then it happens all by itself in wet dreams.

The adolescent penis is the penis at its ultimate power. From here on until the end of life, there is a gradual tapering off. Never again will it be so quick to get hard, so stiff; never again will the orgasms be so explosive and the need for them so insistent. There will also be a loss of independence over time. The adolescent penis needs little or nothing from the outside. It gets hard on its own, without needing physical or other kinds of stimulation. As it ages, it will require more stimulation of various sorts.

Although what I have described about the adolescent penis is typical, there are some that don't fit this picture. Some teenage boys have illnesses or injuries that make erection difficult or impossible to get or maintain. And some have difficulties because of strong feelings such as anxiety, guilt, or disgust.

The penis in young adulthood, approximately twenty to thirty-five, is similar to the adolescent penis, but signs of mellowing may already be present. The frequency of masturbation tends to drop, and wet dreams may be less common. Some men in this age group notice that their penises are not as hard when erect as they once were and that they require direct stimulation to get hard.

As the penis enters midlife, say around ages forty to fifty, some changes are obvious. It may require physical stimulation, either from its owner or his partner, to get hard. It may not get as full or as firm as before. It is easier for it to lose its hardness and, once lost, the hardness may be more difficult to regain. Men often notice and worry about the angle of erection. The erection that in younger years pointed up may now just stick straight out; the one that in previous times stuck straight out may now, though stiff, point slightly down. In most cases, these are just normal changes and nothing to get excited about. The need for orgasm is less pronounced. The force of the ejaculation is less, as is the amount ejaculated. Attending to the penis's conditions becomes more important.

The changes continue as the penis reaches its sixth and seventh decades. Men frequently comment that it doesn't get as hard as it used to. Physical and mental arousal are much more critical. Things that before usually produced erection—seeing one's partner undressed, kissing and hugging, even watching X-rated movies—now may not do so. Penises at this age often take longer to ejaculate and they don't need to ejaculate every time. Every second or third time is fine.

Ejaculation is much less powerful. Semen may seem to seep out instead of shooting out. And once a fifty-, sixty-, or seventy-year-old penis ejaculates, it may be days before it can get hard again.

Many men at this age decide they're over the hill as far as sex goes, or that they need some help. Getting help is realistic for some, but for others all that's needed is the understanding that just because something isn't the way it was twenty, thirty, or forty years ago doesn't mean you can't use and enjoy it. A raging erection that points at the ceiling and that won't quit is not necessary for good sex. After all, many men in their sixties enjoy walking, jogging, and dancing even though they can't move as fast or as far as they did when they were thirty. The senior penis can still give and take pleasure, even though it's not the same as it was decades ago.

As sex therapist Leslie Schover points out, some men do fine with their less-than-Herculean erections until confronted with a new situation: for example, sex with a new partner after a divorce or the death of a spouse. The same erection is now considered inadequate.

The changes I've described gradually continue until the end of life. Like the rest of physical functioning, the erection and ejaculatory processes become less efficient. **But the penis and the rest of the body *never* lose their capacity for pleasure.** There are men in their seventies, eighties, and even nineties who enjoy sex. As do their partners. According to many women I've spoken with, the owners of penises often develop qualities as they age that more than make up for the declining powers of their penises. These women say that older men are attractive sexually because they are more open to emotion and generally more loving, more patient, not as quick on the trigger, and often more sensuous.

The big problem for penises is that they've had a bad press. Perhaps it's more accurate to say that they've had a misguided press. The adolescent penis is the one that's idealized and idolized in the popular media, and it's also the first penis males have sexual experience with. Many men expect a penis of any age to act like the adolescent one.

In other areas we don't have these outrageous expectations. When it's old timers' day in baseball, we don't expect the stars of yesterday to hit and run and pitch the way they did before. And we don't expect a forty-year-old man to run as fast as he did when he won the 100-meter race in the Olympics. But almost every man expects his penis to behave the way it did when he was seventeen or, just as bad, the way he wishes it had behaved when he was seventeen.

To the extent that we can get rid of these ridiculous expectations, accept the penis that we have, meet its needs, and like and enjoy it for what it is— to that extent we can give and receive erotic pleasure as much as we want and for as long as we want. And that, I suggest, is what it's all about.

Am I Normal or What?

Sex is always on my mind. I think about it ten, twenty, or more times almost every day. Is that normal?—*Man, 24*

My lover thinks I'm abnormal because I want sex almost every day. I think she's a little strange because she could do with once a week or less. Is either of us, or both of us, nuts?—*Man, 34*

My wife says it's not natural for me to want anal sex or to experiment with bondage, and I guess I'm not sure myself. Is wanting these things OK? —*Man, 47*

I'm concerned because although I love my wife and we have good sex, I often imagine sex with other women, even when I'm making love to her. —*Man, 55*

BECAUSE SEX IS shrouded in secrecy and loaded with anxiety, people often have questions about whether they are okay. The main concern seems to be whether what they are—or are not—thinking, feeling, and doing makes them different, abnormal, or even weird. This apparently is the main reason for the popularity of books like the Kinsey and Hite reports and others that give statistical data about sex. Readers can check to see if they are in the same ballpark, sexually speaking, as others of their gender, age, and so on.

In earlier times, part of this issue was easier to address, at least in terms of official mythology. Medicine, in league with religion, had long lists of thou-shalt-nots, activities said to be sinful, abnormal, and unhealthy, and only a very short list of what was acceptable. Masturbation, perhaps the most common sexual activity, was definitely not on the approved list. In 1758 a prominent Swiss physician, S. A. Tissot, published a book called *Onania, or a Treatise upon the Disorders Produced by Masturbation*. Needless to say, this was not a celebration of the pleasures of self-love. The idea that masturbation could lead to insanity was promulgated for over two hundred years. The main supporting evidence was the observation that inmates in mental asylums masturbated. Therefore, it was clear that masturbation must have led to their insanity. No one thought of determining the masturbatory practices of those not in mental institutions. The apex of the ideas of masturbatory insanity and sex as disease-producing was reached in 1882 with the publication of *Psychopathia Sexualis* by Richard von Krafft-Ebing, one of the world's leading psychiatrists at the time. He reached the conclusion that not only masturbation but all nonreproductive sexual activity was sick, bad, and abnormal.

Similar nonsense was promoted in America. Benjamin Rush, the father of American psychiatry, proclaimed in the early years of our nation that masturbation (which he called "self-pollution") caused poor vision, memory loss, dizziness, epilepsy, and a host of other disorders, including psychosis. In the middle 1800s Sylvester Graham led one of the first health-food crusades in this country. He thought that bad health was related to sexual excesses such as intercourse more than once a month, masturbation, and erotic dreams, all of which were caused by eating rich and spicy foods. These foods "increase the concupiscent excitability and sensibility of the genital organs." The antidote he prescribed was a vegetarian diet of plain and boring foods, one key element of which was coarse, whole-wheat flour. Although you probably never heard of Mr. Graham, you have undoubtedly tasted a processed and sweetened version of his attempt to reduce sexual excess—the graham cracker.

Graham wasn't the only nut rolling around in nineteenth-century America; many others were also concerned about curbing sexuality. John Harvey Kellogg gained a reputation as both a nutritionist and a sexual adviser. He thought sex the ultimate abomination and remained chaste even in marriage. Masturbation was the worst sin of all, "the vilest, the basest, and the most degrading act that a human being can commit." In his view, it led not only to the usual stuff like tuberculosis, heart disease, epilepsy, dimness of vision, insanity, idiocy, and death, but also to bashfulness in some people, unnatural boldness in others, a fondness for spicy foods, round shoulders, and "acne, or pimples on the face." Kellogg introduced a number of foods designed to promote health and decrease interest in sex, one of which he called Corn Flakes. The rest, as they say, is history.

In the Victorian period it was thought that men had an excess of sexual desire, which they needed somehow to control, and no decent woman had any. Men wanted more sex than their wives but wouldn't get too much because of their partners' reluctance. Presumably no one, except for the seriously deranged, was having a lot of sex. Certainly no one would take things in hand and commit the unholy act of self-abuse, and no one would have sex outside marriage. Within marriage, men and women were supposed to have only the kind of sex that might lead to conception; this usually meant missionary-position intercourse. And that was that.

What people actually did during the period from Tissot to Krafft-Ebing and Kellogg did not exactly match official ideology. We know that homosexuality existed, that prostitution and pornography flourished in England and America, that about one-third of births in colonial America resulted from premarital conception (the Pilgrims weren't half as puritanical as we make them out to be), and that affairs were not unheard of. Masturbation apparently was widespread, as it always has been in human history. It's probable that the main effect of the official ideology was not to change behavior but rather to make people feel guilty, anxious, and bad about what they did.

Needless to say, things have loosened up a bit since then, both publicly and privately. Now almost everything goes and is considered acceptable. A majority of boys and girls have had intercourse before they are out of high school. Although man-on-top intercourse is still the most popular position, every other imaginable position has been tried and many couples regularly use some of them. Anal sex, or sodomy, considered quite depraved in the past, is now an act that about 30 percent of couples have tried and that some do regularly. Another great sin of the past, oral sex, has become quite common; it is a regular part of many couples' sex play. And that ultimate abomination, self-abuse, is engaged in not only by those without regular partners but also by those with. Surveys in the last twenty years also find that a fair number of couples engage in light bondage. As for how often sex takes place, a lot depends on the age of the participants and the duration of their relationship. Sylvester Graham and John Kellogg would certainly do cartwheels in their graves were they aware that a great many people these days have intercourse more than once a month, many of them even more than once a week.

Most experts now believe that the existence of rigid rules regarding sexual normality is itself a kind of sickness. A large reason for this attitude is our knowledge of the incredible range of sexual thought, feeling, fantasy, and behavior. Some people, for example, think about sex a hundred times a day, every day, and others can't remember when they last had a sexual thought. The same is true about behavior, although, to be accurate,

I should say I've never heard of anyone having sex a hundred times a day. It's true that there are only so many convex and concave surfaces on the human body, and only a few protrusions and orifices, but people have been very creative with what they have to work with.

There's actually very little basis for saying that this or that activity, this or that frequency, is bad or abnormal unless it causes harm to a person or a relationship. And it's clear that most of the harmful effects proclaimed by people from Tissot to Kellogg were nothing but rationalizations for their abhorrence of sex in any form.

Of course, there are still folks who are put off by sex, especially by any kind of sex that does not meet their personal notions of acceptability. Nonetheless, these days sexual tolerance is the rule rather than the exception, both among experts in human relations and sexuality and among the general public.

THE ABNORMALITY OF NORMALITY

Concerns about performance and anxiety about sex aren't supposed to be normal. But they're common, perhaps universal, in men. Jim Brown, perhaps the greatest running back in the history of American football, had a reputation as a lover that rivaled his reputation as a ball carrier. In his autobiography, *Out of Bounds*, he complains that even his friends thought he was a superman in bed. But, says Brown, "I was never Superman. I had the same doubts about performing up to expectations that they did."

After interviewing 125 men of all ages for their book *What Really Happens in Bed*, Steven Carter and Julia Sokol concluded that "all men have sexual anxieties." More specifically:

Young men are anxious that their inexperience will show; they are also typically anxious about premature ejaculation and whether they know enough about female anatomy. Middle-aged men are worried that their erections are not as firm, or quickly achieved, as they were when they were in their late teens and early twenties. Older men worry that erections are less frequent, less firm, and more temperamental.

In *The Hite Report on Male Sexuality*, Shere Hite reported that a majority of her seven thousand respondents had concerns about getting and keeping erections and ejaculating too quickly. There is good reason to believe, therefore, that **there's nothing abnormal or unusual about men's being anxious about sex.**

Another place where our ideas of normality are way off base concerns sexual problems. Such problems, most of us think, are rare. But is that really the case? A review of community studies by Ilana Spector and Michael Carey found that about 7 percent of men have chronic erection problems, while about 37 percent suffer from chronic rapid ejaculations. The same review found that about 5 percent of men have difficulty ejaculating with their partners and about 16 percent complain of low sex drive. That's a lot of men with problems, especially since some difficulties—such as a sex drive that's grossly discrepant from that of one's partner's and dissatisfaction with sex even though there aren't any functional problems—weren't even considered.

To add to this, we need to recall that most men *occasionally* don't function as they desire. In Shere Hite's large sample of men, 65 percent answered yes when asked if they had ever had difficulty having an erection when they wanted one, and 70 percent said they had ejaculated more quickly than they had wanted on at least one occasion. I hope the point is clear: **Sex problems are normal and typical.** I know, I know, all of your buddies are functioning perfectly and never have a problem. If you really believe that, I have a nice piece of oceanfront property in Kansas I'd like to talk to you about.

In case you're wondering about women, Spector and Carey found that about the same proportion of women as men have chronic or sporadic problems with sex; these include difficulties getting aroused and having orgasm, painful intercourse, and low desire. For both men and women, it seems, sex problems are not unusual. While I grant it doesn't feel good when you have a problem, it's just part of the human condition. Welcome to the human race.

WHAT ABOUT MASTURBATION?

Although the dictionary definition of *masturbation* is "stimulation of the genitals by means other than intercourse," I use the term as most people do, to refer to sexually stimulating oneself. Common synonyms include "playing with yourself," "self-pleasuring," and "self-stimulation."

Playing with oneself is one of the most common sexual acts. Little children do it—at least until their parents shriek at them to stop—and it has been found in every society studied. In America, the vast majority of boys start masturbating sometime during puberty, and most of them continue to pleasure themselves for the rest of their lives. Estimates are that about 70 percent of married men sometimes stimulate themselves (as do a similar percentage of married women).

Although there is nothing abnormal or unnatural about self-pleasuring, most of us feel ashamed or guilty about it. It seems selfish and too explicitly sexual (you can't pretend you're doing it for anyone else's benefit or for anything but sexual pleasure, and it's thought to hint of immaturity). A real man, we think, would be able to find a partner to have sex with rather than being left to his own devices. If he already has a partner, then why on earth would he want to have sex by himself? A married man in his fifties expressed his concern like this:

> I'm embarrassed about this, but I've masturbated once a week or so all through my marriage. It's not that Grace leaves anything to be desired. She's a wonderful sex partner and rarely turns me down. But there are times when it just seems easier to do it myself. This isn't taking anything away from what we have together, it's just a separate thing. I think she'd be shocked and hurt if she found out and I wouldn't know how to explain myself.

It's understandable that masturbation should make us feel uneasy. Sex by oneself for one's own pleasure—where even the pretense of trying to conceive didn't exist—was always at or near the top of the worst sexual abuses in Western cultures, the mere mention of which was enough to send religious and medical "experts" into a state of hysteria. The terms they used to refer to the act—"self-abuse," "self-pollution," and "the solitary vice"—reflect their attitude. It was only about forty years ago that the American Medical Association and the Boy Scout Manual dropped their opposition to masturbation. Although virtually all medical and psychological experts today consider the activity quite normal, we aren't that far removed from the days when it was considered anything but normal.

Despite its reputation, masturbation actually has a number of uses and benefits.

▲ It's fun, one of the small pleasures of life. What's wrong with making ourselves feel good?

▲ In masturbation you don't have to look your best, and, as Woody Allen put it, it's sex with someone you love. You don't have to concern yourself with anyone else's feelings, desires, or goals. You can do whatever you want for as long or as short a time as you like and get whatever you want out of it. Partner sex, while certainly having advantages of its own, does require that we carefully attend to the desires of our partner and synchronize our behavior with hers, and that's not something one always wants to do.

▲ Self-pleasuring is an excellent way to learn how you like to be touched and stimulated, not only on your genitals but elsewhere as well. This information can then be given to your partner, thus enhancing your sex life together.

▲ Even if you're committed to partner sex as the best way of satisfying your erotic needs, there may be times when you don't have a partner or the partner you do have isn't available because of illness, fatigue, or something else. Why deny yourself sexual pleasure at such times?

▲ As I discuss in detail in the latter part of the book, masturbating in certain ways can help overcome sexual problems such as erection difficulties and rapid ejaculation.

The only sense in which masturbation can be said to be bad is when a man regularly uses it as a substitute for sex with his partner. That is, whenever he feels sexy he satisfies himself and rarely or never wants sex with his partner. Understandably, the partner may feel less than ecstatic about this state of affairs. Usually something else is involved. The man is unhappy about either the partner or relationship, about himself or about sex with her.

Because most of us still feel somewhat uneasy about masturbation, we try to hide it. When a man is walked in on by his partner while masturbating, instead of simply acknowledging what he is doing, he often denies it. "Nothing, just dozing" or "I had an itch [or ache] in my penis and was just scratching [examining] it." Yeah, sure. How much better and easier if he could just say what he was doing.

It's possible the woman may not feel good about what he's doing, just as he feared. She may feel that her attractiveness or skillfulness is inadequate if he masturbates even though she's available.

Such feelings need to be talked about. They stem from our culture's narrow view of sex. As I try to show throughout this book, the only rules necessary for good sex are consent (if you're doing it with someone else, they must agree to the activity), honesty (don't say things that aren't true), and responsibility (it's not right to make babies when you don't want them, to spread disease, or to behave in ways that are disrespectful of your partner). Aside from these things, anything goes. It's perfectly fine to masturbate even though you have a sexual partner, it's fine to masturbate in her presence or with her participation, it's fine for the two of you to masturbate together, and it's just as fine for either of you to stimulate yourself during an erotic encounter together. Just because you have a partner who's available to have oral sex or intercourse or any other sexual activity doesn't necessarily mean you'll always want to engage in that activity with her. There are times when you may simply prefer to stimulate yourself despite your partner's availability.

As far as I'm concerned, the same rules apply to self-stimulation as to any other sexual activities. If whatever you're doing isn't hurting you, your partner, or your relationship, why not just enjoy yourself?

WHAT IS NORMAL SEXUAL DESIRE OR ACTIVITY?

This is a very sensitive topic for both men and women. Bad feelings and name-calling are typical when someone feels his partner wants too much or too little. If she wants less, she's frigid, withholding, unloving, neurotic, and a sexless bitch. If she wants more, she's oversexed, a slut, a tramp, neurotic, and a demanding bitch. As Kinsey put it, a nymphomaniac is anyone who's having more sex than you are. All of these terms are simply ways of saying that you don't like your partner's level of interest. Instead of putting it that way, our frustration and anger result in name-calling and put-downs. In effect, we're saying she's abnormal and ought to shape up.

In answer to the question of what is normal sexual desire, we don't know—unless all you want is a purely statistical report on how often people demographically similar to you have sex. It's not even clear that the question makes any sense. What is normal eating desire or activity? We don't know that, either. Most people eat meals three times a day and have a few snacks as well. Some people eat only two meals a day, and a few eat only one. And there are also people who eat small meals every two or three hours, never having what the rest of us would call a regular meal. We judge not the eating but the results. If you're not obese or anorexic, your arteries aren't clogged, and your health is good, you're okay, whatever it is you're doing about eating. And, unlike sex, eating is necessary for your survival.

I think we need to judge sexual interest and activity, as we do eating, by the results. If it's not causing a problem in your life or relationship, whatever you're doing is okay. We know there are huge variations. Some couples have sex several times a day, every day. Most couples have sex less frequently. Believe it or not, there are also men and women, not all of them priests and nuns, who've never engaged in partner sex.

In my opinion, sex—however defined—is not necessary for survival or for a good relationship. And if you are having sex, a large amount is fine and so is a moderate or a low amount.

A widespread problem these days is the inability of couples to agree on how often to make love. In most of these cases there's no basis on which to say that one partner's desire is abnormally high or the other's abnormally low, but there's plenty of basis to say that the discrepancy is causing huge problems in their relationship.

WHAT ABOUT THE USE OF EROTIC MATERIALS?

The use of erotic pictures, books, and other materials is hardly new. Even in Victorian England, one of the most sexually repressive societies in history, pornographic books and magazines were quite popular. With the advent of moviemaking, erotic movies, often called stag films, appeared. More recently, with the proliferation of VCRs, it has become convenient and common for individuals and couples to watch sexy videos in their homes.

A controversy has raged over erotic materials for a long time. Many religious authorities object to them because they tend to incite sexual arousal, which of course is their purpose. Some feminists object to them, claiming that these materials treat women as objects and cause violence against them. But as other people have pointed out, erotic materials do not discriminate against women: They objectify everyone. Sexual organs and acts are all they focus on. As for violence, the vast majority of erotic films and other materials contain none. You are far more likely to see murder and rape and other kinds of mayhem in PG-13 or R-rated movies than in those rated X. (There is, to be sure, a very small segment of the erotica market that caters to those who are aroused by the combination of violence and sex. But these materials are easy to avoid.)

It's difficult to see how the use of erotic materials can be considered abnormal or sick. It's apparent that most males use them at some times in their lives. How many boys and men can honestly say they've never looked at *Playboy* or *Penthouse*, never read an erotic book or viewed an erotic movie? And millions of women regularly read romance novels that often are hard to differentiate from hard-core sex books. Erotica is not without risk. It can cause the development of unrealistic expectations about ourselves, our partners, and sex itself. But if you remind yourself not to confuse fantasy, which is what erotica is, with reality, I think its use is mainly beneficial. Erotic materials usually turn people on, and often these aroused people want sex with themselves or their partners. How is that bad?

The use of erotic materials is similar in many ways to the use of sexual fantasies. In the case of fantasies, the representation of sexual events is internal; with erotica, it's external—you're reading, hearing, or watching someone else's fantasy, which, of course, may not only turn you on but also start your own fantasies going.

WHAT ABOUT FANTASIES?

Many questions about sexual normalcy have to do with fantasies. A sexual fantasy is *any* mental representation of *any kind* of sexual activity. Many fantasies tell a story and move from beginning to middle to end. An example would be imagining meeting a woman at a conference, taking her to your room, kissing, fondling, and engaging in oral sex, followed by intercourse. But fantasies need not be so full-blown or elaborate. You may, for instance, just imagine one act—a kiss, oral sex, or intercourse—or one feeling, such as orgasm.

Sexual fantasies are entirely normal for human beings, but how we use our minds varies considerably. Some people's fantasies are mainly positive, while other people's are mainly negative. Some people spend a lot more time with their fantasies than others, and usually their fantasies are more elaborate. Some people are willing to fantasize about things that others aren't. They find it pleasurable to fantasize about sex with their partners, other people's partners, animals, and all sorts of combinations. Other people have trouble with such fantasies. They think it's wrong to fantasize about sex at all, about certain kinds of sex, or sex with certain people.

Fantasies serve several purposes. One is that they are an inexpensive entertainment that usually makes us feel good. Even though we're not likely to ever have sex with fourteen Playboy bunnies at the same time, or even sequentially, it can feel very good to imagine doing so. Another purpose is turning us on, really an extension of the first purpose. Whether or not you're fantasizing about sex with your partner, what goes on in your imagination can arouse you to the point that you'll want sex with her or that you'll be more passionate when you see her than otherwise might be the case.

Sexual fantasies can also be used therapeutically. Imagining an arousing activity can be helpful in the midst of sex. If you notice your arousal or erection flagging during erotic activity, conjuring up a favorite fantasy may make a difference. Imagining a sexual activity that you haven't tried but think you might want to can give you a better sense of how you might go about that, and whether you really do want to do it.

Despite the fact that fantasizing about sex comes so naturally and easily to human beings, and despite the helpful purposes it serves, sexual fantasies have not enjoyed a good press in Western culture, which, of course, has traditionally been predominantly antisexual. The biblical injunction "One who looks at a woman lustfully has already committed adultery with her in his heart" sums it all up.

Part of the problem with our culture is that it doesn't make a clear enough distinction between imagining something and actually doing it. The fear has been that if you fantasize about having sex with a neighbor, you'll actually do it. There is at least a grain of truth in this. Fantasy can serve as rehearsal for behavior. Imagining the same thing repeatedly may motivate you to try it out. But in most cases this isn't much of a problem. Real-life obstacles and your own values help keep the fantasy where it belongs—in your head.

People who feel guilty about their fantasies need to remind themselves that there is a big difference between imagining doing something and actually carrying it out. There is no law against imagining forcing someone to have sex with you, and there are both men and women who enjoy this kind of fantasy. Doing it in reality, however, is another matter entirely. There is also nothing wrong with fantasizing about protection-free, worry-free sex with strangers. In the real world, where sexual diseases are commonplace and where conception and bad feelings occur far more often than anyone would wish for, you ought to take the necessary precautions.

Fantasies can also be helpful in determining what you might want in the real world. Perhaps there are some elements of your imagery that you would like acted out. Some men I've worked with, for example, have had fantasies about "zipless fucks"—no words, not much foreplay, just silent, passionate, no-strings-attached fucking. In a number of these cases, they were able to talk to their partners about the fantasies and act them out, much to everyone's satisfaction.

Please don't assume that I mean you should act out everything in your fantasies. I don't mean that at all. Just because you enjoy imagining being whipped and dominated by a woman does not mean you'll actually enjoy the reality of it. Use your common sense and consider whether this is something you'd really like to try and if you're willing and able to go through with it. The real world often exacts prices that fantasies do not. Having sex with your wife's sister may make for a wonderful fantasy. The reality, however, could be quite costly.

Despite the anti-sexual-fantasy position of our culture, most males have and enjoy erotic mental productions. It's typical for boys and men to have fantasies when they masturbate. And from the studies that have been done, it's typical for men and women to fantasize about sex at all sorts of times. But there are still many questions and doubts.

A professional man who consulted me because of guilt about his fantasies loved and was turned on by the woman he lived with, but during lovemaking he often had fantasies of sex with other women. He felt bad about this, as if he weren't being true to his partner. He felt much better after we discussed the subject and I loaned him several collections of fantasies, which make it quite clear that many men and women fantasize about other people while having sex.

Some men readily accept that no matter how much they love and are turned on by their partner, they will continue to be turned on by and have fantasies about other women. But other men, like the man just mentioned, have trouble with this. It can help if they understand that being aroused by other women is typical for men. In fact, I've rarely encountered a man who said he was not turned on by other women and did not have fantasies about sex with them.

Although I can't prove it, I believe that it goes even further than this. My impression is that after the newness of a relationship wears off, most of our sexual turn-ons do not come from our partner. Yes, you may still get greatly aroused by her, particularly if she says or does a certain thing, but I think chances are good that much of the passion you feel and that leads you to want sex with her is evoked by other women or situations. There are many, many attractive women in the world, and you'll run into lots of them through the media and in real life: You'll see them on the street, in your office, on the bus or train or plane, in the restaurant, and so on. There's nothing wrong with getting sexually excited by seeing, hearing, or smelling a woman other than your partner. This is not the same, I hasten to add, as actually doing something sexual with these other people.

Since it's a fact of life that a great many of us get turned on by other people—that the phenomenon is natural, if you will—there doesn't seem to be any point to getting upset about it. As I show in Chapter 15, we can use the arousal generated by other women to better our sex lives with our partners.

Studies of sexual fantasies have found a wide variety of presentations. There are some differences between men and women in the types of fantasies they have most often. As you might expect, men more frequently imagine sex with strangers, sex with more than one person, and forcing a woman to have sex with them. Women more frequently imagine romantic settings and being forced to have sex. There is no basis for saying that any of these fantasies is abnormal or unhealthy.

There is an enormous range regarding the frequency of sexual fantasizing, just as there is an enormous range regarding the frequency of any sexual behavior. Some men have sexual fantasies many times each day, while others can go for weeks without one. My experience is that people to whom sex is a priority have lots of sexual thoughts and fantasies. As long as the fantasizing isn't interfering with your relationship, your work, and the normal chores of life, I can't see how it is a problem.

Some couples find it very arousing to share fantasies. That is, the partners tell each other what they fantasize about, either when they're actually having sex or at other times. These couples not only report increased excitement but also a feeling of greater closeness. As one man put it:

You might think it would make me jealous, hearing her fantasies about sex with other men. But it doesn't. It makes for an incredible turn-on. It also makes for incredible love. I feel closer to her knowing that she trusts me enough to tell me these secrets, things she's never told anyone else. Now I can also share some of my fantasies with her and that makes for even more closeness. I've never trusted any other woman that much.

Despite what I've said, don't rush off to tell your partner your latest fantasy. While the sharing of fantasies can be wonderful for some couples, it is not without risk. Some women are not comfortable with such goings-on. They may feel hurt, insulted, rejected, or jealous if you report imagining sex with someone else. There are also your own feelings to consider. Would you really be comfortable hearing that your partner imagines sex with men more handsome, more muscular, with greater charm or more money or power than you? Realistically assess both your possible reactions and those of your partner before you conclude that sharing fantasies is a great idea. If you should decide to go ahead, do it gradually. Start with a fantasy that is least threatening; for example, one that includes her or of having sex with the girl you first had sex with. Don't get into the fantasies of sex with her best friend, or your neighbor, or with whips and chains, until you feel it's reasonably safe to do so.

All in all, I think sexual fantasies are a natural, healthy, and pleasurable part of life. They're free, readily available, and rarely have side effects that can't be dealt with. It's almost like you can't not have them, so it makes sense to make yours as useful and enjoyable as possible.

THE QUESTION IS NOT IF IT'S "NORMAL," BUT IF IT'S A PROBLEM

Although *normal* is basically a statistical term (what's typical or average), in ordinary usage it has a judgmental and moralistic connotation. That is, there's something wrong with you if you're not doing what most other folks are doing. This connotation mainly serves to increase our anxiety and bad feelings and therefore makes clear thinking and productive decision making more difficult.

If what you want to do makes your life difficult or sets you and your partner at odds, then there's a problem, regardless of how typical your action may be. The incidence of quick ejaculations among young men, for example, is so high that it could easily be considered normal or typical; we're talking about millions of men here. But that doesn't mean that it's not a problem for these men or their partners. Another example concerns the widespread practice of oral sex. If you want to go down on your partner or have her go down on you and she wants no part of either, that's a problem regardless of how common these activities are.

Another example of a widespread practice that is a problem for some people concerns the use of alcohol and drugs in sex, especially among singles. It's not unusual for singles to meet and mingle in bars and at parties where they ingest alcohol and other drugs. While I'm not suggesting there's anything wrong with a social drink to help one relax, it often goes far beyond this. Drugs cloud the brain and often make for destructive sexual decisions resulting in bad feelings, unwanted conception, and disease. And heavy use of alcohol and other drugs over the long run can result in serious loss of sexual appetite and erectile ability. Just because a practice is so widespread that it could be considered normal doesn't mean it's healthy or wise.

There are several ways in which sex can be a problem.

If it's illegal: These days you're not likely to get in trouble with the law about sexual acts done in private with consenting adults. But peeping into other people's windows, exposing yourself, trying to force your attention on women who aren't interested, and anything sexual with children can most certainly lead to the jailhouse. If you're doing any of these things, then you definitely have a problem and should get competent help.

If it's driven or compulsive: Some men's (and some women's) sexual behavior is compulsive. That is, the man feels out of control; he has to fantasize about sex virtually all the time, has to masturbate or have sex with his partner twice each day, or has to have sex every time he can and doesn't care who it's with.

A man I saw some years ago felt he had to have sex three times each and every night with his partner. He didn't feel he had any choice in the matter; he just had to do it. He had already lost several relationships because of this and was about to lose another. As the woman put it: "This is ridiculous. I'm so sore I can't sit down, and I'm so tired I can't stay awake at work."

The trendy term *addiction* has recently been used to characterize such men. Although I have some problems with that term, there's no doubt that compulsive sexual behavior exists and is a source of great suffering for those so afflicted. These men need good professional help.

If it gets in your way: If you are consumed by sexual feelings, fantasies, or behaviors to the point where you can't engage in the usual kinds of social intercourse or can't focus on your work, that's clearly a problem. There are cases where a man felt driven to masturbate five or more times a day. Aside from getting a sore penis, he's also likely not to be able to do his work. The major problem for many of those men who feel their sexual behavior is compulsive or addictive is precisely that it gets in the way of getting on with the other important aspects of life.

If it creates problems with your partner: If whatever you're doing or not doing causes conflicts with your partner and harms your relationship, then obviously it's a problem. This could be the situation when, for example, your partner very much wants you to go down on her but you consider such behavior unseemly or disgusting, or when she wants much longer foreplay than you feel is reasonable or even doable.

Another kind of difficulty that occurs in couples is when, for example, you *always* require a special something in order to get turned on. One woman whose live-in lover could rarely get sexually aroused unless she wore spike heels said this: "It feels like he's in love with the shoes, not with me. Given how he carries on about them, I think he should find a nice pair of shoes to marry." I know of one couple where the man introduced bondage and dominance games early in the relationship. The woman didn't mind, in fact thought them an interesting twist, but as time went on she got turned off completely when she realized the man couldn't get aroused without these activities. She then felt that he was "sick and abnormal."

Men who always use the same fantasy to get aroused (for example, the partner has to be nineteen and has to have a certain build) may condition their turn-on to that type of partner and be unable to get aroused with anyone else. This, of course, can create serious problems in the real world. Similarly, fantasies involving coercion are common among both men and women, but they can become troublesome if you fantasize only about forcing someone to have sex with you. You may be conditioning yourself to get aroused only when coercion is involved, and that will create havoc in a relationship. As long as you enjoy a variety of fantasies, there's no problem.

There are often disagreements in relationships over preferences or conditions that almost no one would consider strange or abnormal. For example, you may feel most sexy in the mornings and prefer that time for lovemaking, but your partner may feel as strongly about evenings. Because of the conflicting preferences, you and your partner are going to have to work out an accommodation. It's important to understand this point. **Just because you and your partner don't have the same preferences or don't agree on when and how sex is to occur does not necessarily mean that anything is wrong with either of you.** It usually means only that the two of you have to negotiate a reasonable solution to your differences.

Fantasizing can sometimes be bothersome in a relationship. For example, let's say that during lovemaking you trip out on a fantasy, and although this increases your arousal and you're having a great time, your partner feels alone and neglected. She doesn't know you're fantasizing; she knows only that although you're having sex with her, you don't seem present. She may not voice her complaint as I have. Instead, she may say that she has trouble getting aroused or maintaining the excitement, or has problems having orgasm. It may only be with further exploration that she can come up with the feelings I've suggested.

Although it seems far more common for women to feel lonely and left out in sex, it happens for some men, too. The reason appears to be the same. The partner gets more involved with her fantasy than she is with you. Regardless of who feels left out, something needs to be done. It helps considerably if the one doing the fantasizing can admit it. There's no need for apologies or feeling bad, just a need to see what's going on and what could help.

Another kind of problem that can arise in a relationship is when the woman gets upset about a man's fantasies or erotic materials. Does his use of them indicate he no longer finds her attractive or desirable? In such situations, a good discussion about her concerns and his feelings is required.

Returning to where we started, with what's normal and what's not, my advice is to forget about the question as much as you can. Focus instead on how you feel about your sex life. If it's not as good as you want, use the information and exercises in this book to make it better. If there are serious problems, decide if the book is enough or if you also need professional help.

CHAPTER SIX

Your Conditions for Good Sex

It doesn't seem right. I know women need fuzzy feelings, the right atmosphere, and appropriate kinds of stimulation. But guys aren't supposed to be like that. We're supposed to be able to get it up and go to it regardless of anything.—*Man, 21*

It's so obvious, it's almost laughable that I didn't see it before. I function better and enjoy more when I'm rested, haven't had anything to drink, and I'm not thinking about work. Wish I'd realized this thirty years ago. —*Man, 52*

THE FANTASY MODEL of sex dictates that men be able to function and presumably enjoy sex without any special requirements. Regardless of how you feel and what's going on between you and your partner, you should be able to do your job.

But the fact is that we all have requirements or conditions. We're accustomed to hearing them from women. In older times a familiar condition was "I can't have sex with you because we're not married." A newer version is "I don't know you well enough" or "I can't have sex with you because you're not interested in a relationship." These women were just stating a necessary condition for them to be able to participate in or enjoy sex. And many of us have heard other ones as well. For instance: "I don't feel like having sex when we've barely been civil all week" or "For me to be able to orgasm, I need this [or that] kind of stimulation."

Certain frames of mind, attitudes toward partner and self, physical and mental stimulation, and a number of other things influence how much we want sex, how aroused we get, how much we enjoy it, and how well we function. And these things are as true for men as for women. Jim Brown put it in his usual blunt way: "Every dick, including mine, has a mind of its own. I never felt like I could fuck any woman, any time. My sexuality hinged on the woman and the situation." Despite what we have been taught, it is not strange or unusual for men to have requirements that need to be met in order to have good sex.

If I was asked what's the most important single thing a man (or woman) could do to have better sex or to resolve a sexual difficulty, my answer would be: Find out what you need and want and make sure to get those things (consistent, of course, with not trampling on your partner's needs). In a very real sense, most sex therapy, most books and workshops on sexual enhancement, and much of the rest of this book can be seen as helping you to determine what you need and how to get it.

The idea of conditions is very simple. A condition is anything that maximizes the chances of reaching a desirable goal: increasing or decreasing sexual desire, getting more aroused, enjoying sex more, delaying ejaculation, getting or keeping erections. When I say anything, I mean exactly that: time of day, how tired or energetic you are, how sick or well you are, how you feel about yourself, how you feel about your partner, what you do, what she does, how much privacy there is, or anything else that makes a difference to you.

It's not surprising that we should have sexual conditions—we have conditions in almost all areas of our lives. Take work, for example. I do my best writing in a dimly lit, totally quiet room with no one else around, just me and my computer. With this arrangement, I get into a kind of trance and just buzz along. I don't do as well in a library or other public place because I tend to get distracted by the goings-on around me. I know a freelance writer who is just the opposite. For months she tried writing at home alone and got nothing done. She needs lots of people around, ringing telephones, and so on. The noisier and busier it is, the better she concentrates and the more she does. Her way isn't better than mine, and mine isn't better than hers. We just have different requirements.

Even with as mundane an issue as getting a good night's sleep, many people have conditions. Some need a firm bed, six pillows, total darkness, and a temperature that would make me freeze. Others have a different pattern. And so it goes in almost every aspect of life. Some people function better socially in large gatherings, others in small groups. Some do better with male teachers or therapists, others with female. Some people get their best workouts in the morning, others in the evening.

Conditions can range in importance from absolute necessities to druthers, things you'd prefer to have but can also live without. For the freelance writer mentioned earlier, working in a noisy, busy place is essential. My requirement for a solitary, quiet place is not absolutely necessary, but it's more than a simple preference. I can get work done in a library if I have to, but I'm not at my best.

In a sexual situation, a condition is anything that makes you more relaxed, more comfortable, more confident, more excited, more open to your experience. Put differently, a condition is something that clears your nervous system of unnecessary clutter, leaving it open to receive and transmit sexual messages in ways that will result in a good time for you.

Despite the importance of conditions, many men have trouble accepting the concept. Conditions remind us that we're not robots, that we're flesh-and-blood human beings with feelings and vulnerabilities. This flies in the face of not only the fantasy model of sex but also most of our training in masculinity. We have no trouble understanding that women have all sorts of needs and preferences. That's how women are. But it just doesn't seem right to us that men should be the same. This is one of the main ways we're supposed to differ from women. We grit our teeth, disregard our feelings (or try to will the ones that are necessary), and do our jobs, including the job of sex. Just give us an available partner, and one way or another we'll be able to have good sex with her.

Because of this attitude, we feel ashamed of any needs and wants we have and try to hide them or pretend they don't exist. But this is destructive. Men are just as human as women, even though we try hard not to show it, and have as many requirements. It is perfectly acceptable to be yourself, to have your own desires, anxieties, concerns, and style. They should not be viewed as deficiencies. Conditions are expressions of our uniqueness and constitute a large part of who we are sexually.

Brad, a man of thirty-six, came to see me with the complaint of "being dysfunctional in bed." It turned out that he occasionally lost his erection or ejaculated very quickly. After doing the conditions exercise that I give later in this chapter, we determined that his "dysfunction" occurred only when he felt that his partner, Lee, didn't care for him.

Lee did not immediately express her complaints and dissatisfactions, but saved them up until she exploded in twenty- or thirty-minute tirades in which she vented all the complaints she had collected since the last diatribe. When an explosion occurred, Brad came away feeling unloved. She, on the other hand, felt much better after having gotten everything out and often wanted to make love immediately afterward. When Lee came on to him, Brad was aware of feeling terrible, but he was so anxious to "regain her love," as he thought of it, that he tried to go along. And that's when he lost his erection or came fast.

He wasn't any happier when I explained it was entirely natural for this to happen given how sad he was feeling (because of his idea that he had lost the love of the woman who meant so much to him) and how much anxiety he had (about regaining her love). His first comment is typical of men; "But I shouldn't let that stuff get to me." It took a while for Brad to learn that it's natural in human beings for "that stuff"—powerful emotions—to get to you. Once he accepted that, we found a solution for his problem.

In their attempt to function like "well-oiled machines," men overlook what they already know: that machines themselves have conditions, including being well oiled. When we're made aware of these needs, we don't get upset, we just fulfill them. For example, we accept that a car doesn't run without gas. If our car runs out of gas, we may get angry with ourselves for forgetting about this, but we don't get angry at the car for needing gas. Computer dealers report that they receive many calls from customers complaining that a printer or monitor doesn't work. The most common reason is that the customer forgot to turn the monitor or printer on. The callers may feel stupid for forgetting to flip the on switch, but they don't kick the printer for needing to be turned on. Yet many men kick themselves for not being able to function sexually even though they aren't turned on.

Rob complained of sometimes not feeling much in sex and being unable to get erect. When we compared such times with times when everything worked out, it was clear that the difference was arousal. When he felt interested and excited, he functioned fine and enjoyed. When these feelings weren't present, he often couldn't get erect or, even if he did, the experience didn't feel very good. In answer to my question of why he was making love when he didn't feel like it, he gave the typical response—he did so in order not to disappoint his partner.

Much like Brad, Rob felt he shouldn't be deterred by his feelings. "Why can't I just jump-start my penis and sexual feelings if I'm not already in the mood?" was how he put it. The answer, simply, is because a man is not a car. Sometimes one can get into the mood by doing the right things—for example, touching one's partner and being touched in return, engaging in loving or erotic talk—and sometimes not. But Rob needed to learn that he couldn't force a mood or feeling and also that it was foolish to proceed in the absence of arousal.

The idea of jump-starting feelings appeals to men because *jump-starting* is a synonym for *willing* or *forcing*, and men have had lots of lessons about being able to force or will things. But it simply does not work in sex. You can't will or force an erection, and you can't will or force erotic feelings. Feel free to try it if you're not sure what I'm saying is correct. What often does work, however, is to figure out what it would take to get turned on or erect (for instance, "If I was feeling more awake and rested [or more sober]") and put that requirement in place. And that's exactly what fulfilling one's conditions means.

For some men, determining and fulfilling their conditions is crucial from the onset of their sex lives. For others, conditions and even preferences don't seem important until later. At first, usually in their teens, twenties, and thirties, they were always or usually aroused, functioned well, and had a good time. Many men, especially when they are young, function automatically, without regard for particular conditions; some of them can function fine even without being aroused. It's not that they don't have needs or conditions when younger, it's just that they can function despite not fulfilling them, much as a young person can function reasonably well without getting as much sleep as he needs. As he ages, however, not getting enough rest will take a heavier toll.

With regard to sex, something often happens—the man and his relationship get older, a sexual experience goes badly, he suffers from job stress or something else—and the system is disrupted. Once this happens, automatic functioning usually cannot be restored, at least not the way it was before. The man has to pay attention to factors he once could ignore. As time goes on, of course, and these factors become a regular part of his thought and behavior, his functioning will become less self-conscious and more automatic. But it will now include some conditions he had previously ignored.

Here are a few common sexual conditions that men have reported to me.

▲ Feeling connected and close to your partner. Although this is often considered mainly a requirement of women, many men need it as well. If you're not feeling connected to her, if either one of you is feeling angry or distant, you may need to do something about it before you can have good sex. I deal with ways of being close and connected in Chapters 10 to 14.

▲ Absence of strong anxiety about performance. You either feel confident about how you'll do or you know that you won't have to pay any great price if things don't go as anticipated. You know that whatever you do and whatever happens, it will be okay with her.

▲ You know you'll get what you need from her in terms of attitude, response, and stimulation.

▲ Not feeling tired, ill, preoccupied, or under the influence of too much alcohol or other drugs.

▲ Feeling positive about the situation before it even starts. You're interested, you know she is, and you're both looking forward to a fun time.

▲ Feeling turned on, aroused, sexually excited. Aside from the absence of performance anxiety, this is probably the most important condition for men. If you want to learn more about this crucial quality and how to increase it, turn to Chapter 15.

Physical stimulation requires discussion. In the fantasy model, men don't require any physical stimulation other than seeing or kissing their partner. They are immediately excited and their penises immediately stand to attention and are ready for action. This matches the adolescent experience of many males: They didn't require any stimulation at all. But this often changes after adolescence. Not only men in their fifties and sixties but also many men in their thirties and forties require direct penile stimulation to get and stay hard and also to get emotionally excited. This is not a "problem," it's just life. If you find you require direct penile stimulation, or any other kind of stimulation, then get it. And make sure you get the kind that feels just right to you.

Foreplay—defined as erotic stimulation preceding intercourse—is usually considered something that man does to get the woman ready for intercourse. And it's certainly true that many women complain they don't get enough of it and many men complain that women want too much. But it turns out that many men need it, too, although sometimes it takes an extreme situation to determine this.

Many years ago when I was a horny student, and long before anyone had heard of AIDS or even herpes, I met a woman at a conference. There was an immediate attraction, and we were soon making out and pawing each other in the hotel lobby. Unfortunately, it couldn't go any further because I had to catch a plane. A few days later she called to invite me to her home several thousand miles away. We were going to finish what we started.

She greeted me at her door wearing only a T-shirt and big smile. She immediately led me to her bedroom and without any further ado took off her shirt, got on the bed with her legs apart, and told me to take her. I still recall my thoughts: "My God, a fantasy come true! But some words, hugs, or kisses would be nice." I tried for the kisses, but she turned her face away and immediately guided me into her. I had an erection because I was young at the time and had been thinking of her ever since her call. So we had intercourse, during which she rejected all my attempts to kiss; although I ejaculated, it wasn't very pleasurable. And it didn't get better on subsequent occasions.

I asked her about kissing. Her words shocked me: "I really don't like kissing or touching. I just like to fuck." In response to my question about the necking we had done at the hotel, she said she was willing to do it there because we didn't have time for anything else and it was clear I enjoyed it. "But here we can screw and don't have to do other stuff."

I felt as if I had landed on a strange planet. I'd never heard of women like this. Although in the past I had sometimes complained about the lengthy foreplay some women wanted and had fantasies about wild women who just wanted to screw, this experience demonstrated that *I* needed foreplay, too. I hadn't yet formulated the idea of conditions, but already I had come up with one of my own. I could function without it, but it wasn't fun (now that I'm twenty-five years older than I was then, I'm sure I couldn't even function without it). In fact, it was so little fun that I cut my trip short and never saw the woman again.

Of course, one can take the position that I'm a wimp, that a real man would have exploited this incredible opportunity to the full. I admit that this idea occurred to me and, as soon as it did, I started to feel bad about myself. But, fortunately, I rejected it in favor of another formulation that has aided me through the years and also been of assistance to some other men.

That idea is that **a real man is *not* someone who can live up to other people's standards and expectations. Rather, he is someone who knows who he is and goes after what he wants and needs, even if some of those wants and needs are not on Harold Robbins's, Arnold Schwarzenegger's, this or that woman's, or anyone else's approved list.** I realized I could have gotten some mileage with male friends by telling them about this wonderful week in another city where I screwed this incredibly attractive woman fifty times without one second of foreplay. But then I recalled that it wasn't wonderful, not even good. I didn't want to get any mileage from that story. It really was okay that I liked kissing and hugging and wanted to feel connected to the women I slept with.

I'm not saying it was easy. A number of times, usually when I was feeling lonely and horny, I was tempted to feel bad about what had happened with this woman. If only I'd accepted her restrictions, I could probably still be in touch with her and occasionally see her for sex. Why did I have to be so damned particular? Any other guy would have been more than delighted by what she offered. What kind of man was I, anyway? But as the months went by, I more and more accepted that it was fine to be myself.

Time of day is another matter that doesn't receive as much attention as it deserves. Particularly for older men, but also for some not so old, the when of sex is as important as the how.

Wendall, sixty-four, was distraught when he came to see me. He had been celibate for almost six years after his wife's death and had practically given up on finding someone with whom to share the rest of his life. But in the last few months he had been seeing Emma, a woman he met at church. Everything was fine except for his inability to get hard with her. Although Emma accepted him as he was and said it wouldn't stand in the way of them being together, he felt it wouldn't be right to marry her unless he could have intercourse.

As we compared sex with his late wife and with Emma, two differences came to light. His wife used to stimulate his penis with her hand during most of their sex play, and Emma rarely did and never for long. The other difference had to do with time. In their later years together, most of the lovemaking with his wife had been in the morning. Because Emma had several times said she was "a night person," Wendall never initiated sex with her except at night.

Wendall had been vaguely aware of both differences before he talked with me, but he didn't give them the weight they deserved. His penis was clearly a "morning person" and required sustained, direct stimulation. He was somewhat surprised: "You mean that's all it would take, sex in the mornings and some hand work from her?" I said I couldn't be sure, but it was certainly worth a try. He left the session a bit skeptical but promised he would talk to Emma about trying the new regimen. Three weeks later he called to say that although his penis wasn't as young as it used to be, the new routine had worked well enough for them to have enjoyable intercourse several times.

Another common condition is the ability to be present; this is the opposite of being preoccupied or spaced out. These days many people are preoccupied by work. Although they're at home, their minds are still going over what happened at work and what they have to do there the next day. This preoccupation about and stress over work can lessen one's desire for sex and also cause functional problems.

What can help with these situations is engaging in a transition activity, doing something—physical exercise, taking a relaxing bath or reading, playing with the kids—that allows you to put work aside and get into a more relaxed frame of mind. The exact nature of the activity is irrelevant as long as it achieves the goal of opening you up to be present with your partner.

It was clear, for example, that obsessing and stressing about work was causing Trevor to lose interest in sex and to start having erection problems. Both he and his wife were upset about this. When I asked him what would help him say good-bye to work for the day, he replied, "Physical exercise and a hot shower." They agreed that when he came home he would turn to these transition activities immediately after giving his wife a hug. He brought his stationary bike in from the garage and put it in front of the TV; the next day he hopped on it when he came home. After a half hour on the bike, he took a warm bath and came downstairs to his wife. "It was like a different person; he was more relaxed and present than I'd seen him in a long time," she reported. Thus Trevor started a habit that is still going strong after more than ten years. The sex problems disappeared shortly after he started on the new program.

Your conditions may or may not be similar to the ones I've mentioned above, but that's not the point. What *is* important is that you find out what you need and then get it.

Before offering an exercise that can help you determine your specific conditions, I want to mention a difficulty you may encounter. Like Brad, Rob, and myself, you may find yourself coming up with things you wish weren't true. Your conditions may strike you as strange, unmanly, old-fashioned, or something else you don't like. Despite this, it is best to write them out and give some thought to them. The vast majority of times, one's conditions are acceptable to one's partner. In general, conditions are much easier to accept and fulfill than to change. With the exception of the rare instance where your conditions involve harm or pain to you or your partner, chances are excellent that, no matter how new or unusual they seem to you at first, you can learn to accept and meet them.

Since what follows is the first exercise I offer in this book, a few words about exercises may be helpful. Although reading can by itself provide you with new information, years of experience with different kinds of self-help materials and psychotherapies have shown that *doing something,* even just writing lists or keeping a diary, is essential for making the kinds of personal changes most people want to make. And that's why I offer exercises.

The best way to deal with an exercise is first to read it carefully one or more times, along with the material that comes before and after it, and make sure you understand what is required. If, after doing this, it seems that an exercise might be useful to you, then just follow the directions.

In this exercise, I use the example of increasing arousal (passion, excitement). But it can be done with any other sexual issue; increasing sexual interest, delaying ejaculations, having and maintaining erections, experiencing more pleasure, and so on. All you need to do is substitute the appropriate word or phrase for *arousal* when reading and doing the exercise.

EXERCISE 6-1: CONDITIONS

Compare two or three sexual experiences in which you were highly aroused with an equal number where you were much less aroused and list all the factors that differ between the two groups. An example might be: "High arousal—I was rested, felt close to Cindy, wasn't preoccupied with work, wasn't in a hurry. Low arousal—I was feeling distant from Cindy, was preoccupied and in a hurry (once I was so involved in a sales talk I had to give the next day that I kept going over it in my mind while I was caressing her and couldn't wait to get back to my typewriter), or was exhausted (like that time I had just flown in from Europe and had crossed five or six time zones; I was totally out of it)." The items in the high-arousal list are your conditions. It's important to be as specific as possible. If you have not had any high-arousal experiences, or if it is difficult to recall them in sufficient detail, use your imagination and list those things you think would be necessary and helpful to be more turned on.

Whether you use real-life comparisons or your imagination, consider all these areas: your physical health; amount of anxiety or tension; use of alcohol and other drugs; how much time you felt you had; whether you were preoccupied with other matters; fears about performance, pregnancy, and disease; your feelings about your partner, especially closeness, anger, or resentment; your feelings about yourself; your confidence that you would not be put down no matter what happened.

When you have finished with your list, put it away for a day or two, then reread it and see if there is anything you want to change. Now go through each item and reword it so that it is specific enough to be put into practice.

Let's say one of your items is "Need to make love earlier. After 10 P.M. I'm tired and into my work mode, thinking about what I'm going to do at the office tomorrow." So what has to happen to make love earlier? Two obvious possibilities come to mind. One is that you talk to your partner and let her know that having sex earlier will make it easier for you to get turned on and result in more pleasure for both of you. The two of you may then need to think about how and when lovemaking can take place. A second possibility is that you decide for yourself how to initiate sex earlier. For example: "When I get turned on at work, I can call

Jan and let her know. If she's up for sex, we can send the kids out to play when we get home, and then take them to McDonald's."

An alternative way of doing this exercise is simply to make a list, over a period of days or weeks, of things you'd like in sex that you're not getting. You should consult both your erotic fantasies and past experiences with your current partner or with others. Are there things you used to do that you miss? Are there things in your fantasies that you'd like to try?

The importance of being specific in your conditions cannot be overemphasized. If they are worded too vaguely, you won't be able to put them into practice. Take all the time you need to determine what your conditions are and how you can fulfill them.

Mario, an ambitious and hardworking lawyer in his mid-thirties, was troubled by sporadic rapid ejaculation. I worked on the exercise with him, and this is what we came up with.

Need to feel Sue wants to have sex with me. I sometimes feel she's just doing it to please me and that makes me tense, which in turn makes me come fast. I'd know she wanted sex if she initiated it, if she said she wanted it, if she physically and verbally indicated her enjoyment, or if she played an active role in physically stimulating me.

Need to know she won't be upset if I do come quickly. Only way I can get this is to talk with her and see if it's okay to come fast sometimes.

Need to be more focused on how aroused or nervous I am during sex. Then I can make the adjustments needed to last longer. A good way to do that is to focus solely on my own pleasure, what I'm doing and feeling. Have to keep in mind to focus on me, not her.

This is a good list, because it is comprehensive and indicates not only what things are needed but also considers ways of getting them.

Here's another list, this one from a man whose main goal was simply to enjoy sex more:

I want to be able to express my "adventurous" ideas, but in order to do that I'd like to know she's not put off when I do it. She's told me it's okay, but sometimes she gets what I take to be a funny look—like

when I suggested she tell me one of her fantasies while we were having sex—that makes me feel ashamed and wish I had kept my mouth
shut.

Also I'd like to know that she's not put off by my expressions of
pleasure. As I've become more open, I've started to do things that
sometimes surprise even me. Like the other night when she was giving me head, I totally got lost in it and realized later that I had panted
like crazy and screamed at the top of my lungs. I think it's okay with
her, but I'd feel better if I knew for sure.

As this man's situation shows clearly, just knowing your conditions may
not be enough. You may have to talk with your partner to determine her
feelings about certain activities and expressions or to ask her to do or not
to do certain things. I discuss effective ways of expressing your needs and
desires in Chapters 10 and 11.

BETTER SEX

CHAPTER SEVEN

On the Road to Better Sex

Had enough bad love. I need something I can feel proud of.
—*Eric Clapton*

"THIS IS STARTING to sound complex," many of you might be saying about now. "Why can't sex be simple?" Sex *is* simple . . . for simple creatures with limited goals. Our primate cousins, for example, apparently have sex mainly to induce male ejaculation and conception. Their sex is very brief—a few thrusts and it's all over—but effective in its narrow aims. We humans could have the same kind of simple sex if we were willing to settle for the same modest ends.

But most of the time we want a lot more. In fact, our goals are quite expansive. We want to satisfy ourselves and our partners (and that satisfaction may be defined differently at different times by each individual), to bring us closer together (to *make* love), to validate our sense of masculinity and femininity, to reflect and generate feelings of excitement and passion, and, for some people, to produce a mystical experience. This is asking quite a bit from what looks like a simple physical activity. The large goals we have in mind for sex make it a lot more complicated than just sticking your thing in her thing and thrusting until you come. A lot is wanted, a lot is at stake. When things reach this level, we are very far from doing what comes naturally and equally far from something that's easy and simple.

The desire to have sexual intercourse is wired into us, but we are equipped with the tools, both physical and mental, to have a more elaborate and interesting kind of sexuality. Developing and using those tools, adding the embellishments that make human sexuality so much more fascinating and satisfying than that of other animals, is the product of intention, effort, and learning. We have already started on the road to better sex in the first section of the book. The chapters in this section continue on that path and focus more directly on what is required. Here are what I consider to be the major requirements for having good sex, which can mean enhancing an already satisfying sex life, making a not-so-interesting sex life more pleasurable and passionate, or overcoming a sex problem.

THE REQUIREMENTS FOR GREAT SEX

1. **Having the kind of relationship in which good sex can flourish.** If you're like most men I've worked with, this one is surprising. They thought I was about to address new intercourse positions or how to find her G-spot and, what a bummer, I'm talking about relating. Like it or not, a good relationship is the basis of all good sex unless your only interest is a one-night stand. Whether your relationship lasts a month or fifty years, what goes on in it aside from sex heavily influences how sex goes. Relationship issues are typically seen as something more important to women than to men, but they are also crucial to men. For there to be good sex over time, or even good sex at any time, there has to be attention, friendship, liking, respect, and trust. There also has to be the ability to quickly and effectively deal with differences of opinion and conflicts. Sex usually suffers when there is tension, hostility, or distance. Much of the material in subsequent chapters deals with aspects of relating. You will do yourself a big favor by paying close attention to this material.

2. **Being able to communicate verbally and nonverbally about all kinds of things, including sex.** An essential component of a good relationship is the ability to communicate generally and sexually. One of women's main complaints about men is our unwillingness to express our feelings, our likes and dislikes. Regarding sex, you need to be able to express your wants and don't-wants, your questions and concerns, and your pleasure, and you need to be able to listen to and understand what your partner is expressing.

One reason you need to be able to communicate is that sex with another person involves physical coordination of a kind that's rare anywhere else. Let's compare masturbation with partner sex to illustrate this point. Our bodies are the most sophisticated feedback systems ever built. When you touch your own body, the process is automatic, self-correcting, and extremely efficient. Continuous feedback between your penis, your brain, and your hand allows the brain to automatically move your hand to achieve the results you want.

Now let's move to your partner stimulating your penis with her hand. Suddenly things are much more complex. Your feedback mechanism still works—you know to what extent you're getting what you want—but your mate isn't part of it. To include her in the feedback loop, you must bring into awareness and put into words what by yourself was done without words and without conscious awareness. "Move your hand up . . . too far . . . down a bit more . . . that's right, and a little harder . . . a little faster . . . that's good . . . harder now . . . faster . . . that's great" and so on. You even have to tell her when to stop stimulating, because she may stop sooner than you want or not soon enough.

The complications increase with other acts. In oral sex, you may have to inform your partner that her teeth are hurting you, that she should apply more or less pressure with her mouth and hand, or that you want her to take more of your penis in her mouth. With a partner, you may want—and she almost certainly wants—certain kinds of stimulation that you ordinarily can't or don't do by yourself (hugging, kissing, touching nongenital areas, expressing feelings orally, and so on). With masturbation, you can do it or not do it, or start and then abruptly change your mind and go do something else. With a partner, you have to inform her of what is happening. And since the two of you won't always be in agreement as to what should be done, there has to be a way of expressing and dealing with the discrepant desires. Partner sex also carries baggage that masturbation usually does not. If you decide not to masturbate today or for the next ten weeks, or if you decide to masturbate every single day, it's unlikely that issues of love, desirability, or adequacy come into play. It's no big deal whatever you do. But with a partner, things are a bit different. Being able to talk, listen, understand, and negotiate are absolutely essential.

3. Understanding your own needs and preferences generally and sexually and being able to assertively express them. Read on to understand the balancing act that's required.

4. Learning, understanding, and being sensitive to her needs and preferences and being willing to fulfill them. I know, it sounds like there is a contradiction between #3 and #4, but there really isn't.

Being only self-centered or only sensitive does not work. The man who only goes after what he wants and pays little attention to his partner will end up alone or with a very unhappy partner. The man who focuses solely on his partner's needs will not get what he wants and therefore be unhappy, and his partner may well be dissatisfied because she's not feeling his strength.

In days of old, sex was mainly an act of male assertiveness. Having an orgasm inside a woman was what he wanted, and it was far from clear what she might want or what he might be able to do for her. Many men thought women wanted nothing in sex but engaged in it only because they wanted something else that sex could bring—conception, a steady boyfriend, a happy husband—or because they had been tricked into it. For men who weren't cads, the main aspect of sensitivity was not harming the woman—in other words, treating her gently and using protection against pregnancy and disease.

The view of women as nonsexual came increasingly under attack in the nineteenth and twentieth centuries, until it was finally accepted that women are indeed sexual creatures. Men should strive not only for their own satisfaction but also for their partner's. Since men were still seen as more sexual than women, and since they had more leeway to gain experience, it was their task to open up women to the joys of sex.

The research of Kinsey and that of Masters and Johnson added influence to this view, showing that women were capable of not only enjoying sex but also of orgasm, maybe more orgasms than men. This was an important step forward, but one result was that men felt more pressured to perform because somehow the message was that they had to "give" their partners orgasms. Some men became so focused on ensuring their partner's pleasure that they forgot about their own.

In the new male sexuality I hope we are constructing, the satisfaction of both partners is paramount. The man has to assert his own wants and preferences, but also be sensitive to his partner's. It is not his job to give her orgasms, but it is in his interest to understand her desires and to fulfill them to the best of his abilities. It behooves men to learn as much as they can about the similarities and differences between the sexes, a topic I address in Chapter 8.

Being assertive and self-focused is just another way of saying that you know your conditions, go after them, and thoroughly involve yourself in your own pleasure. You want sex now, so you try to interest your partner. You like to kiss this way, so that's what you do. You like to touch her breasts that way, so you do it. You like intercourse in such a position, so that's what you go for. And while doing these things, you're immersed in your sensations and experience, fully present and alive to what is happening. A good lover is assertive in these ways. He knows what he wants, or is willing to find out, and he goes after it without apology or guilt.

But a good lover is also sensitive to his partner's needs. You notice if she doesn't seem interested in exactly what you want or suggests something else, and you're flexible enough to try to combine both of your desires to make for a mutually satisfying experience. And you don't use guilt or other types of coercion to get what you want. A good lover is attentive to his partner's breath, sounds, and movements, and notices what works and doesn't work for her. He also listens carefully when she says what she likes. If she doesn't spontaneously voice her likes and dislikes, he asks. Bad lovers don't ask, don't listen, and don't remember.

A good lover takes the time and energy to use his knowledge to make sure his partner enjoys sex as much as he does. He also knows that sex isn't necessarily over when he's satisfied. Maybe she wants something more. A good lover would not be open to the charge a woman made about her new boyfriend: "He's one of these selfish or unconscious men. When he comes, it's all over. I have to go, 'Knock, knock, can I have a turn, too?' " A good lover is also sensitive enough not to pressure his partner to perform to boost his ego.

It *is* difficult, perhaps impossible, to be both sensitive and self-absorbed at the same time. The trick is to be able to be both, but at different times. If you want her to go down on you, for instance, ask her to. That's being assertive. But if she says no, accept the no with good grace and find out what else you two can do. If she never wants to stimulate you orally and that kind of stimulation is important to you, talk to her about it and see if something can be worked out. If she wants you to go down on her, you hear her request and then either do as she wants, say you don't feel like it now, or tell her what your objection is and work something out. If you want her to initiate more, you say so, but you also listen sympathetically if she tells you why this is difficult.

There can be times when sex is mainly for her and times when it's mainly for you. During these times, there should be no problem knowing what to do. If it's for you, then get into your self-absorbed mode and get exactly what you want. If it's for her, then focus entirely on what she wants.

Of course, there are other times when it's mainly for both of you. This requires some shifting back and forth. Perhaps you like to kiss her breasts quite hard, but she likes that only after some softer touching and kissing. So you would do it the way she wants until she's ready for you to do it your way. If she likes slow and gentle intercourse and you prefer it fast and furious, you could do it her way for a while, then your way. Or there can be occasions where intercourse is done her way, other times when it's done your way.

We have already started on the self-centered side by determining your conditions in Chapter 6. Chapter 11 deals with how to get them met and how to be assertive in your communications. In that chapter and in most of the ones that follow, I switch back and forth between the two poles of sexual happiness: assertiveness and sensitivity. I realize it's a bit of a balancing act, both for you as reader and me as writer, and for all of us in real life. But it is a balancing act that must be mastered if we are to have truly wonderful sex.

5. **Accurate information about your own sexuality, about your partner's, and about sex itself.** This means getting away from the myths and unrealistic expectations discussed in the first section of the book and being able to learn about your own sexuality and that of your partner. Much of the material in the following chapters is designed to help you garner the information you need.

6. **Having or developing an orientation based on pleasure (arousal, love, lust, and fun) rather than performance.** In other words, holding to some version of the definition of good sex given in Chapter 3 and being willing to work and focus on arousal (excitement, passion), the key to good erotic feelings.

IT'S OKAY TO BE WHO YOU ARE

It is important that you try to enjoy the journey to better sex and that you feel as good as possible about yourself as you undertake it. Being a man, I'm well aware that sometimes it feels like we're made out to be the bad guys: everything we do is unhealthy and wrong, everything we want is somehow not the right thing.

I don't think there's anything wrong with men's style in love and sex or with women's style. The problem is that there are differences, and we're all going to have to learn about one another and to accommodate the differences. There's always room in all of us for change and growth.

We men have taken a lot of heat in recent years for our attitudes about sex. We are told that we are obsessed with sex, especially sex without love and commitment; that we push too hard for it and in inappropriate ways in both new and old relationships; and that we pout when we don't get what we want. Such attitudes, we are told, are immature and maybe downright sick. But I think the criticisms themselves are wrongheaded and destructive. Males can't help having their attitudes, which are probably due at least as much to physiology as to learning. Sex, after all, is life-affirming, and there's no point in feeling bad about that.

Sex is not only life-affirming but life itself. I find it fascinating that so many people who take such great joy and pride in the birth of a child find it so hard to acknowledge, let alone celebrate, what made that new life possible. But a thrusting, sperm-shooting penis in a vagina is exactly what it took. If we felt better about sex, we might find male attitudes easier to accept.

I think there's a lot to be admired in men's, especially boys' and young men's, attitude toward sex. They are wonderfully curious, enthusiastic, and exuberant about it, and they're willing to pay an enormous price to pursue the subject.

A number of times I have watched a group of two, three, or four boys at a bookstore looking at *Playboy* or *Penthouse*. The only word that comes to mind to describe what I saw is *charming*. There's something truly wonderful about it, a lot of what I can only call good energy. I rarely sensed any disparagement of women. The same was true in my high-school days when we boys passed around novels with explicit sexual descriptions; there was desire, curiosity, and great enthusiasm, but really no ugly feelings toward girls or women. With testosterone virtually running our minds and bodies, we wanted to learn everything we could about the doing of sex, and we looked forward with great excitement and anticipation to the acts themselves.

What does present a problem is that the girls these boys pair up with are coming from a different place. While most boys report mainly positive feelings about their first sexual experience—if nothing else, at least relief that they finally had it—many girls don't feel so good about it. It's as if sex happened to them while they were thinking of something else. Aside from anything else, the boys feel good because they got something they wanted. The girls, on the other hand, don't feel as good because they did something they aren't sure they wanted to do. Perhaps it is true, as so many parents and others have charged, that we ought to do something to stop boys and young men from putting so much pressure on girls and young women. But there's an equally valid case to be made for allowing females to take a more lively interest in sex. Why should girls and women who are sexually active have to worry about their reputations when boys and men don't? But making this kind of change assumes that we really believe willing participation in sex is life-affirming and healthy.

A lot of these differences between men and women are things that both sexes have taken heat about. Women are often criticized by partners for their relative lack of interest, not initiating enough, wanting too much foreplay, and taking too long to get aroused or to orgasm. Men have been scolded for just about everything. I think the criticism is unfortunate and gets us nowhere. In a sense, everyone is doing what comes naturally, whether *naturally* is defined as what's built in or as what's acquired over the years through learning.

While it is true that we have to learn to accommodate one another, I don't think blame and accusations or feeling guilty is going to help. We have to feel good about ourselves if we're to have decent relationships and sex. A man should not have to feel guilty for looking at or fantasizing about younger women, for desiring sex without love, or for anything else that he is. But, on the other hand, neither should he denigrate his partner. It's fine if you have fantasies about the college girl next door, as long as you keep them fantasies, but it's something else if you make comments about her in front of your lover that imply your lover is inadequate. It's fine if you sometimes want a quickie—perhaps you can arrange it with your partner—but it is not fair to complain that you can't have them all the time or that she takes too long to get turned on.

The male ways of expressing love and sex are really okay. And so are the female ways. The better we understand and feel about ourselves and one another, the more likely we will be able to make the changes we desire in our sex lives and elsewhere.

Some Things You Should Know About Women

Has anyone ever come up with an answer to Freud's famous question of what do women want? If so, I'd sure like to see it. —*Man, 51*

ALMOST ALL THE men I have worked with—in therapy and in courses and workshops—have wanted to know how to be better lovers for their partners. This is an admirable goal, and we know from surveys it is one held by the vast majority of American men. It is no longer the case that men can feel like good lovers without satisfying their partners.

In the final analysis, being a good lover for your partner means knowing her—her tendencies and preferences, her likes and dislikes—and also yourself. And this brings us to the fascinating topic of sex differences, because at least some of her tendencies and some of yours are due to the fact that you are a he and she is a she.

Since the beginning of time, men and women have been attracted and charmed by one another, and also frustrated by trying to understand and deal with one another. We complain: Why do women want to talk so much? Why are they so emotional and such nags? Why are they so weird about sex? What in God's name do they want? From women come a different set of complaints: Why are men so withholding? Why are they so focused on sex and so unromantic? Why can't they remember a birthday or anniversary? From both men and women comes the cry "Why can't they be more like us?" The common phrase "the war of the sexes" indicates the strength of our feelings.

One could easily get the impression that men and women are totally different, as this man's statement implies: "If the first space visitor arrived from Mars, and was male, I'd have more in common with him than with

any woman on Earth." In fact, since we are all humans, we are more similar than different. We all breathe air, walk upright on two legs, use language, think, feel, eat, eliminate, sleep, and so on. If it were possible to
quantify everything, we'd probably conclude that women and men are 90
to 95 percent similar. But it's that remaining 5 to 10 percent that's so fascinating and causes all the trouble.

Even in something as fundamental as the use of language, there are differences between the typical man and the typical woman. Though men
and women use the same words—*intimacy, love, making love, sex*—they
don't necessarily mean the same things by them. As Deborah Tannen
demonstrated brilliantly in *You Just Don't Understand*, the definitions of
even simple terms like *talk* and *conversation* depend heavily on whether
you are a she or a he.

We saw in Chapter 1 that girls and boys specialize in different areas.
Boys learn to achieve and perform in the outside world, while girls get
more practice dealing with feelings, communicating, and relating. We also
saw that males and females come to sex from different angles, girls approaching via love and sensuality, boys more from lust and a desire to
prove themselves. While men and women both want love and sex, they
have separate styles of loving and being sexual.

These separate styles result in no end of misunderstandings, confusion,
and conflicts. Here is a common example:

HE: Everything between us was so tense after our spat on Sunday. I
    thought if we made love, things would get better.
SHE: How can we make love? We haven't talked in days.

The differences between the sexes affect our perceptions and understandings of ourselves, our partners, and our relationships and make us
feel bad about all three. It can help enormously to understand and accept
these differences. The more you can understand and accept your male tendencies, the better and the less guilty you'll feel. The more you can understand that your partner is acting as she is not to thwart you, not because
she's neurotic or passive-aggressive or a nag, and not necessarily because
of anything you've done, but simply because this is the way women tend to
be, the better you'll feel both about her and about yourself.

As you read the following material, please keep in mind that I am not
trying to provide a blueprint for satisfying women. Nor am I saying that
all women are the same. But the following points are ones that many
women agree with. In fact, I developed them after doing two separate sur-

veys of women regarding what makes a man a good lover; most of the quotes and examples come from those studies. Discussing the material with your partner can be beneficial. Even if she doesn't agree with some of the items, you will learn what's true for her, and that's the only important thing.

Please also keep in mind that I do not believe and am not saying that one way is better than another. The point is to promote understanding, not to pass judgment. If we can be open and withhold judgment, we can understand one another better, learn from one another, and enjoy one another more. There are, of course, exceptions to every single item. But the existence of an exception, or even many of them, does not necessarily invalidate a rule.

▲ **Women's style of love is different from men's.** A man feels he is showing love by working to support his partner, spending time with her (watching TV, playing tennis, walking, taking trips, and so on), having sex, giving her help and advice when she has problems, and doing chores like fixing the car and the back door. This style is called side-by-side intimacy. With the exception of sex, it's the same kind of closeness men have with one another. Shared activities, not personal discussion, is the main theme. Women, on the other hand, prefer face-to-face intimacy where personal sharing is the main theme, and this is what they do with their women friends.

Given who men are, it's not surprising that they haven't been articulate about what they're doing, but they can put it into words when pushed. A forty-eight-year old accountant had this to say after his wife complained he never said he loved her and didn't share his feelings:

What's so important about words? Words are cheap. It only counts when you put your money where your mouth is. Every tax season, the busiest time of my year, I spend several evenings doing taxes for all of her relatives and several of her friends. I barely know some of these people, and some have complicated returns. I don't get a cent for this. I don't want to do their taxes. I wish they'd get their own accountants. I do them only out of love for my wife. Why can't she understand that's what love is?

In one study, when a man was told to increase his affectionate behavior toward his wife, he washed her car. He was surprised to discover that neither his wife nor the researchers viewed car washing as an affectionate act.

I have related this story in a number of talks and always gotten the same reaction: Virtually all of the women in the audience have a good laugh, and it's clear most of them believe the man is a dumbbell. What they fail to see, however, is that he's not stupid, only naive; he's expressing love as he knows how to do it. I'm sure he had better things to do than wash her car, and washing it was a genuine act of affection. And I'm sure his wife liked having a clean car. But to her it was a favor, not an act of love.

In recent times, the female definition of love has triumphed. Face-to-face intimacy is the standard against which men are judged; not surprisingly, they come out on the short end.

Both sexes need to understand the validity of both sides. Men have to understand the value of personal talk and sharing feelings. But men also need to articulate and stand up for their style of loving. Sharing activities, including sex, can also be healthy and beneficial. The advice and practical help men offer their partners is not to be sneered at. Given who men are, having sex with their partners often is a real act of love, one of the best ways they know to give love.

Because how men see things and act is so foreign to women, they need to explain themselves. The man who washed his wife's car, for example, needed to realize that she might not see it as an act of love, and he needed to look for a way of explaining what washing the car meant to him. It can be done.

▲ **Women attach great importance to words and talking.** Big surprise, right? Aside from affectionate touching, this is the main way they relate and want to relate. Needless to say, men are a bit different. I got an important lesson in this matter from my son when he was nine years old. The two of us had been eating dinner and talking for about twenty minutes when he said: "I'm getting bored. When are we going to relate?" When I responded that I thought we had been relating, he replied: "No, we've only been talking. I mean real relating. Let's wrestle." It's clear that for him, and for many males, talking has nothing to do with relating. Action is what's important.

Women tend to be different. They love to talk with their lovers, and they tend to believe a relationship is working to the extent that they can talk. Even if there are problems, being able to talk about them suggests there is hope. When talking is rare or full of tension, women tend to lose hope.

Talking about what? you ask. Almost everything—your day and her day, your plans for tomorrow and hers, your hopes, pains, and fears, and hers.

But not quite everything. Women generally do not enjoy long conversations about things—cars, computers, and tools—and most women are not crazy for a lot of talk about sports. If these are among your favorite topics, you need to find some male friends. Women most certainly do not like these subjects to be brought up in the midst of serious, romantic, or lusty conversations.

Women love talk that includes compliments and appreciations and words of love. Here's what one fifty-seven-year-old woman said:

> I adore men who can speak up in all ways, and I especially like men who freely express their like, love, and lust for me. If I've spent two hours putting on my face and getting ready for a big night out, I love to hear how good I look. I know my aging body isn't what it used to be, but I still have some good points, and I like a man who notices and says so.

And from another woman, thirty-seven:

> I guess I know Rolph appreciates and loves me, and it's obvious he depends on me a lot, but it wouldn't hurt to have him say it once in a while.

I discuss compliments and appreciations in several later chapters. While on the subject here, however, let's not forget specifically sexual compliments. This is one place where we can heal one another. So many women feel bad about their bodies. Most women in America have breasts that they consider to be too small, too large, or too droopy, and butts and thighs they imagine to be too big, too fleshy, and too jiggly. If you like your partner's parts and tell and show her consistently that you do, in time she will see them in a new way, as this woman did:

> I've always hated my butt. I thought it was humongous and was always careful not to let my lovers see it in broad daylight. When Aubrey said he loved it, I thought he was bullshitting. I mean, who could like such a thing? But he persisted in wanting to look at it, play with it, and tell me how it turned him on. Over the years I've started to see my butt the way he sees it, and I feel much better about it now. When he wants to have me from the back, instead of cringing like I used to and lobbying for an alternative position, I just put my butt up there for him and even wiggle it with some pride.

▲ **For women, sex has meaning only in the context of a caring relationship.** Surveys show that both men and women prefer sex in a loving relationship. But men also tend to view sex as a good thing in and of itself, regardless of whether it's part of a loving relationship or if the participants have any other feelings for each other. For most women, sex devoid of some kind of relationship and close feelings is not appealing.

In one study among college students, 85 percent of the women said emotional involvement is a prerequisite for engaging in sex "always" or "most of the time," whereas 60 percent of the men said "sometimes" or "never." In response to the question of what would be the primary reason for refusing to have sex, all of the women answered "too soon in the relationship" or "not enough love/commitment." Forty-six percent of the men, and none of the women, said they would never refuse to have sex regardless of anything else.

This difference is well illustrated in comparing the different erotic materials men and women favor. In the material men like, plots are flimsy and character development and relationships virtually nonexistent. Pornography focuses on orifices, organs, and positions, with vaginal sex, oral sex, and anal sex (and sometimes more than one of these at the same time); sex with one person, two people, and whole villages; sex with strangers, friends, and relatives; voluntary sex and forced sex; private sex and public sex—in short, sex in every combination and permutation. But the novels women like are about love and romance. There is sex, sometimes spelled out graphically, but sex with love, not just the conjunction of body parts.

What we can learn from all this is why casual sex usually has such little appeal to women. In order for them to want and have good sex, there has to be some kind of relationship in place, or at least the promise of one. And the relationship has to be in good shape. As a forty-two-year-old woman said to her husband in my office: "If I'm not feeling good about you or our relationship, the door to sex is closed." She did not mean this in a threatening way, just as a statement of fact. Another woman, close to sixty, said something similar to her husband of over thirty years: "Things have been so bad between us about [problems they were having with one of their grown children] that making love is the last thing on my mind."

▲ **Women like men who are fully present and accounted for.** Virtually every woman I've talked to said that they can't abide men who seem spaced out or somewhere else when they're together. As the comments below make clear, women want someone who is alive in the moment with them, who listens, who talks, who pays attention.

I've had it with unconscious men. They're not quite there when talking to you because their eyes are roaming around the room looking for someone prettier, they're not quite there when at home because they're trying to see around you to the TV, and they're not even all there in sex. God knows where they are then.

I knew my husband was a keeper shortly after I met him. On an early date we talked about favorite junk foods, and I mentioned a kind of chocolate I especially like. The next time we got together, he brought me a whole box of chocolates, exactly the ones I had mentioned. I thought, "My God, a man who's conscious and listens." Didn't take me long to realize that he's almost always where he is and not like so many others who seem perpetually spaced out.

▲ **Women appreciate men who listen to them and take them seriously.** Listen to her and take her words seriously, especially when she says no and when she requests a change in what you're doing. If she says she doesn't want sex tonight, or that she doesn't want to do a certain thing, make sure to guide your behavior accordingly. If she says she doesn't want you to blow in her ear, then stop blowing and make sure to remember her preference. Many women feel they don't get listened to sexually (and generally), and it drives them crazy: "I've told him a hundred times I don't like him blowing in my ear, and here he is doing it again!" If there's a big conflict about what she says—for example, if blowing in ears is important to you—then understand what she's saying, tell her your thoughts, and see if something can be worked out. But don't pretend you didn't hear her. Learn to listen; better yet, learn to enjoy listening.

Whatever you do, absolutely abide by her sexual rejections. If she says she doesn't want sex now, it's fine to try to persuade her. But this must be tempered by an ability to hear her rejections and back off. Women are enraged by men who can't take a no seriously and graciously.

When my husband is hot to trot, he just keeps coming on. First he tries verbal persuasion and, if that doesn't move me, he escalates: I don't really love him, I don't care about his needs, that kind of thing. If that doesn't do it, he gets demanding—I have a duty to have sex with him—or tries the old his-work-will-suffer-if-he's-carrying-around-all-this-tension routine. If none of this succeeds, he stops talking to me for a week. I really hate this shit.

I like a partner who can be sensitive to my needs while still being true to his own. I like to have my requests listened to and not to be forced into doing things I don't want. In short, I like an equal relationship rather than a one-sided one.

▲ **Women are more receptive to making love when there's an ongoing romantic/erotic connection.** Many women report that their men seem to be "seriously fragmented" or "compartmentalized." One of them went on to explain:

Men amaze me. One day he's watching the Forty-niners on the tube and I'm reading a book in another room. Suddenly he appears and asks, "Do you want to fool around?" How did he get there? We haven't been having any problems, but we also haven't been close in days. I like sex, but this is way too abrupt. I'd have needed some nice talk or touch in the last few days, or even some talk about sex, or else some of that stuff now. But no, he had somehow made the leap and was ready for immediate action. And then, I suppose, he would have gone right back to the game. I can't do that!

Having an ongoing romantic/erotic connection means at least three things. One is regular sex. Your sexual encounters don't have to be tightly scheduled, but it does mean that the last time you made love shouldn't be so long ago that you can't recall when it was. You want to keep the momentum going. Another part of an ongoing connection is regular romantic or erotic talk. This means that you remind yourself and your mate of the erotic component of your relationship with words when you're not making love—sexual compliments and appreciations, happy recollections of what you did sexually last time, last week, or last year, excited anticipations of what you'll do next time, sexual innuendos, and so forth. The last part of the connection is regular erotic touching. This means that at least some of your kisses and hugs are intended to be and feel sexual. There is a big difference between a peck on the cheek or a closed-mouth kiss and a sensual open-mouth kiss with tongue play. There is a big difference between a hug where only chests and heads connect and one where pelvises talk to each other.

A beautiful woman I know who has enjoyed a wonderful sex life for many years with her husband had this to say when I discussed this topic with her: "Tell the men connection is the most important thing. Not just chitchat and catch-up talk, but talk and touch that's laced with eroticism. Keeps the juices flowing. Then there's really not much making needed in making love. Everything is already in place."

▲ **Unlike us, women use words to bridge the gap.** A common conflict in couples is conveyed by the example I gave earlier in the chapter where the man reaches out sexually after a rift and the woman can't respond because they haven't talked first. Yes, it's the old talking thing again. Women generally are more comfortable reaching out with affectionate touch and words. Then, after some closeness is established, maybe there is sex. Men, on the other hand, being less comfortable with words, tend to reach out sexually.

Each way works some of the time; neither way works all the time. You and your sweetheart have to find what's acceptable in your relationship. If you know she would rather talk but that's hard for you right now, maybe you can say something about it ("I know you'd probably like to talk now, but I think I would feel more like talking after making love"). If that sounds like it would never work, listen to this sixty-six-year-old woman:

All my life I was convinced I was right on this, that it's impossible to make love without having closeness first. But my second husband, who's quite able to express himself, explained that sometimes we talk too much and being sexual might be a better way. He was so persuasive that the next time we had a fight and he reached out sexually, I went along. As our lovemaking went on, I started to respond in my usual ways. We had a very good time and afterward had a helpful talk about what had caused the fight. From that and subsequent experiences I learned that sometimes making love is the best way to get close.

▲ **Women are more aroused by words and touch than by what they see.** Although the human species generally depends heavily on sight, and although women are also capable of being aroused by what they see, this is more common with men. With men, it's as if the optic nerve is directly connected to the penis. Male fantasies, for example, include more visual content than female fantasies, and men tend more to focus on minute details of their fantasized partner's physical appearance.

One young and articulate woman put quite clearly the differences between men and women:

> I swear we're from different planets. Men see a pair of legs or boobs they like and they're turned on and ready to go. They don't care if she's a nice person or if they'd want to be with her longer than screwing would take. I'm not like that and neither is any woman I know. There's no kind of body or body part in itself that can make me want sex. I have to get to know the man and see what else is there. If I keep getting stuff I like, then I start to turn on.

I realize that in recent years women have enjoyed going to clubs where men engage in stripteases for them. But women go for different reasons and have different reactions than men. For them it's a "fun night out with the girls" that has very little to do with sex. One woman said, "It was wonderful, hooting and hollering and being coarse." In response to the question of whether she got sexually aroused, her surprised response was, "Why would I?" This is not the answer one would expect from a man at a strip show.

Because they are so visually oriented, men generally prefer young, physically attractive women. In sexual materials that appeal to men, the women are almost without exception young and beautiful. Women seem more flexible with respect to age and physical characteristics. In romance novels, for instance, the hero is often older, sometimes much older, than the woman. Other qualities, such as those that indicate the man might be a good mate, seem more important.

We need to understand that seeing a naked male body, even an aroused naked body, doesn't necessarily turn women on the way seeing a naked female body turns us on.

One night Burgess, one of my clients, stood on the bed and did a sexy dance and strip for his partner, Alicia, who was sitting naked on the floor. He got very excited looking at her and dancing. As soon as the dance was over, he grabbed her and tried to enter her. He was surprised by her shocked response. They were not in good shape when I met with them a few hours later. He told her, "I was very aroused dancing for you. And you seemed excited, too. I don't understand the problem." She replied, "I liked your dance—it was fun. I assumed we would make love. But no way was I ready for you to come in me right after the dance. What about a little foreplay?" Looking at and dancing for her was all the foreplay he needed. She needed more.

▲ **Affectionate touching is very important to women.** This is seen in how much they touch their women friends and how much they touch and want to be touched by you. They like touching of all sorts. It's a way of expressing many things—caring, support, love, lust—and they like to be touched here, there, and everywhere. Women are perturbed that touching is so often seen as sexual by men. As one woman put it: "I'd like to just snuggle sometimes without him thinking we have to go on to sex. Why do men take every kind of physical contact as a sexual advance?"

Men are often a bit different in the touching department. Touching is merely a means to an end, and they go for the important goals—genitals and orgasm—as quickly as possible. This is a good impulse to learn to resist. It will help both of you if you learn to enjoy nonsexual touching and sensuality. I'm sure you love a back rub. There are many other kinds of nonsexual touch that you can also learn to enjoy.

Women often take a man's way with touching as predictive of other things, and they are much more likely to be receptive to lovemaking if there has been a lot of nonsexual touching first. As one forty-one-year-old woman said: "Hey, if a guy can't snuggle, what's the point of having sex with him?" Experiment with hugging, cuddling, bathing together, foot rubs and back rubs, stroking and brushing her hair, and so on. Like the women quoted below, your partner will appreciate it—and you probably will, too.

> I go for sensual guys, the ones who enjoy kissing (and not just passionate kisses), holding, hugging, and caressing. I love to touch and be touched, and I just can't be with a man who can only slap you on the back or fuck you. With a guy like that, being fucked is what it feels like, and I don't need that.

> Affection is what I crave. Touching is important *all* the time.

▲ **Women tend to prefer a gradual approach to and in sex.** While many men don't need much in the way of foreplay and are ready to stick it in almost instantaneously, most women are usually not this way. They tend not to like immediate and exclusive concentration on genitals. A life-long bachelor summed up the sex difference this way: "I've concluded that in sex, women are more interested in the foreplay and afterplay, while men, or at least this man, is more interested in what happens between those two events."

In a study of sexual fantasies, women were much more likely than men to focus on nongenital caressing and touching and much more likely to take their time getting to explicit sexual activity. For the men, on the other hand, intercourse or other genital activity was right there at the very start of their fantasies.

Women also like gradualness and tenderness rather than the rough, almost violent encounters that are a staple of pornography.

> I absolutely cannot tolerate men who go for my breasts or crotch right away. What does it take to get them to understand that's not a turn-on to me or any other woman I know? None of us are prudes by any means, but we like to move gradually into sex, not be smashed into it.

As the song goes, women like men with a slow hand and a gentle touch. You have nothing to lose by starting slow and easy. Allow her interest and desire to build. As arousal develops, more vigorous activity can follow.

▲ **Women like men who express themselves during sex.** Although men are supposed to be the big talkers when it comes to sex, many women report that their partners rarely say or express much of anything. A great many women comment that after years of being with the same man, they have no idea what their husband likes most in sex or if he even enjoys it. As surprising as it may sound, scores of women have told me that their men are so unexpressive in sex that the only way they know he's had an orgasm is when he stops moving.

So learn to express yourself. If you've been missing your lover and thinking about how much you want to kiss her, fondle her, make love with her, or whatever, tell her. If you don't know what you like best, experiment and find out. I can't tell you how many women complain that they can't find out what their lovers want in sex.

> I like for men to tell me what feels good to them and what they like for me to do sexually. It not only helps me know what to do but it also makes it easier for me to tell them what I like.

> I try to find out by asking, but no matter what I do, all he says is, "It feels great." It's like talking to my five-year-old; no matter what I ask, the answer is always "Fine." I'd like to know specifically what he most likes and doesn't like.

Many women interpret this lack of a differentiated response to mean that the man is withholding information or that he isn't interested enough to give a relevant answer. So pay attention and express your desires and pleasure. If you like what she's doing to you right now or what she did to you yesterday, tell her. Use words, sounds, and movements to convey your enjoyment.

I like a guy who lets it all hang out in bed—and, come to think of it, elsewhere, too. I like it when he laughs during sex, or screams in ecstasy—it makes me feel good about the effect I'm having on him— or lets all his emotions come out when he's coming. Some guys are like robots or dead people. I can't even tell if they're having a good time.

▲ **Women like men who understand that women's orgasms are more problematic than men's.** One reason that men like sex so much is that their having an orgasm is virtually certain. Only a small number of men have problems having orgasm in partner sex. For women, on the other hand, difficulties reaching orgasm are a major complaint.

Part of the discrepancy is explained by the fact that the traditional script, where intercourse is the main event, favors men. This is a way in which men come easily but most women do not. Even with oral or manual stimulation, men orgasm more quickly and easily than women.

Women like men who understand that their partners can't necessarily come with two or three minutes of stimulation. They like men who take an interest in their orgasms and are eager and happy to do what is necessary to get them there.

One reason I fell in love with my husband is that he was the first guy ever who said when we were first in bed, "Please tell me how I can give you pleasure." I thought I had gone to heaven. I'd never been orgasmic with a man before, because even though I knew what it took, I didn't know how to tell them. He gave me the permission, and it's been wonderful ever since.

Some guys are real nice and make it clear they want me to enjoy the experience as much as they do. They're willing to take their time and do what I need. Other guys, though, expect me to come as quickly as they do. They're real impatient, and I always have the sense they aren't enjoying giving me a good time. That's not my idea of fun.

▲ **Women want to be emotionally and physically close after sex.** Since women view sex as part of an emotional connection, they want to keep connecting after the sex is over. They want to cuddle, to talk, to stay connected in some way, at least for a moment or two. Even if the sex was planned as a quickie, it's important to take a little time to stay connected. Otherwise, the women are likely to believe that, having gotten what you wanted, you no longer have any interest in them. This feeling is certain to lead to trouble.

Some men are uncomfortable with this. They want to go directly to sleep or jump up and do something else. A smart lover will avoid these impulses most of the time. Even if you're very tired, even if there are things to do and places to go, there's always time for a moment or two of cuddling and sweet nothings, as these women point out:

> Going to sleep right away is okay sometimes, but usually I need a little loving after sex. I want to savor the experience. Makes me feel very close and peaceful in a way that sex itself doesn't.

> For me, the buildup and the afterwards are at least as important as the actual sex. It's just a wonderful sense of connection that I have to have.

▲ **Women like men who are honest.** Despite the fact that many men have lied to get sex, it is not acceptable, at least not to any women I've talked with. It's not okay to say you've had a vasectomy when you haven't, that you'll use a condom when you won't, that you love her when you don't, that you're disease-free when you're not or don't know if you are, or that you're not married when you are.

Lying in order to have sex comes from the childish idea of conquest—scoring no matter how or what the cost. If you're not the right person for her, why not just accept that fact and move on? If the circumstances aren't right for her now, why not see what can be honestly done about them, or just wait for another opportunity?

> I want a man to level with me and let me make up my own mind. A number of men have lied, especially about not being married or involved with anyone else, and I always felt bad when I found out. It's a terrible feeling. On the other side, last year on vacation I made it with a married man I met in Paris. I was charmed by him, especially his

honesty. I thought it out after he told me he was married and decided I wouldn't mind spending the next two weeks with him. We had a great time.

Honesty is crucial. I will never, repeat, never, see a guy again if I learn he's lied to get me in bed.

▲ **Women appreciate men who take an interest and participate in the preparations and protections that make good sex possible.** It's as much your responsibility as hers to get the children to bed, to ensure privacy, and to make sure that no unwanted conception occurs and that no disease gets passed on.

Some men act like they're doing you a big favor by giving you their cock for a while, so everything else is up to me. I no longer put up with that. A good lover shares the load. He asks or says something about contraception, and if we decide I'll use something, he takes an interest in it and helps pay for it.

That's one of the main things that attracted me to my husband. He was one of the first men I'd been with who brought up protection and had condoms with him. After I decided to go back on the pill, he offered to pay. When I asked why, he said that since I was taking them for our mutual pleasure, he wanted to do his part. Can't help but like a guy like that.

▲ **Women like men to admit to their own sexual concerns and problems.** Women are much more willing, in almost all areas, to admit ignorance and to look for ways of making things better. But since so much rides on a man looking like he doesn't have questions or problems, especially in the sensitive arena of sex, it's very difficult for us to admit even to ourselves that there's a problem.

Yet it is crucial to be able to acknowledge difficulties. If you're having trouble with desire, arousal, erections, or the timing of your orgasms, why not say so? It's not that she won't notice if you keep silent, so why not get the issue out on the table and have a discussion about what should be done?

I don't mind if a guy has problems. Hell, we all do, and I've got my share. What I can't stand, though, is when he pretends that he doesn't or tries to blame them on me. I want to say, "Hey, be a man. Say what's what and let's see what we can do about it."

The only time that men's sexual problems become real problems is when the man uses it as a way of distancing himself from me by withdrawing or berating himself, refusing to accept my acceptance of the situation.

In short, women appreciate men who are honest, responsible, present, and attentive; who talk and listen; who go after their own desires and yet are sensitive to their partner's desires; and who know how to have a good time. I take up most of these topics in greater detail in the chapters that follow. If you pay attention to these chapters, you'll be well on your way to being a good lover for your partner and yourself. And in Chapter 16 I deal with ways of physically stimulating your partner.

CHAPTER NINE

What Is This Thing Called Relating, and Who Needs It, Anyway?

I've heard it from every woman I've been with: "Talk more on a personal or feeling level." But whenever I think I'm doing it, they say I'm not.—*Man, 46*

My wife was definitely right about this. You have to spend time sharing thoughts and feelings to be able to clear the air and just keep up with one another. I didn't believe this when I was younger, but things are much better now that I do.—*Man, 56*

ALTHOUGH RELATING OR connecting is not what men have been trained for, we have a great deal to gain by improving our abilities in this area. This is not only what women want but also what almost all experts say is essential for good sex.

I think, however, that there's a lot more to it than just more or better sex. Here are some of the benefits you might derive.

▲ **Get more of what you want, feel more in control of your life, and feel better in general.** A great many men are not getting their needs met in their relationships and in sex, either because they aren't sure what their needs are or because they can't express them appropriately. Not getting one's needs met leads to frustration, anger, and a sense of hopelessness. It can make a world of difference to be able to express yourself and have some control over your relationship.

Often when a couple comes to therapy, the man says he doesn't have any needs and that he's there only because of his partner's complaints. But at some point I'm able to help him look more closely at himself, and it turns out there are all sorts of things he's missing. One man, for example, was very dissatisfied with his career. But he put off discussing this with his wife and doing anything about it because he feared she might not be supportive. So he continued to do work he disliked and felt very discouraged about ever being able to change. When he finally was able to talk to her, she was both understanding and supportive. Another man had some ideas about adding spice to his sex life but for years didn't bring them up with his lover because of a vague anxiety that she might not agree. The partners of these men are often shocked at what they hear: "I had no idea you felt like this. Why didn't you tell me sooner?" If you want to get more of what you want, good communication is essential.

▲ **Enjoy better health.** There's a host of evidence that we men keep too much bottled up inside and pay for it with unnecessary stress and stress-related diseases and problems.

▲ **Improve your relationship.** Your partner will appreciate what you're doing and be happier as a result. Women complain more about their men's unwillingness to talk and listen than any other thing. Fully 98 percent of the several thousand women in Shere Hite's study *Women and Love* said they wanted "more verbal closeness with the men they love." Specifically, "they want the men in their lives to talk more about their own personal thoughts, feelings, plans and questions, and to ask them about theirs." Almost every single woman I've talked to, in therapy or out, agrees.

When you do relate more, not only will you have the satisfaction of making your partner happier but you'll also reap the many benefits of being with a more contented person.

▲ **Avoid serious relationship distress.** When people in relationships feel unable to connect easily and comfortably, the results are almost always unpleasant and sometimes dreadful: irritability, angry blowups, constant tension, affairs, and even divorce.

When men don't listen or talk, the results can be shattering. Brian had been married to Sharon for twelve years. The relationship wasn't the same as it was at the beginning, but Brian thought it was solid. Then he came home one day to find a note saying Sharon had moved out and wanted a divorce. Brian felt like he had been hit by a thunderbolt. When he came to see me a week later, he kept repeating that he had had no idea Sharon was so unhappy. He was absolutely shocked at her leaving. As he talked, it became clear that Brian hadn't been paying attention. Sharon had countless times expressed her dissatisfaction: her desire for more time together and better communication and, in the last few years, for marriage counseling.

Brian had heard her complaints—he was able to tell me about them—but they hadn't registered. And Brian isn't alone: In one study of divorce, fully 25 percent of the husbands were surprised when their wives said they wanted a divorce.

Because of the way men have been trained, many of us are almost unconscious in our relationships. If you want a decent relationship and good sex, it's important that you learn not to be unconscious. Rather, work on being present, on listening to the complaints and suggestions you get, and on expressing your own. When you do this, you and your partner will probably understand each other better and be able to work out some difficulties that previously seemed insurmountable. This will allow you to feel close and hassle-free more of the time and avoid some of the blowups you've had in the past.

▲ **Be in a better position to work on and resolve any sex problems you or your partner have.** Almost all sex therapists agree that before a couple can work productively on a sex problem, they need to feel close and get their relationship in as good an order as possible. Otherwise, trying to resolve the sexual complaint can be difficult or impossible.

▲ **Increase your ability to deal with other people.** Many men report that the skills in these chapters have benefited them in dealing with their children, with people at work, and with relatives and friends.

I hope I've said enough to spark your interest. We men have a lot to gain from improving the ways we connect with the people we love. I realize that the process of accomplishing this will take time and effort, and you'll feel awkward and uncomfortable at times. I wish I had a way around this, but I don't, and neither does anyone else. But from my experience, both personal and professional, I'm fully convinced the costs are well worth it.

In this and the following chapters on relating, I use both sexual and nonsexual examples. If you've understood what I've said earlier about the association between good sex and good relationships, you know why the nonsexual illustrations are here.

Here are the requirements—I think of them as the "glue" for keeping relationships vital and happy. Without them, there is no relationship or none worth having.

1. Spending quality time together regularly so that you can relate. This time is just for the two of you and does not include time you spend with children, relatives, and friends. When couples are courting, they typically spend a great deal of time together, getting to know each other and having a good time. Although I can't confirm it, I have heard that some men were even willing to miss *Monday Night Football* in order to be with their sweeties. Then something strange happens as they move in together or get married. They start taking each other for granted. They spend less time focused on one another and more time doing other things. Typically men get more involved in their work and the friends and hobbies they took time away from during the courtship. The result in many relationships is a sense of distance on one or both sides, less happiness, and often less sex as well.

I'm sure you're not happy to be reading about this. Everyone I know is afflicted by busyness and feels great pressure to do all the things they think they have to do. To hear that you probably should be putting more time into your relationship may feel like another burden, yet there it is. There are no good relationships that do not involve and require lots of quality time together. I knew a self-employed man who was away five days a week virtually every week, being home only on Saturday and Sunday. While courting his fiancée he had largely given up his favorite sport, but at a certain point he wanted to get back to it. She went ballistic when he called her during the week, informed her of this, and asked which day she wanted to spend with him. When she responded she wanted both days, he said that wasn't possible because he wanted to start spending most of one day every weekend playing golf. Trying to placate her, he mentioned that he was calling her before his golf buddies and giving her the choice of days. She was not placated, and he was not pleased.

He also wasn't pleased when I suggested that if he was gone five days of every week and wanted a decent relationship, he might have to consider significantly reducing the amount of time he wanted to spend playing golf. He looked at me with a combination of anger and sadness and asked in a quiet voice, "Why can't one day be enough for her?"

The answer is simply that, like it or not, good relationships take time, more than most of us expected. But we should know better. Anything we want to do well takes a lot of time—work skills, staying physically fit, parenting, and so on. Human desires are infinite, but time and energy are not.

Very often you can't have everything you want. You have to give up one valued goal in order to achieve another. Maybe you can't work as many hours as you have been, go to as many meetings as you do, take as many classes, or entertain as much and still have the kind of relationship and sex life you want. Something has to go, maybe several things.

The man in the example above had several choices. One was to play golf on his business trips, so he wouldn't have to do it at home. Another was to play golf Sunday morning, but only for two or three hours and spend the rest of the day with his partner. Another was to rearrange his work so he could be home more often. Yet another, God forbid, was to give up golf altogether. Or, if golf was that important to him, give up the relationship. As it was, he didn't have to decide. His fiancée realized that there wouldn't be much relating if she married him, and so she left.

At least two kinds of time together are important. One is regular dates when you do what people usually do on dates: eat in or out, dance, take walks or bike rides, attend movies, plays, or musical events, and so on. Every couple I know who has a good relationship does this. They have certain days and times reserved for their dates, and when on a date they don't bring along work. They most certainly do not do what I've seen a number of people do since the invention of the cell phone—talk on the phone while on a date in a restaurant or in a movie theater. These regular dates should be supplemented by getaways of various lengths. Most couples get along better and have more sex when they're away from home, so it's a good idea, even if you have young children, to spend a night or two away from home as often as possible.

If you're not already doing this, it would help if both of you pulled out your appointment books and wrote in times to be together for the next few weeks and then to keep those dates as if your lives depended on it. Although there's no rule you have to make love, you should plan to have fun. And there's to be no work done, no calls to make or take, and no chores. Every couple needs at least one or two dates a week. Without this, there is no relationship.

Another kind of time together that is needed is shorter visits every evening, or almost every evening, when you check in and catch up on each other's day. These visits need not be long—sometimes five or ten minutes will do it—but they do serve to keep you up to date and in touch. I realize you have to take care of the children, make and eat dinner and clean up, go over your to-do list for tomorrow, and take the dog for a walk. But can you also find a few minutes to catch up with your beloved? Some couples do this while walking the dog.

2. Get to know and keep learning about one another. An important purpose and outcome of spending time together is to really know each other. Consider these questions: Do you know your mate's birthday? The thing she'd most like to do on a day off? The project, person, or activity she's most concerned about these days in her work? The project, person, or activity she most likes about her work? Her best friend(s)? Her worst nemesis? Where she hopes things will be in five years? If you can't answer these questions accurately, I wonder if you really do know her. I'd be willing to bet she can accurately answer these questions about you. Women usually can because they pay attention.

How do you determine these things? Simple: by asking questions, listening, and paying attention.

Here is a simple exercise that can help. For the next month, every day before you separate for your day apart, ask her what she's most looking forward to that day and what she most fears. When you get together for your time together in the evening, ask about these things (for instance, "How did the meeting with Madge go?" or "Was the new boss as bad as you thought?"). If you do nothing more than ask these questions daily, I guarantee you'll learn a great deal about your spouse, and I can almost guarantee she'll be appreciative. By the way, if you realize you don't know the answers to the questions I posed above, or aren't sure, why not just ask her? It's amazing what you can learn by asking.

3. Administer lavish doses of C and A (compliments and appreciations). I'm astonished by how many couples rarely say anything nice to each other. All the nice things that were said during courting ("You were so funny at dinner tonight," "You look so hot in that outfit," "That was an incredible insight you had," and so on) seem to have been forgotten, and now we have either silence or criticisms. Many women weep when they tell their friends or therapists how long it's been since their men paid them a compliment.

If you want a great relationship, compliment your wife as often as possible. What about her do you find beautiful, striking, attractive, exciting, fascinating, or sexy? What makes you glad to be with her? There's no such thing as overdoing it in this department. I've never heard a woman complain that she can't take all the compliments and that she's ready to rush out and have an affair with someone who doesn't tell her good things.

I address compliments and appreciations in more detail in Chapter 10, but for now you might want to take it as an assignment to give your partner at least one specific compliment or appreciation every day for the next two weeks.

4. Be liberal with physical affection. Compliments and appreciations are one way of showing your interest and affection. Physical touch—

holding hands, cuddling, hugging, kissing, rubbing her thigh in the car or the theater—is another and equally important.

5. Be present. There's no point spending time with your partner or touching her if your mind's not in the same place as your body. You have to attend to and be present with your partner if it is going to count.

Some people think being present is a mystical concept. Trust me, there's nothing mystical at all about it. If you have children, you know how often they're not present when you talk to them. Being present is the opposite of withdrawing or spacing out. It means being fully attentive and present—listening to yourself and her, and expressing yourself as appropriate.

This is the old '60s idea of "be here now." Whatever you're doing, do it. If you're talking to a woman at a party, look at her. Don't let your eyes keep roaming around the room as if you're looking for someone better. If you're having a talk or getting affectionate, don't turn on the television or keep glancing at a magazine. If you're being affectionate or sexual, don't bring up extraneous matters. Talking about sports or business does not work in the bedroom, although I've been surprised to hear how many men bring up these subjects.

Men are superbly attentive when they first meet you. But after we're an item, their attention span seems to reduce to four seconds except when they're working or watching sports. It's infuriating to try to talk to someone who's glancing at the TV or a paper.

I like a man who's all there when we're together, especially in bed, really focused on us and what we're doing. I don't like guys who space out and I don't know where they are. It's like they're marching to a different drummer, and since I have no knowledge of the drummer or the beat, I feel totally abandoned. They can drum their own song when they masturbate. When they're with me, I want a duet.

All of us frequently put out what relationship expert John Gottman calls "bids for contact." That is, we try to get the other person to pay attention to us. The direct bids are easy to spot—for example, "I need to talk to you." The indirect ones, however, are just as important and not so easy. For instance, when your partner says, "Looks like it's going to rain today" or "There's a deer in the backyard," we have to assume she's trying to engage you in a conversation. A man who is present or conscious notices these bids and responds accordingly by turning toward his partner and accepting the bid or, if necessary, explaining why he can't at that moment. The unconscious man doesn't notice or, even if he does, just continues with what he was doing.

6. Take your partner's feelings, ideas, and opinions seriously. Many men don't take women seriously in bed or outside it and are dismissive of their feelings and ideas. This is a sure route to a miserable relationship and sex life. I know very few men will jump up and admit, "Yeah, that's me, I don't really care what she wants or says," but I've witnessed it in therapy thousands of times. The woman offers an opinion about anything—what school to put the children in, where to spend the family vacation, what to do in bed—and the man continues on as if she hadn't spoken at all.

Check yourself out on this issue. One good way is to ask your partner whether she feels you take her seriously. If so, that's great. But if she says no, you might want to do something about that. Listen to her ideas, see what value they contain, and accept the ones that make sense. Even if you think your idea on what school the children should attend is better than hers, don't just dismiss hers. Tell her what you see as the advantages of your plan and why it might be better than hers. Have a discussion with her, always treating her ideas with respect, and observe the results.

7. Take complaints and anger seriously but with equanimity. Gottman determined in his research that healthy relationships were greatly facilitated by the man's not getting upset about—that is, not taking personally—his mate's anger. I say more about this in Chapter 12, on listening, but suffice it to say here that it helps to take her anger simply as information. There's something she really wants you to understand. If you can listen and understand without getting angry, defensive, or crazy yourself, that's excellent.

8. Enjoy carnal delights together. Lovemaking is another "glue" that keeps a relationship strong. There's no need to say more about it here, because it's the topic of this entire book.

Expressing Yourself

Learning to be more forthcoming about my personal feelings has not always been easy because I was brought up in a family where mum was the word. For several months I had to remind myself to say something personal to Dana before I left the house every morning, and every evening when I came home. But the payoff has been terrific—she is very appreciative of this openness—and it's gotten easier over time. Now it's kind of automatic and the result is a much stronger marriage.—Man, 39

OKAY, NOW LET'S talk about talking. Despite what some women think, it's not true that men don't have or don't express feelings. Men can get very emotional—excited, enthusiastic, sometimes ecstatic—about sex, closing a deal, winning the woman of their dreams, and cheering on their favorite athletic team. They also can get very emotional—upset, gloomy, angry—when their team loses, when they don't make the big deal or win the woman, and when they don't get sex. But basically a man is someone who is in control of himself, including his feelings, and doesn't let them carry him away.

Certain feelings aren't acceptable for men at all, including ones related to caring and love or their lack. These are difficult because they make the man seem or feel dependent on women. Men are, of course, exceedingly dependent on their relationships with women (in many ways more so than women are dependent on relationships with men), but it's hard for us to admit it because of what we've been taught about masculinity.

Another set of feelings that men won't acknowledge includes those suggesting weakness, including fear and hurt. These strike at the strength that's supposed to be the essence of masculinity. No man wants to feel, or others to think, that he's confused, overwhelmed, intimidated, or feels neglected or despondent. There is no end of stories of men being called wimps, sissies, girls, and pussies by other men because they manifested any of these feelings.

Because anger is one of the few feelings men believe they can have, it's often a mask for other feelings, especially the ones that suggest weakness. It's much easier for men to deal with anger than these other emotions.

The result of the prohibition on experiencing and expressing feelings is that men often lose track of them. That is, they don't know when they're feeling love or sadness, and they don't get much practice expressing most of their emotions. Strange things can happen when one doesn't feel or express much.

Rod, a forty-four-year-old executive, is an extreme example. He learned as a child that expressing any emotion was unacceptable, and he became a virtual robot. He says he has never been angry; neither has he felt love or strong sexual arousal. In situations that would make almost anyone angry, he feels "mildly annoyed" or "slightly irritated." He's attracted to women in a mild sort of way but has all manner of problems with them and with sex. He sometimes doesn't get erections. When he does, he usually can't ejaculate. Whether he ejaculates or not, there isn't much feeling. Then there are the physical problems. His blood pressure is off the charts, even though there's no family history of high blood pressure and even though he exercises and eats carefully. His exercise program is often on hold, however, because he's had back and neck problems for many years. And he's always having accidents when walking, running, and driving. Though Rod's situation is extreme, it gives some clues as to what can happen when emotion is constantly blocked.

Because men are not trained to be aware of emotion, many of us don't notice feelings even though they may be apparent to observers. In my practice, it happens many times that a woman says her man is feeling a certain way (angry, irritated, fearful, or something else, even joyful) and the man denies it. I don't want to imply that women are always correct in their reading of men's feelings—that is not the case—but I do know that in such situations very often the men come to realize that they were indeed feeling as their partners said they were. In sex, partners often pick up on the man's anxiety before the man himself does.

If determining your feelings is difficult, attending to the two main indicators of emotion—what's going on in your body and what's going on in your head—can be very helpful. Therapists and partners usually pick up on body language. When a client clenches his fists and maybe his teeth as well, I suspect he may be angry even if he denies it. I can't be certain, of course, but if he consistently manifests this behavior when a certain topic comes up, I know it's worth asking him to consider what he's feeling. Let's say you know that in certain situations your heart pounds, your neck, back, and shoulders feel tight, your stomach is upset, your hands are sweating, or you're holding your breath or breathing shallowly. These things in themselves don't necessarily indicate emotion. Maybe your heart is racing because you've been exercising; maybe your stomach is upset because of something you ate. But if these phenomena, singly or in combination, occur regularly in certain situations, ask yourself what emotion might be behind them.

Your mind is also full of clues about what you may be feeling. Research in the last thirty years strongly suggests that to a large extent emotion is generated and maintained by our thoughts. You may not be aware of being anxious, sad, or depressed, for instance, but if you're having thoughts of losing someone important to you or failing at an important task, you should ask yourself what emotion you might be having. Recurring images of hurting someone may indicate anger, hurt, rage, or frustration.

The examples I've given so far have to do with what most people consider negative emotions. But positive feelings are also indicated by your mind and body. If your usually tight neck muscles are not tight when you engage in a certain activity or are with a certain person, if your body feels light and generally good, or if you usually have positive thoughts and pictures about that person or activity, that may be a sign of relief, comfort, enthusiasm, joy, affection, or even love.

To get a better idea of where you are and what you want to do about knowing and expressing emotion, consider the following questions: Do you know what you're feeling much of the time? When a lover asks what you're feeling, do you usually know, or are you at a loss? Has a woman friend or lover ever told you that you're not in touch with your feelings or that you don't express them?

GETTING IN TOUCH WITH EMOTION

Learning about your feelings is basically a matter of paying attention to your inner world. The simple exercise that follows can help.

EXERCISE 10-1: LOGGING FEELINGS

For the next two or three weeks, carry a small notebook or some index cards in a shirt or jacket pocket wherever you go. As many times as possible during each day—at least eight to ten times—ask yourself what you are feeling. You should pay attention to the two indicators of emotion discussed earlier: your body and your mind. Jot down in your book the day and time, the stimulus for the feeling if you know what it is, and the feelings(s). Feel free to use whatever shorthand you like. An entry in your book might look like this: "Mon., 10 A.M.: Read that Bob died of heart attack. Feeling sad. Also scared."

For best results, vary the times when you check in with your feelings and where you are when you do so. Make sure you check your feelings before and after sex and before and while you spend time with your children. You might also want to take in some movies or plays. Actors and directors are masters at manipulating emotion. They want to get you to feel pride, anger, sympathy, fear, sadness, and many other feelings. Since they are working at evoking feelings in you, this is a good way to check on your range of emotions.

If you don't know what you're feeling or aren't sure, take a moment and see what happens. Don't settle for "nothing," "don't know," or "neutral." These are not feelings. Make a guess.

Whenever you feel angry, ask yourself this: "If I weren't feeling angry, what would I be feeling?" Try to determine if the anger is just that, or whether it's a disguise for another feeling.

There are a couple of traps you need to beware of. Feelings usually consist of only one word. If your expression of feelings consists of more than a word or two, check to make sure you're really talking about feelings. If your sentence would make as much sense if it started with "I think," then you're *not* expressing feelings. But work backward. If what you said was, "I feel my wife should assert herself more at work" (which is *not* an expression of feelings), this may mean that you feel sad because it seems your partner is being taken advantage of on the job or that you're frustrated because you can't help her.

Another trap is to assume that you can have only one feeling at a time. In fact, you may feel several things at once, some of which seem contradictory. There's nothing wrong with that. Often by talking about your feelings, you will get clearer about which is the dominant emotion.

After a week or two, take a few minutes to go over the feelings you've written down. Do you experience a wide range of emotion, including the feelings that men have trouble with? Do you basically have the same feelings all the time? What kinds of feelings are missing from your list?

FEELING STATEMENTS

In order to talk about feelings, we want to do more than just label them. We want to create statements about them. These statements include not only the name of the emotion but also what it and the event that evoked it mean to you. Here's how a feeling statement about it might go (with the feelings underlined).

It <u>scared</u> the hell out of me that Bob died. He was my age. Really hit me: life doesn't go on forever. Made me very <u>concerned</u>. I haven't been taking care of myself. I'm carrying at least twenty extra pounds and haven't been exercising. The <u>fear</u> is motivating. I'm going to call my doctor for an appointment right now.

I'm also <u>sad</u>. I wasn't <u>close</u> to Bob, but he seemed like a nice guy. Very sensitive and kind. I'm <u>sorry</u> I didn't get to know him better. It's been typical of me to get close to the go-getters and not pay much attention to those like Bob. But the <u>sadness</u> I'm feeling suggests that I <u>miss</u> having friends like Bob, guys who aren't going to set the world on fire but who are decent and interested in me as a person, not as an account.

A feeling statement can be more or less elaborate than this illustration. But it must contain more than the simple "I'm sad" or "I'm feeling down." Sometimes, however, you may not know more than what you're feeling. In that case, it can be worth it to say something like this to your partner or a friend: "I've been feeling very sad and low the last few days and have no idea what it's about." Of course, this is itself a feeling statement. If you're open to an exchange, it may well be that the questions your friend or partner asks may help you figure out what's going on.

EXERCISE 10-2: CREATING FEELING STATEMENTS

Here you want to develop a statement about your feelings, something that you might want to express to others.

Go over several of the items in your book and create feeling statements about them, as in the illustration I just gave. Your statements don't have to be as elaborate as that one, but they should have at least a few sentences in them.

You can also practice creating feeling statements when things come up in your life. Everything from the trivial to the monumental can serve your purpose: someone cutting you off on the highway, a piece of good or bad news in the mail, a news event, or the promotion, marriage, divorce, or death of someone you know. The more you practice identifying your feelings and creating statements about those feelings, the more comfortable you'll feel doing this and the more ready you'll be to express these statements to your partner when you choose to do so.

And make sure to go over some recent activities you did with your partner—making love, planning or taking a trip, dealing with a disagreement, and so on—and create feeling statements about each.

TO EXPRESS OR NOT TO EXPRESS

Being more aware of your feelings is useful in itself because it helps you zero in on what's going on with you in a way that no amount of thinking can do. But since our primary concern here is connecting with another person, the main question now is when to express your feelings to your partner. All the rules are simple common sense. What purpose will be served by telling her (or not telling her)? What harm or benefit may result to you, to her, to the relationship? For example, if your partner has bought a piece of clothing on sale that cannot be returned and you don't like it, clearly no purpose is served by telling her, so it's probably best to keep your dislike to yourself.

Expressing Negative Feelings

You may believe, like many men, that you are being virtuous by not expressing negative feelings to your partner. You don't want to burden her with your anxieties, concerns, complaints, doubts, and so forth. While that's an understandable sentiment, there's also another perspective. Chances are excellent that your partner senses something is wrong. But she doesn't know what's going on and is probably thinking that your mood is the result of something she's done. If that's true, she can't do anything about it because you're not talking. Even if it isn't true, she's still in a funny place that isn't helping her or the relationship any. She can't get close to you and she doesn't know what's going on. There's also the point that it may help you to share what's on your mind. Just talking about a painful experience or feeling can make you feel better. And perhaps she can do or say something to comfort you. This is how people get to know one another better and feel closer. According to psychologist and marital therapist Dan Wile, this is what true intimacy is: each of you telling the other the main things that are on your mind and in your gut.

Expressing Compliments and Appreciations

With positive feelings, there's not as much to think about. It's rare, for example, that expressing appreciation, affection, excitement, happiness, joy, love, or passion carries much risk. We're talking about your partner now, of course, not the boss's wife. Ayala Pines's research into what she calls "marriage burnout" demonstrates that the more appreciation is expressed in a marriage, the less burnout there is. If you're not expressing such emotions to your partner, you really need to ask yourself why.

It's amazing how often a woman will complain about not hearing something such as "I love you" or "You look terrific" or something of the sort and the man will respond with "But I do love you" or "You certainly did look terrific." But why didn't he say it spontaneously? Why does the woman have to fish for compliments and expressions of love? The rest of this discussion assumes that you do love your partner and find her attractive but just aren't expressing the feelings directly. If you don't like or love your partner, or you are so angry with her that you're not even sure if you do love her, you probably need to get competent professional help.

Human beings need to be appreciated and complimented. We all need our daily quota of strokes. When we don't get enough, we are irritable and out of sorts. When we do get enough, we're more pleasant to be with, more amenable to working things out, and can endure a great many things that otherwise would have us climbing the walls. Yet it's amazing that both at home and at work so many of us—men and women—feel unappreciated, unnoticed, and unliked.

If you have trouble expressing compliments or words of love, the next two exercises can help.

EXERCISE 10-3: EXPRESSING APPRECIATION OR COMPLIMENTS

Spend some time over the next week thinking of things you like and appreciate about your partner and jot them down. Most of the time you won't actually have to do any thinking; you'll be aware of saying things to yourself like "I'm glad to have her help with X," "She really looks great," "She's such a joy," or "She's got a great sense of humor." Write these thoughts on a piece of paper.

At the end of the week go over your list and ask yourself how many of these thoughts you expressed in words to her. Be careful with this. Many men believe they've expressed a compliment when in fact all they did was say it to themselves. Make sure you actually said it to her. If there are compliments you didn't give her, would you be willing to express more of them? What would it take?

If you're willing, just do it. Not all at once, but when it's appropriate. For example, if you appreciated the help she gave on some task, even if that was two weeks ago, why not tell her now? If she looked beautiful when you went out last weekend, why not tell her now? If you appreciate her intelligence, decisiveness, humor, mothering skills, cooking, or anything else, why not just say so?

Give yourself a goal of giving her a specific number of compliments in the next three days, maybe two or three of them. Keep track of how many you give and what they were.

Then ask yourself what good feelings you have about her that you're not letting her know about. If there's no compelling reason for your silence, see if you're willing to break it.

You might also want to determine if your compliments are limited to just one or two areas. Are you, for example, complimenting your mate's beauty and sexual abilities but not her intelligence and sense of humor? Women love being treated as sex objects by the men they love, but they detest being treated as nothing *but* sex objects. Feel free to compliment her looks and sexual competence, but make sure to mention other qualities as well.

You should do this exercise every week for a month or so, until you get into the habit of expressing your positive feelings.

Now to the famous phrase "I love you." Few words mean as much to a woman, yet a great many women claim they don't hear it at all or as much as they'd like. What's fascinating about this is that upon hearing the complaint, the men usually respond immediately with "But of course I love you." The problem is not with a lack of love but with a lack of expression.

EXERCISE 10-4: SAYING "I LOVE YOU"

For the next week, every time you feel that you love your partner, tell her. If she's not there, call and tell her. If you can't reach her, leave a message on her voice mail or tell her later: "I was in a meeting today but had a hard time concentrating. All I could do was think of how much I love you." Another option is to write your feelings down on a piece of paper and leave it where she'll find it. Don't get fancy: "I love you" or "I adore you" is all that's needed. Other phrases such as "I'm so glad you're in my life" or "Marrying you was the best thing I ever did" will be taken as synonyms for "I love you" by some women but not by others.

If you can't do what I've suggested above—that is, tell her you love her—then write your feelings on a piece of paper when you have them. Do this for several weeks, and at the end of each week go over what you've written. Then close your eyes and imagine yourself telling her these things. Many men find that after a week or two of this, it's much easier to express their love directly to their partners.

GETTING IT OUT OF YOUR HEAD

Much of what I've been saying in this chapter can be summarized this way: Get your feelings out of your head or body and make them public. As I mentioned earlier, men frequently think or feel what their partners want to hear but don't express it. So most of the time it's a question not of finding things to say but simply of getting out what's already there.

A related issue doesn't have to do so much with feelings as with just keeping your partner up to date with what's going on in your world. One couple I counseled came to see me very upset about what had happened the day before.

Tracy had called John at work, and although he didn't sound particularly glad to hear from her, she started telling him about her day. A moment later he screamed at her to stop bothering him and hung up. In our session, John explained that when she called, he'd been frantic—two of his company's largest clients were visiting, and a report was due before five o'clock. Tracy's call made him feel that she didn't care about his hectic schedule. The truth was that Tracy was very considerate of John's time and work, but he hadn't said a word to her about how that day was special. If he had only told her, she wouldn't have called.

If Tracy and John had been having the nightly debriefing sessions I mentioned in Chapter 9, this incident would not have occurred. He would have told her the night before what this day looked like.

When something changes in your schedule or in your mind that might affect your partner, why not tell her? It's a good idea, because not doing so can result in unnecessary upset and arguments.

WHAT ABOUT TEARS?

Crying is a natural way of expressing feelings associated with losing someone or being reunited with someone we thought we had lost or might lose.
But it can also be a way of expressing great joy or nostalgia. I suspect that
when someone doesn't cry at certain times—for example, on learning of
the death of a loved one—some serious suppression is going on. While I
don't think you have to cry to be a good person, I do believe that being
able to do so is one sign of being in touch with and able to express certain
feelings.

All babies cry, and it's not unusual for five- and six-year-old boys to
shed tears. But you don't see many ten-year-old boys cry, and it's rare in
the popular media to see or read about a male of any age crying. The message, although perhaps delivered earlier, starts getting through around
age seven or eight: "Big boys don't cry." The message often comes from
parents, but also from peers and is certainly reinforced by them. An eight-
year-old boy who cries during a game or at school is going to find out very
fast that such behavior is unacceptable. It's fascinating and quite sad to
watch eight- and nine-year-old boys when they are hurt, disappointed,
fearful, or in grief. You can see the tears well up and the lip trembling, but
you also see them fighting back the tears, trying not to look at you, biting
their lips and, as novelist Jonathan Kellerman so aptly put it, "straining for
macho."

And that's all it takes for many males. They may never again cry, not
when a friend or their parents die, not when they return from a war to see
their wives and children after years of absence, not even when they are so
sad or lonely or heartbroken that they're thinking of killing themselves.

You can release the ability to cry if you want to. What's required is to remove the blocks that are in the way. Being in a safe setting, or with a safe
person, makes a great difference. Many men, for example, cried for the
first time in years when they participated in encounter groups popular
during the 1960s and '70s, or in group therapy or men's groups. Many
men have cried for the first time in years when they were in a relationship
where they felt safe. They knew it was acceptable to cry in such places, that
they wouldn't be put down or considered less manly for doing so.

What these men accomplished in groups and relationships can be done
on one's own by deciding that crying is okay and by looking at how you
stop yourself from doing it. A common obstacle is fear, not only of not being manly but also of not being able to stop crying if you start. Since men
aren't accustomed to their own tears, they often fear being overwhelmed

by them. That fear is not realistic. You usually can stop the crying when you want; even if you can't, you eventually do get "cried out" and the tears stop of their own accord.

Here is one man's account. He decided in his forties that not being able to cry made him an incomplete human being. He felt bad that he hadn't cried when his mother died a few years earlier—he had felt sadness and desolation then, but wouldn't let himself cry. He set himself the task of sitting down one night at home and thinking about his mother. If the tears were there, he wanted to let them out. They were, and he did.

This was the first time I've cried since I was a baby. It was frightening at first. Felt like a tidal wave of tears and I thought I might drown in it, but I made an amazing discovery. Crying actually feels good. It's a way of handling sadness, and you feel better as a result. I somehow feel more complete about my mother than I have before. She was very good to me and a wonderful person. It's fitting that her son cried for her. When I feel like crying in the future, I'm going to let it happen. No more stomping down the tears like I've done all my life. If someone doesn't like it, that's their problem.

EXPRESSING YOURSELF SEXUALLY

Many women I've talked with complain that men don't express their sexual passion and pleasure. The specific complaints range from men who don't initiate sex with passion and enthusiasm to those who don't express pleasure during sex and, perhaps most surprisingly, those who are so quiet during orgasm that their partners aren't sure if they have come.

My take on all this is that it has to do with the general flattening of affect in men because of what we've been taught. Because we learn that any expression of emotion is suspect, and any indication of being carried away by feelings is even worse, many of us keep a tight rein on all our feelings. Even though sex may feel great, we tend not to let it show. This is unfortunate in at least two respects. One is that we cheat our partners. By not letting them know how much we appreciate, desire, and enjoy them, we rob them of feeling desirable and knowing how much pleasure they bring us. We also rob ourselves, because the expression of desire and pleasure can add to our own arousal and enjoyment.

Many of us are unaware of how inhibited we are in these areas. I have watched many times while men listened in disbelief as their partners reported they didn't feel desired (even though the men initiated sex) and didn't feel the man enjoyed sex. These men were simply unaware of how little they let their feelings show.

One way to check into how expressive you are in sex is to ask your partner. Does she know when you're really hot for her? Does she know how much you enjoy making love with her or when she does a certain thing? Is she aware of how beautiful and sexy you find her? Is she aware of how much you enjoy your orgasms? Another way of checking is to look into yourself. When you desire her, are you letting all of your desire show, or are you doing some heavy editing? An example of editing would be feeling that you really want her but saying only something like "Would you like to make love?" Why not show her and tell her what you're actually feeling? And during sex, are there any feelings, sounds, and movements that you're bottling up?

One man whose partner complained about his inexpressiveness told me this when we were alone: "I know there's a lot I'm keeping to myself. I really do enjoy sex, but I'm afraid I'd sound like a squealing pig if I let it all show. This doesn't quite fit my image of myself, and I'm not sure how well she'd accept what I might do." What he didn't know was that his wife had had a lover before him who did let it all hang out, and she'd loved it. "I loved seeing him so uninhibited and out of control," she said, "and it made me feel so powerful that I was the source of all this pleasure."

I have never heard a woman complain that her lover was too uninhibited, that he made too much noise, that he showered her with too many compliments, or that he expressed too much pleasure. When you think about it, it's clear that we love to see others express pleasure, especially when we're the source of it. We delight in babies who squeal and squirm with joy when we touch them. And the main standard many men have of judging good lovers is how "wild" and "uninhibited" the women are. Maybe there's a moral here.

If you want to be more expressive in sex, just attend to the difference between what you're feeling on the inside and what you're exhibiting on the outside. If there's a sound, a word, or a movement that wants to come out, why not let it? If you have concerns about how your partner might react, why not discuss this with her first? As you express more, I'm sure you'll find that you and your partner's enjoyment will increase. Decorum has its place, but not in the bedroom.

And don't forget about talking about sex after it's over, minutes later, hours later, and even days later. Such talk provides guidance to your partner and can help the good feelings continue long after the act is over. The kinds of expression during and after love play can vary from general comments about what went on to more specific feedback:

"Saturday morning was special. You're terrific."
"I feel so good and so close to you. I love making love with you."
"That was wonderful. I especially liked it when you licked my nipples at the same time you were playing with my penis."
"You have the most beautiful breasts in the world. I love looking at them, touching and rubbing them, licking them, sucking them."
"You are, without a doubt, the best blow-job giver in the Western world."
"I keep thinking about last night. It was great. I'd like a repeat performance ASAP."
"You drove me crazy when you squeezed my balls while I was coming."

Of course, "I love you," if sincerely meant, is never out of place.

Regular practice with the exercises and ideas in this chapter can make a dramatic difference in how well you express yourself and the quality of your relationship. Men have a lot to gain by being more expressive.

The Power of Asserting Yourself

I know I'm supposed to be able to assert myself—that's what men do, right?—but I've never been good at it. —*Man, 33*

I'm fine at the office and in public. No trouble saying what I want. But at home, especially in bed, it's like I'm mute. I don't know what I want and can't express it even when I do. —*Man, 42*

All my life I've gotten into trouble because of my pushiness. People get turned off by how I try to get my way. —*Man, 64*

BEING ABLE TO express what you want and go after it—meeting your conditions—is an absolute essential if you want good sex. This is supposed to be something men are skillful at, but I've not been impressed with the ability of men to get, or even to express, what they want in personal relations.

Of course, no one ever gets everything he wants, and all of us must compromise and sometimes do things we aren't thrilled with. But an assertive person expresses his desires and tries to get what's right for him. He does not regularly go along with a situation not to his liking and withdraw in silence or express his anger in inappropriate ways.

I have certainly seen men act aggressively, intimidating and bullying their partners. They sometimes get their way, of course, but they cause immense damage to their relationships and aren't happy with what they get; they recognize at some level that it wasn't given freely. Although most onlookers would agree that these men have lots of power in their relationships, I have yet to meet one who felt powerful. They often feel just the opposite, powerless. Hank, for example, comes on very strong. He doesn't ask, he demands. His girlfriend often has sex with him, and does other things as well, when she doesn't want to because there doesn't seem to be a choice. The result is that she's turned off sexually and has been seriously thinking of leaving. And Hank isn't happy with the sex he's been getting. He wants a more enthusiastic partner. Yet he has difficulty understanding that the way he expresses himself is a turn-off to her.

Other men are sensitive and empathic, but they are not strong or assertive. They don't seem to have much energy, enthusiasm, or skill for getting their own needs met. They are similar to aggressive men in that they feel no sense of control in their relations with women. Roger often wanted sex with his wife, but he rarely got it because before suggesting it to her he carefully considered her mood and situation. If she seemed tired or busy, if she said she'd had a rough day, or if she was reading a book or watching TV, he didn't initiate sex. Needless to say, Roger felt frustrated a lot of the time. Even when he had sex, he didn't get what he wanted. He accepted whatever his wife offered and never bothered to tell her that he wanted something else.

To help you determine if you need help with assertiveness, consider the following questions:

▲ Can you tell your partner that you need more time for yourself (to be with your friends, read, exercise, or whatever)?

▲ Can you tell her you want to spend more time with her?

▲ Can you let her know about something she's done (or not done) that upsets you?

▲ Can you let her know that you are not in the mood for sex even though she is?

▲ Can you let her know clearly when you do want sex?

▲ Can you indicate in a clear way that you don't want intercourse but would like some other form of sex?

▲ Can you indicate exactly what kind of stimulation you want?

▲ Can you let her know that certain feelings are getting in the way of your sexual interest, arousal, or functioning?

▲ Can you ask her how she likes to be stimulated?

▲ Can you say clearly that you want to stop in the middle of a sexual event?

▲ Can you initiate a conversation with her about things in your sex life you'd like to be different?

▲ Can you, when there is disagreement, understand the validity of her position as well as your own and work toward a resolution that satisfies both of you?

If you answered yes to some or all of these questions, I have another one for you. Can you say and do these things in ways that do not leave her feeling blamed, disliked, humiliated, or undesirable? If you can honestly answer yes, you are one of the fortunate few. These are situations that men find difficult to handle. If you have trouble with any of these items, you could benefit from developing your assertiveness skills—so as to get more of what you need, not go along with things that make you uncomfortable, and do so in ways that do not intimidate or crush your partner.

Assertiveness is not rudeness, bullying, or aggression. Being assertive does not mean that you won't consider your partner's needs or satisfy her. It does mean, however, that you are going to pay serious attention to your own needs. It does mean that you will express your desires directly and try to get what you want.

So often in sex today the situation is that each partner is focused primarily on satisfying the other one. Each is looking out for the other and neither is taking care of his or her own needs. A lot of mind reading and guesswork is involved. No one wants to appear selfish, which we've all been taught is a very bad thing. While such altruism may sound virtuous, the result is usually somewhat less than satisfying for both participants. If both could start paying more attention to getting their own needs met—a little selfishness, if you like—sex would be much better for both.

When people become more assertive, they tend to get more of what they want and to be happier as a result. One additional benefit in sex is that people who are more assertive are more turned on, which feels good not only to themselves but to their partners as well.

THE ISSUE OF ENTITLEMENT

Some men don't feel they are entitled to get what they want. This has been said before, but usually about women. The fact is that many men have exactly the same problem. Part of this comes from the performance or work ethic: A man is someone who does what he's supposed to do. No one said that taking time for yourself or enjoying yourself was part of being male. Now that we have a new rule in sex—the man's primary job is to satisfy his partner—there's an additional reason to focus on her enjoyment rather than your own.

You have every right to be assertive. You have every right to try to get your relationship as you want it and to try to have sex when you want, where you want, and how you want—provided, of course, that you go about this in ways that honor your partner and allow her to have her own preferences and opinions.

If you think this sounds self-centered or selfish, ask yourself why. Why don't you have the right to say what pleases you? What's selfish about that? What's wrong with a man telling his partner that he'd like to go out more (or less) with friends, that he'd like sex on the floor (or on the sofa or in the car), that he'd like this kind of stimulation or that?

See if you can get yourself into a mind-set where you realize that being assertive not only is *not* bad but is actually good for you, your partner, and your relationship. In the traditional model of masculinity, assertiveness was a given; it was assumed a man would stand up for himself and get what he needed. I think this is one part of the old model we need to keep. There's very little to say against it and a great deal in its favor. Many women are trying to be more assertive. I think that's good for them and for us. But we need to respond with our own assertiveness. That way, each of us can look out for him- or herself *and* the other, thus creating healthy relationships.

"I JUST CAN'T DEAL WITH HER"

An important reason that men aren't assertive in their relationships is that they simply don't know how to deal with their partners. Here are two examples.

No matter how I put it, whenever I say that I want something, she takes it as a criticism and cries. I can't handle that, so I try to comfort her and get things back to where they were. I either forget what I was trying to get or just give up on it.

My impression is that when I've asked for something, she starts talking about something she's not getting. I feel criticized and am happy to drop the whole subject before we get into a fight.

Many of the men I work with hadn't even tried to get what they wanted. They feared the consequences illustrated in these examples and didn't want to risk finding out if they were right.

Notice that underlying both of the statements is the fear that being assertive will make matters worse. There's no question that going after what you want can make matters worse, at least for a while. But there's no necessary link here, no reason assertiveness has to make things worse, and certainly no reason why things should usually get worse.

"BUT I DON'T KNOW WHAT I WANT"

A great many men, in discussing assertiveness, come up with this: "I don't know what to ask for; I don't know what I want." My response is that saying you don't know what you'd like to do tonight or on your day off, where you want to travel, or what kind of sexual stimulation provides you with the most pleasure is an interesting kind of statement to be making about yourself. If you don't know the answers to the questions, you can find them. All you really need to do is pay attention and use your mind. Try different things (in your mind if you can't try them in reality without great cost or effort) and see what feels best. That's all there is to it.

Regarding sex, you can also use your imagination to help determine the kinds of things you might like. What kinds of acts and stimulation do you use in your favorite fantasies? Do you want to try any of these with your partner? Try different things with her. You can touch her here and there, this way and that way, and get her to do the same for you. You can try this act and that one. You can try it in the living room, the dining room, the kitchen, and the hallway. Find out what you like best.

"BUT MEN ARE ALREADY TOO SELFISH"

Some women object to my thesis that men need to be more assertive. Their argument is that men are selfish and always get what they want while the women don't get anything. I think the problem is that we're talking about two different groups. There's no question that some men, like Hank, are too self-centered, are too aggressive and demanding, and barely even recognize that their partners also have needs. They need to learn to be more sensitive to their partners and become more assertive rather than aggressive. But there's also no question that a great many men, like Roger, are far less assertive than is good for them. Both the Rogers and the Hanks of this world can benefit from becoming more assertive and either less passive or less aggressive.

TAKING CARE OF YOURSELF

Asserting yourself is part of a larger idea: being good to or taking care of yourself. We men are always so busy doing our tasks and performing that we rarely take sufficient time to get what we need and enjoy, and this is directly related to the problems we have in relationships and in sex.

The following exercise will give you the opportunity to do some things that please you.

EXERCISE 11-1: DOING THINGS YOU ENJOY

This week do one or two things that you really want to do and that are fun for you. The only criteria are that you enjoy them and they not be work-related. They may or may not involve other people.

Here are some examples of what some men did with the exercise. Jake loved spending time with his two girls, although he rarely did so because he "didn't have the time." So he took them on a picnic on Sunday, followed by a children's movie. He had a ball. After years of not reading mysteries and science fiction because they were a "waste of time" (even though he really enjoyed them), Lou bought some books and started reading. Bernard took a week off from work and went alone to visit a friend in Florida with whom he had served in the army; he had long wanted to make this visit but didn't because he felt it wasn't fair to leave his wife for a week. James, who loved children although he didn't have any, volunteered for a community organization that helped tutor disadvantaged kids.

Your activities may or may not be similar to these examples. As long as you enjoy them, you're doing the right thing.

Do one or two enjoyable things per week as long as you follow the programs in this book. I hope you'll continue taking time for yourself long after you have forgotten this book.

ASSERTING YOURSELF WITH YOUR PARTNER

The next exercise, developed by sex therapist Lonnie Barbach, is the best I know to help you learn to assert yourself in a variety of situations.

EXERCISE 11-2: YESES AND NOS

A *Yes* involves attempting to get something you want from someone, something that you ordinarily would not allow yourself to ask for. The assignment lies in the request, not the response. Even if your request is rejected, you have done a Yes by asking. Examples of Yeses are: asking someone to give or lend you something, like a ride, a book, or an audio tape; asking someone to spend time with you or listen to something you want to say; asking for a certain type of date or sexual activity.

A *No* is a refusal to do something that you don't want to do but ordinarily go along with. If you habitually loan money to a friend not because you want to but because you fear what he will think of you if you refuse, turning him down would be a No. We all do many things we don't want to do. Some of them are necessary (like paying your bills) since the consequences of not doing them are serious. But there are many other things we don't like that we don't have to put up with. The Nos will give you an opportunity to turn some of them down. Being able to say no is crucial in sex, as going along with things you don't like in sex is one of the best ways not to get turned on and to lose interest in the whole subject.

Before doing Yeses and Nos, it's a good idea to read the next section on principles of assertive communication.

SUGGESTIONS FOR DOING YESES AND NOS

1. Do two Yeses and two Nos the first week, then three of each per week. As you do them, you'll discover what is easy and what is difficult. Start with items that are easy, even trivial, and gradually work up to ones that are more difficult.

2. Since sex is a hard issue for many men, don't do sexual Yeses and Nos until you are comfortable doing them in other areas.

3. Use your common sense. There are situations where the consequences of being assertive may be serious. For example, don't get too assertive if an armed thief demands your money.

4. Continue doing Yeses and Nos until you feel confident of being able to get what you want in sex. This may take anywhere from two to twelve weeks. Since this exercise takes only a few minutes a week, it is simple to do while you continue with other exercises in the book.

POSSIBLE PROBLEMS

1. You try to do too much too soon; this is the most common problem in doing the exercise. Remember to start with relatively easy items. Since this is an important exercise, do it in a way that will allow you to progress and feel good about it.

2. You feel bad about being rejected. You will undoubtedly get turned down some of the time when doing Yeses. If you are getting rejected almost every time, this means you are asking for too much or from the wrong people, or in such a way that defeats your aim.

3. You feel guilty about being assertive. For most men, guilt diminishes in fre-

quency and intensity as they get more practice using their assertive skills. It can also help to reread the section on entitlement earlier in this chapter.

The Yeses and Nos exercise will provide you with many chances to try different approaches to getting what you want and evaluate their effectiveness.

PRINCIPLES OF EFFECTIVELY ASSERTING YOURSELF

Gottman's research showed that happy couples talk differently than do those who end up divorced. Partners in happy relationships assert themselves, express anger, and sometimes raise their voices and even yell. Yet they do not fight dirty—they do not belittle their partners, they do not generalize their criticisms, they do not engage in name-calling, they are not sarcastic or contemptuous—and there are lots of positive comments even in the midst of conflict. This is not utopian; happy couples actually communicate in this way.

It makes sense that we all should attempt to do what successful couples do. Since it works for them, it should also work for us. Here are some principles of effective assertion and effective communication generally. (I realize rules are hard to remember when you're upset but my clients have found it helpful to read or hear them frequently. They say that doing so gives them reference points. They also find it helpful to do lots of mental rehearsal with the rules, that is, going over in their minds past communications that did not work out and doing it in new ways according to the principles given below.) I think the principles can be fairly summarized like this: Conduct yourself in a way that maximizes your chances of getting what you want. That means, at the very least, treating your partner in a manner that helps her be receptive to your ideas.

1. **Keep in mind that, no matter how aggrieved you feel, you're dealing with your beloved, not an axe murderer.** Yes, you feel she hurt you or betrayed you, and you may not feel a lot of love for her right now, but nonetheless she still is the woman you care deeply for. Sometimes looking at her can help because you can see that she too is having a hard time with the situation.

2. **Be careful what you say when you're upset or angry.** This is a controversial point. Many therapists encourage people to get their upset and

anger out whenever possible. But, as Carol Tavris documents in her wonderful book *Anger,* unleashing anger doesn't work.

When you're experiencing deep pain or are furious, you're not dealing with a full deck. Your cerebral cortex, the civilized and thinking part of your brain, is not functional. Instead, what's running you is your amygdala, a very small and primitive part of the brain that manages emotion. That's not a lot of intellectual equipment. When people lash out in anger, they say provocative and stupid things, which encourages the listener to respond in kind. The result is usually all-out war or stony silence.

You have every right to express what's bothering you, but you have a much greater chance of being heard and getting all or some of what you want if you wait until you're not in the heat of anger. Until then, it's best to keep your mouth closed—but I hasten to add that this is not the same as sulking. Maybe you should meditate, take a walk, or hug the dog until you calm down at least a bit.

There are times, of course, when your emotions will get the best of you and you will lash out. It happens in even the best of families. When that happens, you need to repair the damage as soon as possible (see Chapter 13).

3. Focus on your feelings and desires rather than hers. "I'd feel more loved if we had more sex" works better than "You never want sex" or "You don't like sex." This is the "I language" that's been promoted so vigorously by communication experts in recent years. Saying "I feel this" and "I'd like that" is less likely to make the listener feel defensive than are blaming or accusing statements such as "You always do this" and "You're responsible for that."

4. Keep your criticisms focused. In other words, don't generalize. If you're angry that she didn't pick you up when she said she would, you have every right to say that. But under no circumstances call her irresponsible or untrustworthy or say you can never count on her. That's attacking her personality rather than her behavior. Stick to what actually happened.

Try not to tell your partner what she thinks or feels in a negative way; for example, avoid statements like "You're afraid of intimacy," "You don't care about me," or "You're being irrational." And steer clear of moralistic judgments or name-calling. Watch for words like *withholding, compulsive, hysterical, neurotic, sick, prude, slut,* and so on. These tactics almost invariably lead to countercharges and defensiveness, which is exactly what you don't want.

Don't bring up the past. If you're complaining about your partner's being late yesterday, there's no need to remind her that she was also late for your first date twelve years ago.

Stick with one complaint or problem at a time. People find it easier to hear about one thing they're doing that upsets you than two or three or twenty things. The more different complaints or problems you bring up at a time, the greater the chance that your partner will feel overwhelmed and discouraged, and get defensive.

At this point you may be wondering what is a good way to express your anger about her not picking you up as she promised. It's easy—just do it. "I'm pissed that you didn't show up when you said you would. I left a meeting early to get there and then waited in the rain for an hour. I couldn't call you because I had no idea where you were. I don't like this one bit." You have expressed your anger, no doubt about that, and let her know exactly what is upsetting you, yet you haven't called her names, haven't destroyed her character, haven't resorted to contempt or sarcasm. I would say, "Well done."

5. Show your understanding of and empathy for the listener's position to whatever extent possible. "I know you had a busy day and had to pick up the kids before coming to get me, but I'm still pissed." The more she feels her position is understood, the less need she will have to explain, defend or justify herself.

6. If there's something different you want for the future, say so clearly. "From now on, when you're going to pick me up outside after picking up the kids, I'd like you to call me at the office after you already have them. That way, there's no risk I'll be standing in the rain again."

7. If possible, make it your problem rather than hers as much as possible. It's usually a matter of perspective, anyway, so why not express the perspective that's most likely to get her to listen? You may think that her lateness is a crime against humanity that would bother any sane person. But that's not the case. I know people whose partners are frequently late and it doesn't bother them at all. They take the behavior into account and bring something to read or even come late themselves. So you can use this information to make your presentation more effective. "I'd like to talk about your coming late to things. I don't know why, but it bothers me terribly [this is what I mean by making it your problem rather than hers]. I get upset when you're not here within five or ten minutes after you say you'll be. And I go absolutely crazy when you're not here within half an hour. Is there anything we can do about this?"

Her willingness and ability to hear you can also be increased significantly if you acknowledge your contribution to the problem: "I realize my working so late has made you feel neglected" or "I know it didn't help matters when I called you frigid."

"Something bothers me about these items. They're too nice, too considerate. I thought assertive meant being strong and really socking it to her. But you're very concerned about her feelings and reactions."

Assertiveness is not about having a temper tantrum. That's assertiveness only for a two-year-old. If you're so angry that you want to explode at your partner and don't care about consequences, be my guest. Just be aware that this type of behavior is not assertiveness and that you're going to have to pay for what you say. Being assertive is about effectiveness, about maximizing the chances of getting what you want. It is strong in that it directly puts forth your desires, but it is also considerate because by being respectful, understanding, and willing to negotiate, you are far more likely to get what you want.

EXAMPLES OF ASSERTIVE COMMUNICATION

You want your partner to stop complaining about you in public. When the two of you are alone, you might say something like this: "I enjoy going out with you, but I have a complaint. I really dislike it when you criticize me in front of Roger and Chris [saying what bothers you]. I don't think our finances are any of their business, and I don't like airing our problems in public. I realize you may be frustrated because I haven't been eager to listen to your complaints at home [showing an understanding of her position and taking responsibility for your actions]. But I want to change that. I want to hear what's bothering you, and I promise I'll listen and respond [saying what you're willing to do to help], but please, not in front of other people."

You want to figure out what your partner expects from you. Let's say that, following her requests for more personal expression, you've made a concerted effort to be more expressive, and you believe you've made big strides. Nonetheless, she continues to complain. You're tempted to say: "What the hell do you want from me? You say I don't talk enough, so I try my best and talk more, and you continue to be on my case about it. Will you ever be satisfied?" This guarantees she'll be defensive and that things are going to get worse. Here's a better way: "I'd like to talk about your expectations about my expressiveness, okay? I agreed with you that I needed to say more about what's going on with me, and I've worked very hard at it for the last few months. I believe I've made a lot of progress. But you still criticize me for not speaking up. That troubles me. I don't know if you don't notice the changes I've made, if the things I do say aren't exactly what you want, or if your expectations are different from mine. I'd like to get your perspective on this." You're now asserting yourself in a way that most people would find easy to listen to. Instead of attacking her, you're asking for a better understanding of what's going on with her.

You want to stop feeling neglected and have more time with your partner. "Honey, I need to talk to you about something I'm feeling, okay? I'm feeling very neglected lately. I know you love me [your acknowledgment of her love will probably prevent her from having to defend it], but it seems like you don't have much time for me. I know your job and school take up lots of time and energy, but I feel left out. I mainly see you when you're too tired to go out, too tired to talk, too tired for sex. Is there anything we can do about this? Maybe we could schedule one night a week when I'd have you all to myself with no homework and no calls to return." A concise statement of the problem from your point of view says clearly what you're feeling, shows an understanding of her position, and suggests a possible solution for her consideration.

You want more time alone. Balancing time together and time alone is tricky for many couples. Individuals vary considerably, with some needing more alone time and some needing more togetherness, and it's usually the case that the partners in a relationship don't have exactly the same requirements. Making the necessary adjustments and compromises takes both assertiveness and consideration. Here's how a conversation might start when you've decided you need more time alone and you're concerned about your partner's reaction: "I'm having a problem I'd like your help with [making it your problem and asking for help—both good ways of disarming defensiveness]. I've realized I'd like to go fishing by myself, but I'm concerned you'll hear that as negative, as meaning I don't want to be with you." Her: "Well, I do." "I was hoping there's a way I could talk to you about it so you wouldn't take it that way. Last week I saw some kids fishing, and it reminded me of how much I used to enjoy it. After a few hours being by myself in the sun, I used to feel so at peace, like a mystical experience. I was sad that I haven't been fishing in years, that I haven't had that wonderful feeling. I'd like to have it again." Given the nonthreatening way you put this, it's going to be difficult for her to feel angry or negative about the request.

You want to feel better about oral sex. "I'd like to talk to you about a problem I'm having with sex [making it your problem]. I know you don't like to swallow my come [acknowledging her position], but I feel terrible when you immediately grab the towel and spit it out. It makes me feel dirty and rejected. I'm not asking you to swallow [saying this will probably prevent her from having to justify her unwillingness to swallow], but I'd like to work out something that wouldn't feel so bad."

You want more feedback in sex. "We've kidded around about how quiet you are in sex, but there is something about it that bothers me. Is this a good time to bring it up? It doesn't bother me that you're not a screamer, I don't need that, but I don't think I'm being as good a lover as I could be because I'm not getting the feedback I need. It's hard for me to tell if you're enjoying what I'm doing or if I should do something else. So I often feel confused, not sure if I should continue or change. Is there any way you could let me know how what I'm doing affects you?"

You want more immediate feedback in sex. "I would enjoy sex more if I felt you really wanted me and really got off on what we're doing. I know you've told me many times how much you enjoy our lovemaking, but I'd like something different. I'd like to hear how much you're enjoying it when we're actually doing it. I'd like to feel and hear your pleasure. Some of the things you've said out of bed would mean a lot more to me if you said them in bed. And I wouldn't mind some of the sounds and movements you make when we're dancing."

You'd like your partner to initiate sex more. "I think our sex is pretty terrific. But it would be even more terrific for me if you initiated it more often. I can't describe how exciting that feels, that my woman wants me and is coming after me. Is there something we can work out about this?"

You don't know exactly what you want. All you know for sure is that you've been feeling out of sorts and want to talk. "I've been feeling out of it—kind of down, not really excited about anything or even interested— the last week or so. It would help if I could ramble on a bit about what's going on. Okay with you?"

Being assertive means directly going after what you want in appropriate ways. It means avoiding the extreme position of being so passive and compliant that you don't get your needs met, and also avoiding the other extreme of being so overbearing and aggressive that you trample on the rights of others. The middle position of assertiveness, however, is by no means a thin line. There are many, many ways to express appropriately what you want and what you don't want, and you can find those that feel most comfortable and work best for you and your mate.

CHAPTER TWELVE

How to Be a Better Listener

My buddies and I agree that the worst four words you can ever hear from your wife are "We need to talk." That's enough to scare the shit out of any man. —*Man, 44*

I know I'm a better listener than I used to be, but let me tell you, it wasn't easy. The easier part was remembering to listen up during regular conversations. Much harder was remembering not to space out when she was angry or critical. But I'm doing much better, and the results have been terrific. It was definitely worth the effort. —*Man, 53*

PEOPLE IN RELATIONSHIPS complain all the time about not being heard. Women are the chief complainers, but statements like "My wife doesn't understand me" are also common. I think men do have a special problem regarding listening to personal talk. They often believe it's not important (just "women's stuff"), or they feel free to tune out because it's something they don't want to deal with. This makes their partners furious, and they often attempt to make the man pay attention by repeating themselves endlessly or yelling. Then the man accuses them of nagging. Obviously, this is not a recipe for a happy relationship.

You can learn to be a better listener. Being a good listener can make a critical difference not only in your relationship and sex life but in every single aspect of your life that involves other people.

There are several barriers to listening that apply particularly to men.

▲ **Not realizing listening is important.** No one ever said that being a good listener is an important part of masculinity, so we tend to discount it. We feel free to listen with less than full attention when our partner is trying to tell us something.

▲ **Assuming and fearing that understanding is the same as agreeing.** Some men believe that if they say they understand what their partner says, she'll take that to mean that they agree. That isn't the case at all. You don't have to agree with your partner. It's often the case in relationships that the partners don't agree, and while the lack of agreement can cause problems, most of the time these can be ironed out. What's important is hearing and understanding. People are usually receptive to working out an arrangement if they feel understood. If they don't feel understood, they aren't receptive to much of anything, because all their energy is tied up in trying to get understood or in dealing with their feelings about not being understood.

▲ **Not understanding the feeling that's expressed.** Communications consist of at least two parts: content (what is said) and affect (the feeling[s] behind it). Because we men haven't been trained to give much importance to feelings, we're more likely to get the content and miss the feeling, meaning that the speaker will not feel understood. The feeling is usually more important than the content.

Let's say your partner is feeling neglected. Ideally, she would just say so. But that's not always how it goes. So without mentioning neglect, she accuses you of having an affair. Her feeling of neglect is the issue, but it's easy to miss that and get caught up in defending yourself against the accusation. The problem is that proving you aren't having an affair will settle nothing. She'll still feel neglected.

▲ **Judgmentalism—criticizing the speaker's feelings or position.** Your partner says her boss takes advantage of her generosity, and you tell her she's overreacting or that the situation isn't as bad as she thinks. Now she has to persuade you that it's exactly that bad.

Another example of judgmentalism is commenting that her feelings aren't logical, maybe because she expresses two seemingly contradictory emotions. But feelings have their own logic. It's common to have contradictory feelings. Love and hate come quickly to mind. One can experience both of these emotions at the same time toward the same person, especially a parent, child, or spouse. Feelings aren't neat and clean, like a balance sheet or a syllogism.

▲ **Trying to fix things rather than just listen.** Since men are trained to be problem solvers, when we hear of a difficulty we immediately set out to make it right. It's hard to remember that there's often nothing to fix. Your partner may just want a listener. It's common for a woman to say, "I just wanted to tell him about a problem I'm having. But before I even get it all out, he's already got four things for me to do to make it better. I don't need him to solve my problems. All I wanted was a sympathetic ear."

This does not mean you have to forgo giving advice entirely. Offering practical advice is something many men are good at and many women appreciate. But it's crucial to listen carefully first. She may be especially interested in what you have to say now that she believes you have all the essential information.

HOW *NOT* TO LISTEN

Following these rules is guaranteed to enrage your partner and to cause serious damage to your relationship.

▲ Let her know you don't want to listen. Tell her that you have better things to do, complain that you don't want to listen to the same old stuff again, or ask, "Do we have to talk about this?"

▲ When you do get around to listening, do it halfheartedly. Keep glancing at the TV or at a newspaper as your partner talks. This will let her know that you aren't interested and are hoping she'll finish as soon as possible.

▲ Interrupt frequently with irrelevant questions and topics. This will reinforce her sense of not being taken seriously.

▲ Make lots of judgments about what she's saying. Tell her she's having the wrong feelings, that she's not being logical, that she's misread the situation, that she's handling it wrong, and so on.

▲ Give unrequested advice. Tell her exactly what she should do to resolve the problem.

The key to effective listening is what's called empathy: the ability to understand what's being said from the talker's point of view. This requires that you try to get into her shoes and see it from her perspective, not from your own. You might want to recall an experience where you expressed something and the other person seemed to understand exactly what it was like for you. Wasn't that a powerful experience, and didn't it give you a feeling of comfort and freedom? The comfort results simply from having the understanding. Humans need that. The sense of freedom comes from not having to defend or justify what you've said. It's been accepted, and that frees you to explore the issue further, to come up with solutions, or just to leave it alone. That's what everyone wants.

RULES OF EFFECTIVE LISTENING

1. **Remember that your one and only job while listening is to understand** *her* **experience, feelings, attitude, or point of view.** While listening, your point of view is not relevant. You can express your side later if you want, but only after you've understood what she is saying.

2. **Give her your full attention.** Turn off the TV, put away any materials you have in your hands, and look at your partner. This is very important, because it gives her a sense of being listened to and helps cut down on anger and defensiveness.

3. **Ask questions to encourage her, to help her along, and also to gain clarification for yourself.** For example, ask, "How did you feel about that?" or "What happened next?" When we are asked questions about an event we are relating, it not only helps but also assures us of the listener's interest. Other ways of encouraging her to continue include "Oh," "I see," "Mmm," and similar sounds, and gestures like nodding or touching her.

Asking questions about her experience can also defuse tension and hostility. Most of us are accustomed to hearing denials and angry statements when we're lodging a protest or criticism; anticipating such responses adds to our anxiety and anger. But when we are greeted with something like "Can you say more about what I did that upset you?" a lot of the negative feelings evaporate.

4. **Try to understand the feeling behind what she's saying as well as the content.** She may tell you directly (for example, "I'm so angry [or upset or disappointed or sad]") or you will get clues from what she says, her tone of voice, and her demeanor. If you're not sure what emotion she had or has, ask: "How did that make you feel?" or "What was that like for you?"

5. **Demonstrate your understanding.** Perhaps the best way is by acknowledging and validating her feelings: "I can see why you're so angry" or "That's really frustrating" or "That's so annoying." It's important that you acknowledge the feelings *she's* having, not the ones you're having. If you talk about your feelings at this point, you're taking attention away from her, and that will probably make her upset.

There's no question whatever that these rules are hard to follow. Even the best listeners don't always apply all of them. Despite that, they are important. The more of them you use, and the more often you use them, the better listener you will be.

Here's an example of how *not* to do it:

HER: I'm so upset, I feel like quitting my job. Fred got on my case be-cause the Jones report wasn't done today, even though it's not due till next week.

YOU: Fred's an asshole, and you should tell him what to do with his report.

This is risky because you're unnecessarily interjecting yourself into her situation. She may not think Fred's an asshole and may resent your giving advice she hasn't asked for. You are not seeing the situation from her perspective.

Another way of *not* doing it would be like this: "I'm sure Fred will realize his mistake and it'll all be okay tomorrow." This doesn't work because the hidden message in your statement is that she's having the wrong feelings: She shouldn't be upset. This is not likely to make her feel understood.

Here's a better way:

HER: I'm so upset, I feel like quitting my job.

YOU: You're really upset. What happened? [simply acknowledging her feeling and encouraging her to continue]

HER: Fred got on my case because the Jones report wasn't done today, even though it's not due till next week.

YOU: That's enough to upset anyone. [validating her feeling]

HER: It wouldn't have been so bad except that he did it in front of Lucy and Jane. It was embarrassing to be scolded in front of them.

YOU: Wow. That really made it worse. [again, just acknowledging what she's saying]

HER: Yeah, it was pretty bad. But I feel a little better now. [followed by a silence]

YOU: Have you decided what you want to do about this? [gives her encouragement to express any plans she's considered, but also allows her to say that she's been too upset to consider what to do]

HER: I think I need to talk to Fred. Usually he's fine, but he gets so stressed out by deadlines that he loses it and acts like an ass. . . . Yeah, I definitely need to talk to him about this.

YOU: Sounds like you have a plan. [acknowledging her plan]

In this example, you didn't seem to do a lot. Yet chances are she'll feel it was a good discussion and will be grateful to you for listening. She got something off her chest and decided on a plan of action. You helped facilitate it without judgments, without interference, without giving advice. What you did may have been what allowed her to come up with her plan.

Some people wonder why it's okay for the woman to call Fred an ass but not okay for the man to call him an asshole. The reason is simple: It's her show—she can call him anything she wants. But it's not your job to tell her what Fred is or isn't.

The best way to become a better listener is to practice listening as often as possible, employing the above rules as much as you can. Opportunities for listening are usually close to hand. Someone is always trying to say something to you: your lover, child, boss, colleague, a customer or client, someone sitting next to you on the plane or bus, and so on.

EXERCISE 12-1: LISTENING

When you feel like it, but at least twice each day, make it a point to really listen for a few minutes. It might be when you know someone is going to talk to you—a client is coming in at ten o'clock to discuss a problem, or your partner says you need to talk—or when someone has already starting talking to you. Your goal is simply to try to understand what is said from the speaker's point of view. So put on your listening hat and apply the principles suggested earlier.

If you are someone who listens better at work than elsewhere, you want to discover how to transfer your work skills to a different environment. When you're going to listen to someone not connected with work, find a way of getting into your best listening mode. There may be some behavior connected with your work listening mode that you can use; perhaps you have a way of clearing your mind of other things. If so, then do the same mind clearing before listening to your lover or child. Another way is simply to tell yourself, "I want to listen to June the same way I listen to our largest customer." These aids may seem awkward at first, but they get much more comfortable and effective with regular practice.

The results of this exercise can be astonishing. One man said that after years of what he considered nagging, he finally understood what his lover meant by wanting more intimacy and the legitimacy of her request. Many other men report having new understandings of their partners and of increased closeness as a result.

LISTENING TO COMPLAINTS AND ANGER

"What am I supposed to do when she's shrieking and making it sound like I'm the worst bastard who ever lived?"

Being able to listen nondefensively to criticism and anger is crucial in a good relationship. But this is where lots of men have trouble. Who wants to hear complaints and bad news? Such a reaction is understandable; I feel the same way. But I also know it's smart to listen to bad news.

Even though it doesn't feel good at the moment, a complaint or criticism is a gift. Instead of taking her love or sex elsewhere, your partner is sticking with you, alerting you to a problem, and handing you an opportunity to rectify it. Many of our best-run businesses have learned to look at complaints in this way and require their top executives to spend time each month reading letters of complaints and taking phone calls from those with problems. Most relationships would benefit from a similar policy.

It is crucial when listening to complaints or anger that you stay present and do not tune out. How you do this is up to you. You have at least one way of doing this. I know this because I'm certain you don't space out at work when your boss is angry or has a criticism. If you can be present for your boss, you can do at least as much for the woman you love.

When people are critical or angry, they want to be heard and understood. What they don't want is criticism in return, denial of their perceptions or feelings, or attacks on their position or personality. So don't add fuel to her fire. By simply listening and not attacking her, not defending yourself, and not withdrawing, you help keep her anger where it belongs—on the specific behavior or issue that set it off.

But what else can you do? A great deal. Anything conciliatory will be of benefit. Asking questions, for example, is an excellent way of disarming anger. Rather than slamming her back or withdrawing (both of which can be taken to indicate a lack of interest in her feelings), you can ask her to tell you more: "I'm sorry you're so angry. Could you say more about what I did that upset you?" Another resource is empathy, showing that you understand what she's saying. Yet another is to agree with what you can agree with. Sincere apologies are yet another. All of these approaches are elaborated on in the chapters that follow.

I can't guarantee that her anger will immediately evaporate if you use some or all of these methods. It probably won't. She'll still be angry over whatever it was, and you may have to hang in there until she calms down. But you won't be making matters worse, and your conciliatory gestures will help her calm down and deal more constructively with what's troubling her.

NAGGING

One of the most common complaints men have about women is nagging. "She's always on my case" or "She's the biggest nag since my mother"—these are the words men use to register this behavior, which bugs the hell out of them. The best way I've found to look at this issue is to understand that nagging represents usually desperate attempts on the part of a woman to get what she needs. She wants her man to listen to and understand her, to express his feelings, to discuss an issue, to make certain agreements or to live up to ones he's already made.

The men usually feel overwhelmed. They work hard, they're tired, and they don't want to hear about something that they're doing wrong or that needs work. Unfortunately, there may not be a good alternative. **The best way to stop nagging is not to let things reach that point.** That is, listen to what your partner has to say, and deal with those things that can be dealt with, no matter how difficult that may be. If she says, for example, that sex has become boring, you might want to swallow your pride and do your best to find out what she means, then decide with her what should be done about it.

A good way to prevent nagging is to be honest. A lot of nagging is simply an attempt to get a man to open up. During a session in my office, Judy said she thought Dan had had a bad day at work. He immediately denied it but not in a way that persuaded either her or me. Then Judy started in with what he would later call nagging: Did he have a bad time with a customer, was it the sweltering heat, was his back bothering him? After she, with some help from me, convinced Dan to say what was going on, it turned out that indeed it had been a bad day. But his unwillingness to open up to her right away had pushed her, because of her concern, to nag him. He could have prevented the nagging by simply being honest.

Another good way to prevent nagging is to live up to your agreements. If you make agreements you don't keep, you can be sure that nagging is what you're going to get.

Yet another way to prevent nagging is to be willing to get outside help for the problems the two of you can't solve on your own. There are lots of kinds of help that may be required. Some couples I've seen needed to hire child care or house-cleaning services. Neither the woman or the man could do any more, and the only good solution was getting someone else to help. Other couples needed financial advice. Yet others needed psychotherapy or sex therapy.

Men are much less willing to go for psychological help than women. It's difficult for a man to acknowledge that he has a relationship or sex problem that he can't resolve on his own. One dramatic case comes to mind. In this couple, the woman had been begging the man to get help for his very quick ejaculations for over fifteen years. During the first years of their marriage, he wouldn't even hear her complaint. Then he acknowledged a problem existed, but it was hers: If she didn't take so long to come, his lasting longer wouldn't be an issue. By the time he finally came to grips with reality and they came to therapy, it was almost too late. Her anger had built to such a point that she was never able to fully let go of it even though he was now eager to get the help he had so long resisted.

As I talked with this man, he mentioned time and again how difficult it was to live with such a nagger. What hadn't occurred to him in fifteen years was that his behavior gave her no choice. If he had simply admitted the problem and sought help, there would have been no reason for nagging.

My best advice is: Don't be like this man, or like the man who wouldn't admit he'd had a bad day. Don't cause your spouse (and yourself) to suffer for fifteen years just because you don't want to hear about a problem. Sooner or later you're going to have to deal with it, so you might as well skip the suffering and get right to it.

If you think your partner is a nag, why not ask yourself what she's talking about? If you have any doubts you have it right, why not ask her?

For example, you could begin this way: "I'm concerned about the housework business. You keep bringing up that I don't do my share, and I barely hear you anymore. It's not good for us. Would you please tell me exactly what you want? Then let's talk about it."

Let's say she says something like this: "John, it's not just about sharing the housework. I'm worried about us. We seem to be drifting apart." That is a wake-up call. She's saying the relationship is in trouble. You may feel like hell and want to run away, but, believe it or not, you're being handed a gift.

Here's one way *not* to handle it effectively: "Look, I know I've been busy. But things will be better after the Christmas season. You'll see." All you're doing is shutting her up and making light of the complaint. The only sure things anyone will see is her increasing anger and a worsening of the problem.

Here's an even worse way: "Damn it! I'm tired of your telling me something else is wrong. Just leave me alone." I won't even comment on that one except to note that it's quite common. But suppose you actually said it and later realized you were wrong. No need to feel embarrassed or alone. Many of us have done it. What you need to do is admit your mistake and tell her you'd like to listen. "I made a mistake last night when you said we were drifting apart. It scared me and I blew up. I'm calmer now and would like to hear what you have to say."

YOUR CONDITIONS FOR EFFECTIVE LISTENING

Each of us can be a better listener under certain circumstances than under others. You need to determine how you can listen best and take steps to get what you need. Most people, for example, find they don't listen well when they're tired, angry, or in a hurry. So they need to assertively say this isn't a good time: "I know we need to talk, but I'm too bushed to give you my full attention. Could we talk about this in the morning?" Or "I want to hear what you have to say, but I'm so pissed about what happened at work I really can't concentrate. Can you wait until I've taken a bath and calmed down?"

Suppose you'd like to listen to your partner but she talks in ways that make that difficult. Maybe you need to tell her something like this: "I know you're upset, and I really want to hear what you have to say. But it's very difficult for me to listen when you call me names and belittle me. I promise I'll listen attentively if you tone that down."

If she can't or won't stop, you have every right to call a time-out (see Chapter 13). When the two of you regroup and are calmer, assure her of your desire to listen, but let her know the circumstances under which you can hear the best.

LISTENING TO SEXUAL COMPLAINTS AND FEEDBACK

It's not easy for men to listen to sexual complaints. We like to think that we're good lovers, so anything suggesting we're not hits us where it hurts. But at the same time, it's necessary that we do learn to listen. Let's say your partner tells you that you come too fast. It's important that you hear what she's saying instead of your own fantasies or nightmares—for example, "I'm not man enough for her" or "She's going to leave me." Hearing such things will probably cause you to become upset and defensive. So you reply with something like, "Well, if it didn't take you a week to come, it wouldn't be too fast." Now both of you are hurt and angry, and you're heading for trouble.

A better way would be like this: "That's upsetting, but tell me more about it." You want to find out all the specifics about her complaint and what she wants.

> HER: I know I won't have an orgasm with intercourse, but I really like having you inside me, and I feel frustrated that you're in and out so fast. I'd like it to be longer.
> YOU: Let me be sure I understand. Although you're not looking to climax that way, you're frustrated that we don't have longer intercourse.
> HER: That's right. It feels so good, I want it to go on longer.

Now that you understand the gist of her comment, you can try to get more information.

> YOU: When you say longer, what do you mean?
> HER: I don't know—maybe twice as long as now.

This is crucial information that you learned only because you were able to hear and understand what she said earlier. It may be that what she's saying sounds fine to you. In that case, you need to let her know: "That sounds reasonable. I'd like that, too." Now the two of you need to talk about how to reach the goal you've agreed on.

It's equally important to let her know if you don't agree or don't think change is possible. For example: "I'd love to be able to last longer, but I've been coming fast all my life. When I was with Joan, I went to a shrink for over a year and it didn't help. I don't know what to do." Your statement, as discouraging as it sounds, leaves the door open for further discussion. For example, she may want to bring up going to a therapist who specializes in this kind of problem. Or maybe you have something to offer: "This book I'm reading has exercises that the author says have been helpful. I'll show them to you if you like. Maybe they can work."

Let's turn to the subject of listening to sexual feedback, which may or may not be a complaint. Many men appreciate hearing what their partners like and don't like in sex. It saves them the effort of making assumptions and wondering if they have it right. But some men get into a snit because they feel bossed around. As one man said: "It's always 'a little slower, a little more gently, do this and do that.' It's like she's directing traffic." These men often take the woman's suggestions as criticisms and feel bad because what they were doing wasn't right.

Many women are perplexed about giving sexual feedback. They know they need to say what they want, but they fear hurting their partner's feelings. It's immeasurably easier for them when the partners encourage and welcome information. It's much harder when what they say is not received well. The partner of the man quoted above had this to say: "He doesn't know what I like, but he doesn't seem to want to learn. I tell him in the most gentle ways I know, but he takes everything as a criticism. What am I supposed to do?"

Men have been trained to believe that they should somehow know what a woman needs in bed. If they don't, that's a negative statement about their masculinity. But, like all the other myths, this is ridiculous. There is no way of knowing how to please a partner without learning from her. No matter how many women you've had sex with and no matter how many books you've read, the only way to know what this partner wants is from her.

Some men who've heard this have objected, saying they had experiences where what they did was exactly what the woman wanted. Other men have reported stories from partners who said that a former lover knew exactly what to do. I don't deny that it sometimes happens like this; the man's style and preferences exactly or very closely match the woman's and all is fine, as if by magic. But you need to understand that this is rare. In most cases, sexual and otherwise, learning is necessary.

Feedback is something to be thankful for. When your partner tells you to touch her like so, or that she likes this or that, she's telling you what she needs for a good sexual experience *with you*.

It's possible, of course, that your partner is speaking in ways that are hard to hear. Or, perhaps because she's anxious about hurting your feelings and how her comments will go over, she may not communicate very clearly. If you object to the manner of her speaking rather than to the content, it's perfectly acceptable to let her know how you could hear better.

Otherwise, you have no choice but to get over your feelings of being criticized and listen. Unless you listen carefully to what she says and act accordingly, the chances of good sex are seriously diminished. Virtually all of the women I've talked to say that listening to, understanding, and acting on the woman's suggestions are important aspects of being a good lover.

That's what they want rather than a man who can anticipate their every desire or automatically know what they prefer.

If you're not sure you understand what she wants, having a longer talk about it and getting a demonstration can be of great help.

GETTING A DEMONSTRATION

Let's say your partner wants longer kisses or a particular way of being touched. Although you may be able to repeat back her words exactly, you may still not know what she means. For example, your understanding of "long" or "gentle" may be very different from hers. It happens all the time. The woman tells the man to touch her more softly. He shows his understanding by saying, "You want a softer touch," and then proceeds to touch her in a way that is soft by his definition but not by hers.

Even the seemingly simple word *kiss* can present problems. There are many different kinds of kisses, and it's by no means clear that you have the same kind of kiss in mind when your partner says she'd like more kissing. Is she talking about a peck on the cheek, an affectionate kiss, an all-out passionate kiss? It's important not to assume that just because she said "more kissing" and you repeated back "more kissing," the two of you are talking about the same thing. You may be, and then again you may not be.

Asking for a demonstration is very helpful, which is what the next exercise is about. I use the example of kissing because the first few couples I used it with were having trouble with kissing, but the exercise works well with many activities: genital and nongenital stimulation, hugging, holding, intercourse positions and movements, and even back rubs.

EXCERISE 12-2: KISSING (OR WHATEVER) SEMINAR

Time Required: 2–10 minutes

Tell your partner you'd like help with kissing, because she's been complaining about it. "I'd like to learn to kiss the way you want, but I need help. Would you tell me exactly what you want and then show me? I want to get this right."

Listen to her explanation and check your understanding by summarizing what you hear her say. When she agrees that you have it, have her kiss you that way. (If the issue is touching rather than kissing, you can have her demonstrate on herself as well as on you. You can also have her guide your hand with hers when you touch her.) Then you do what she's been doing and ask for feedback.

Use that information when you try again. Don't expect to have it perfect right away. Pay attention and take your time.

The exercise should probably not last more than ten minutes. End it when you're both feeling good, even if you still haven't mastered what she wants. You can always arrange another seminar later.

POSSIBLE PROBLEM

You can understand and do what she wants, but it's not what you want. Kissing her way is not your favorite way. One possibility is to try it her way for a time—say, a few weeks—to see if you get to like it more. If not, the two of you may want to agree to have more my-turn, your-turn sex, where sometimes it's done mainly for her and sometimes mainly for you. When it's done for her, you kiss her way. Another possibility is to kiss both ways during sex, sometimes her way, sometimes yours.

LISTENING TO REPORTS OF SEXUAL ASSAULT

By now it should come as no surprise to hear that millions of American women have been victims of incest, molestation, or rape. These assaults are a leading cause of sexual problems in women. If your partner was a victim, it's important to be able to listen to her if she wants to talk about it. Of course, she probably won't tell you if you're not already a good listener.

You may well find that her story stirs up all sorts of feelings in you, but it's crucial not to let them overpower you. This is definitely one time where her feelings are far more important than yours. What you mainly need to do is listen, encourage her to say as much as she wants, and be supportive.

Whatever you do, do not explicitly or implicitly criticize her behavior now or in the past. You may believe that she shouldn't have gone out with that guy in the first place, shouldn't have been walking in that area alone at night, or should have fought back harder, but do everyone a favor and keep these ideas to yourself. She's had a horrible experience and needs you to be there for her. Don't give advice unless it is requested, don't make judgments, and don't try to fix her. You are not her doctor or sex therapist, and you shouldn't try to be. If she needs professional assistance, she should get it from a professional. It is also counterproductive to get crazy and threaten to kill the man who assaulted her. Such macho posturing works only in the movies. Besides, if you get angry, she'll be torn between dealing with her own feelings and dealing with yours. She was the one who was assaulted. Don't take the attention away from her by getting carried away with your feelings.

You'll need all the empathy you can muster in order just to be there with her. It's possible that talking will bring back strong feelings, and she may shake, scream, or cry. Try not to think you have to do anything about her feelings and behavior. The only thing you can do, aside from listen, is to hold her, if she wants to be held, and assure her of your love and support. If she doubts her desirability, you can reassure her of it, but that's all. If at some point she wants to be alone, then let her be alone.

It may well be that she'll want to talk about what happened a number of times, not just once. If that's the case, be there for her as often as she needs. If you keep two words in mind—*understanding* and *support*—you should do fine.

Tools for Dealing with Conflict

We're grinding each other up into mulch each time we fight. There's got to be a better way.— *Man, 35*

We almost got divorced numerous times. It took us until we had been together over thirty years to work out ways of being nice to each other and to work out differences. What a shame it took so long.— *Man, 67*

CONFLICT IS AN inevitable part of close relationships. How it is handled determines to a large extent how well relationships and sex go. In this chapter I discuss a number of ideas and tools that can help keep conflict to a minimum. I have given examples of some of them in previous chapters, but I want to get into more detail now. They aren't panaceas— unfortunately, there are no panaceas—and they cannot by themselves undo the effects of years of neglect, distress, and abuse. But these suggestions and tools can help discussions and negative feelings from getting out of control.

Keep two things in mind whenever you deal with or think about your partner and while you read the following material. One is your overall goal with her, which I assume is having a loving relationship. The more you focus on this goal, the less you'll give in to temptations to berate or criticize her, or to withdraw from her physically or emotionally.

The second thing to keep in mind is that even though it may not seem that way, you always have choices. No matter how badly certain conversations have gone in the past, no matter how upset you've gotten when she said or did a certain thing, it doesn't have to be that way now. You can choose to listen more empathically, to greet a complaint of hers with a request for more information rather than a countercomplaint, to phrase your comments in a more constructive way, and to call a time-out when things are going badly. These choices are always available, and every important change starts with choosing to do one thing differently. The smoker decides not to have a cigarette after dinner, the drinker not to have a drink before. If you pay attention, you'll notice many opportunities for doing things in ways that will help you reach your goal.

PREVENTIVE MEDICINE

The first thing, of course, is to keep bad feelings to a minimum and to take care of whatever needs taking care of before it becomes an international incident. If you have followed the advice in the preceding chapters, you have already taken several giant steps in this direction. By spending plenty of time being close and having fun with your mate, and by keeping up on each other's feelings, interests, and concerns, you are developing and maintaining a loving friendship, and that bond in itself helps keep anger and nastiness from arising or getting out of control.

By doing these things, you are ensuring that each of you feels valued, loved, and attended to. Not having these feelings is precisely what causes conflict in many relationships. And by keeping in close touch with one another, there is ample opportunity for each of you to bring up concerns and complaints while they are still easy to manage.

Another important preventive measure is keeping your word. Not keeping agreements is a huge source of contention in many relationships. By only agreeing to do what you in fact can do and by sticking to your word, you will eliminate a great deal of conflict.

The rule is the same in business and in relationships: Don't agree to anything unless you're certain you can and will do it. If you don't want to do what your partner requests, you need to be assertive and state your position; then the two of you need to see what can be worked out. While there are a number of reasons all of us sometimes fail to keep our agreements, men have a special one: We often agree just to stop the conversation, to "get her off my back." While this is understandable, it's going to cause trouble because she's going to be even more upset when we don't keep the agreement.

So if you're asked to do something, first make sure you understand exactly what it is. The best way is to check your understanding with her. If the two of you agree on what's to be done, take a minute to imagine yourself doing it. In her presence or not, imagine yourself doing exactly what the two of you are talking about. Then you need to seriously consider whether you can and will do it—and also whether you need any help in doing it. All of this will take time, anywhere from a few seconds to minutes or longer. But it's important to take the time you need. When you talk to her about your thoughts, you should close the discussion with a summary of what the agreement is. This is handy to prevent misunderstandings. Here's an example of the whole process:

> YOU: I find myself in a strange place. I agree with you that it's your body and I shouldn't touch you in ways you don't like. So I'll do my best not to touch your breasts roughly. But I can't guarantee never to do it. What feels rough to you comes from a strong feeling of lust. I'm not sure I can always catch this impulse before I grab you.

Depending on what she says, you might want to ask for her help:

> YOU: I think I can do it most of the time. But there may still be a few occasions when I don't catch myself in time. I may already be squeezing your breast before I remember. It would help me a lot to know that you're not going to get upset if that happens occasionally. Maybe you could just remind me of what I'm doing.
>
> HER: I'm willing to call it to your attention if you forget occasionally, but I want to know that you're taking this seriously.
>
> YOU: I am. I want to touch you the way you like. I'm going to follow through on this, and I appreciate your willingness to remind me if I forget.

You're right if you think she's going to be watching your progress with this, especially the first few times. You need to take whatever measures are necessary to make sure you carry out your agreement. Little aids can be a big help; for example, writing a note in your appointment book about what you agreed to do, or even putting a similar note on the bathroom mirror or on the nightstand next to the bed. Another aid is mental rehearsal. The more you imagine yourself touching her breasts in ways that are acceptable to her, the better the chances that you'll do exactly that.

You can count on it, however, that you won't always remember. Rather than assuming this won't happen, it's best to plan how to deal with it when it does, which is what the man in the last example tried to do.

UNDERSTAND THAT NOT EVERYTHING CAN BE RESOLVED

A huge source of bad feelings and hostility in relationships is failing to understand and accept that most issues in a relationship—any relationship—cannot be resolved. Understanding this surprising fact can prevent a lot of unnecessary frustration and conflict.

According to John Gottman's research, only about 30 percent of the differences or problems in a relationship can be fixed or resolved. The remaining 70 percent are deeply rooted in the different personalities and histories of the partners and have to be accepted. You already know the kind of thing I'm talking about: one partner is more of a night person, the other a morning person; one more sedentary, one more active; one more interested in sex, one less so; one more outgoing, the other more introverted; one more organized, the other less so; one more a spender, the other more a saver; one more impulsive, the other more restrained; one neat, the other messy.

When you choose a romantic partner, you're also choosing the problems that you'll have to face for as long as you're with her. Most of them cannot be fixed, and it's highly unlikely any are going to disappear.

What's needed in these situations is to find ways of accepting and dealing gracefully with the unresolvable differences. You need to be able to talk about them, because they come up all the time, but to expect an end to them or a resolution is to court serious relationship distress. As one of my clients put it, only half jokingly, after years of work with a number of respected therapists: "I guess I need to accept that this ain't gonna change, ain't gonna be different, no matter how many shrinks we see. The week before we die I'll still be wanting more sex than she. So now it seems the big question is, how do I handle this in a way that helps our marriage instead of hurting it?"

That's a good question, but the answers are beyond the purview of this book. Suffice it to say here that you need to learn the difference between resolvable and unresolvable problems, to resolve those that can be resolved, and accept and be able to manage or regulate those that can't.

KEEPING IN TOUCH

In the first edition of this book, I suggested that couples have a regular time each week to discuss their feelings about the state of the relationship. The reason for the suggestion is that a major problem in relationships is feelings, complaints, and issues that don't get dealt with. They get swept under the rug but continue to cause trouble. It can help immeasurably if couples have a definite time each week where each partner feels free to bring up anything he or she wants. This prevents anything festering for more than a week.

You can still do this if you want, but I have found that it's not necessary provided the couple spends a fair amount of time together each week and takes at least a few minutes each night to catch up with one another. With this kind of togetherness, they can bring up complaints, concerns, or anything else whenever they want.

You and your partner can choose either way, but my experience is that you have to have one or the other.

Despite what I've said about preventing and minimizing conflict, it cannot be entirely eliminated. Even the happiest couples sometimes get furious with each other, sometimes can't talk to each other, occasionally even wish they were alone or with someone else. I hope you feel relieved to know that even in the happiest couples, there is anger, there are loud voices, and there is distance—but not frequently and usually not for long. And therein lies a tale. The rest of the chapter deals with ways of not getting too far away from civility and sanity, and for healing the hurts as quickly as possible.

CALLING TIME OUT

Taking a time-out is perhaps the big gun—the biggest gun short of getting professional help—in romantic relationships, and it should be used whenever necessary.

It makes no sense to continue with conversations that have parted company with sanity. If nothing else works and things are falling apart—that is, the conflict and negative feelings are increasing, both of you are angry or yelling and not listening, and your pulse is racing—you can always call time out to stop the craziness from escalating further. This signals that the two of you need to take a break and get into a better frame of mind before continuing. It can do a lot to prevent conflicts from getting unmanageable.

John Gottman has demonstrated that when people's pulses go over about 100 beats per minute, they are overwhelmed and not exactly at their best. The part of their brain that makes them human is being short-circuited and they are doing their thinking, if it can even be called that, with the same little part of the brain that a snake or mouse has, and I'm sure you don't see many truly civilized snakes or mice. There is simply no point in going further at this juncture. It's better to put a stop to the activities and to find your humanity again. Gottman also found that men get overwhelmed in interpersonal confrontations sooner than women—which is why they often try to leave the situation—so it may well be you who needs to call most of the time-outs.

If you like the idea of calling time out when things are getting out of hand, you should discuss it with your partner and get an agreement to use it. Either of you can say "time out" whenever you feel that discussion is turning into argument. The harder part is for the other partner, the one who didn't call time out, to stop talking or screaming immediately. But this has to be done for the exercise to work. Once a time-out is called, there is no more talking. Each of you does something to calm down: take a walk, do some work, think things over, or whatever you like.

There are two important considerations regarding what you do during the time out. First of all, put a frame around it. That is, if you are going to leave the room or the house, don't just walk out, because that will probably cause your partner to feel more anger and perhaps to feel abandoned as well. Tell her what you're doing and when you'll be back. For example, "I'm going to take a bath to try to calm down. Be back in thirty minutes," or "I need to take a walk. I'll take the dog with me. I'll be back by ten-thirty." Of course, you need to be back when you say you will.

The other important thing about a time-out is what you do in your mind. Gottman found that many men walked around the block muttering to themselves, "I don't have to take this crap." In other words, they kept reinforcing their bad feelings and came back in worse shape than when they left. This is not a good idea.

The goal of a time-out is to calm yourself and get into a more loving space regarding your spouse so that you can work out the problem. Telling yourself that she's a mean bitch or that you don't have to put up with her isn't going to help. On the other hand, reminding yourself of the good times you've had with her, her qualities that you like, admire, and love, and things like this can help immensely. Even leafing through a newspaper or magazine for half an hour can help. When you're feeling better, you should consider how you might say what you have to say in more constructive ways.

How long should a time-out last? Five or ten minutes is usually too short to allow yourself to calm down. A half hour to an hour, or sometimes an hour and a half, seems to work best for most people. The sooner the two of you can reconnect and get to a more harmonious place, the better for all concerned. Often it's best to do what's necessary to feel close again, which may mean tabling discussion of the troublesome issue for a while. Once the two of you are feeling close, you can get back to it.

We now move to several measures that can help when you're in the midst of confrontation.

AGREE, AGREE, AGREE

In any relationship there will be disagreements about certain issues. But the more agreement there is, the easier it will be to solve the problem. In many cases, the real issues don't even get dealt with because the partners get into conflict about peripheral matters.

Say your partner's very upset, claims you don't love her, and accuses you of having an affair, but you're innocent of the charge. Since she really blasted you, you probably come on just as strong. "That's the stupidest thing I've ever heard. I'm either at the office or here. When the hell would I have time for an affair?"

The real issue, I suspect, is not about affairs. My guess is that she's concerned about the way you've been relating to her. Maybe you haven't shown much interest in spending time or having sex with her. She's worried about what this means and may be angry as well. So instead of saying, "I'm worried about us. We seemed to be drifting apart," she accuses you of having an affair. Since you're being attacked, you defend. And you know you're right. You're not having an affair, and you tell her so.

But now she's in a bad situation. It would be terrific if she could realize she didn't say exactly what she wanted to and make a U-turn. But maybe she can't. So she may feel that she has to defend her accusation. She may therefore reply that she doesn't know where you go on Sunday mornings when you say you're playing golf or what you do on all those business trips to Boston. You may now feel you have to deny her accusation once again and perhaps account for your time in Boston.

But let's say you caught yourself and decided to try something different. Is there anything in what she's saying and implying that you could agree with? It makes no sense to agree to an affair if you're not having one, but are there reasons for her to think that you might be having one? In other words, can you understand what's going on with her? Suppose you said this to her: "I can understand why you think I might be having an affair. We haven't been close lately." This amounts to agreeing with her concerns. Imagine the effect on her. She doesn't have to defend or prove anything. Now she can get to what's troubling her. And you haven't lost anything. Rather, you've gained an opportunity for a serious conversation with your wife about what's going on in your marriage.

Take another example. Your partner says: "You never do your share around the house. I'm sick of it." A typical defensive reply would be to tell her she's wrong and enumerate all the household tasks you've recently done. Then she'll be forced to deny them ("Like hell you take out the garbage every week; you took it out only once last month") or claim that you still don't do as much as she does ("Big deal! So you take out the garbage. Do you know what I do every week?"). We are clearly headed for an unpleasant experience.

But suppose you decided to try something different and said this in response to her first statement: "It's hard to admit, but you're right. I don't do as much as you." This will probably stop her in her tracks. Now you can have a useful conversation about household chores, a common source of disagreement in couples.

I'm suggesting you seriously consider agreeing with your partner's complaints and criticisms and thereby allow the two of you to get to the serious issues. Don't allow yourself to get hung up on and defensive about whether you "never" do X, "always" do Y, or her choice of words. Since she's probably angry or upset, you can bet her words won't be tactful or precise.

"I object. This is the weirdest thing I ever heard. Why should I agree with my partner if she's wrong?"

I understand that what I'm saying can sound very strange. It sounded strange to me when I first heard of it years ago, and I was reluctant to hear more. I was especially concerned because it seemed as if I was being asked to lie. It helped me to understand that was not the case.

The real request is to find something in your partner's criticism that you can agree with. Maybe it seems surprising, but there almost always is something. No matter how outrageous her statements, no matter how exaggerated, there's usually a strong element of truth somewhere there. In the illustration above of the man charged with having an affair, he wasn't in fact having one. But he had been very distant from his wife, so there was reason for her to think that maybe he was. He did not agree that he was having an affair, which would have been a lie, but rather to understanding how she could think he was, which was true.

Many people find it easier to agree with feelings than with content. After all, if your partner says she feels X, Y, or Z, there's little room for disagreement. Acknowledgment of her feelings can help: "You're really upset with me" or "You're angry about what happened tonight."

Even better is if you can validate her feelings: "I understand why you feel that way" or "You have every right to feel that way."

Probably best of all is if you can validate her feelings and some of the content as well. "You're right. I was nasty to your sister. I can see why you'd be upset."

Although I've ranked these kinds of agreement in terms of good, better, and best, all are helpful. Any agreement is better than no agreement, and the greater the agreement, the less the chance of defensiveness and arguments.

Go over some arguments you've had with your partner and consider when you could have agreed with something she was saying. Then think over some complaints she's likely to make in the future. This isn't difficult. Most people can determine in advance what their partner will soon criticize. Then decide how you could agree with at least some of what she's saying to make for a more constructive discussion about the issue.

Therapist Dan Wile makes the important point that trying to find a way to agree is useful because it counteracts our natural tendency in such situations to distort in the direction of disagreeing. Agreeing with what you can agree with focuses on the similarities between you and your partner rather than on the differences. This can put both of you into a more relaxed and positive frame of mind, so you can better work on what you truly disagree about.

APOLOGIZE

Just as there is incredible power in agreeing with your accuser, there is incredible power in apologizing for something you did wrong or for the hurt you caused. But many of us men have difficulty saying "I'm sorry." We've had little permission to acknowledge errors and to apologize. It makes us feel weak and less manly, and that's unfortunate.

If apologizing is hard for you, you might want to consider doing something about it. When you feel you were wrong, when you feel you hurt someone, you should draft an apology in your mind, rehearse it, and then consider if you want to give it. No matter how awkward you feel, I think you'll be pleased with the results. And try to remember that there is nothing weak about apologizing. It takes a strong person to be able to say he's made a mistake or feels bad for what he's done.

Apologies are often parts of agreeing with your partner ("You're right, I was late. I'm sorry") and making U-turns ("I'm sorry I got so defensive. I can understand why you're angry"). The apology validates what she has been saying (that you were late, that you hurt her feelings, and so on), and this automatically puts her in a much better frame of mind.

Although it's essential to be able to apologize for your behavior, there is at least one circumstance where an apology not only won't satisfy your partner but may actually inflame her further. This occurs when you continually do the same offensive thing and continually apologize for it. She will—correctly—believe that you're just using apologies as a way to contain her anger, and this will make her angrier.

Each of us at times treats our loved ones badly and each of us at times hurts the ones we love. I think a strong man is one who recognizes these facts and quickly apologizes for the harm and hurt he has caused.

REPAIR ATTEMPTS AND U-TURNS

One of the main differences between happy and unhappy couples, according to John Gottman's research, is that while happy couples experience conflict and bad feelings just like everyone else, they quickly repair the damage, and this usually means making a U-turn.

In driving, a U-turn consists of turning around and going back the way you came after realizing you were going the wrong way. In conversations, a U-turn is slightly different; here you head off in any new direction once you realize that the way you are going is leading to trouble. You are trying to repair the rift that is developing.

Anytime you are aware that one of you is being defensive, that you're getting sidetracked by issues of right and wrong, or that the conversation is getting out of control, consider a U-turn. A U-turn has the advantage of allowing the discussion to continue without interruption. If it works, you may not need a time-out.

A U-turn can be almost anything that puts the conversation back on a better plane. One example we just covered: Stop defending yourself and agree with the portion of your partner's comments that you can agree with. Apologizing for something you did is another kind of U-turn, as is apologizing for being defensive.

One day in my office a man was trying to express his anger over his wife's sharing information about his sexual preferences with her best friend. What he said was, "You always tell Katie everything." She, of course, immediately started to defend against his overly general terminology, the "always" and "everything." He then felt the need to justify his use of those terms. Both were getting angrier by the second, and the conversation was drifting further and further away from reality. A repair attempt could have easily rectified the situation. He could have said, for example: "I'm sorry, I used the wrong words. Let me take back 'always' and 'everything.' I'm just angry that you told her about my liking for anal sex. I'm afraid she'll tell her husband and he'll kid me about it."

Now we're dealing with the real issue and can go on with the conversation. But this was almost lost as they started to get into a dispute over whether she tells Katie everything. It's sad, as in this case, when lovers get into conflict over trivia and lose sight of the real concerns.

Anything positive, anything conciliatory, can be effective in repairing the damage and setting the two of you on a better course. Something I once did is a good example. My sweetie and I were getting into a heavy argument, when I blurted out, "I'm sad we're banging at each other like this. I love you so much." She responded by saying how much she loved me, too, and that broke the ice. After a long hug, we were able to discuss the problem—which, of course, was so important that I can't even recall what it was—in a much more constructive way.

A client I saw recently told me that he's often able to soothe himself and his partner in the midst of a dispute by saying simply, "I wish we could get back to the loving couple we were this morning."

UNDERSTANDING AND FORGIVING YOUR PARTNER

We now move to a special kind of situation, when you believe that your partner has said or done something so heinous that you're entirely justified in your ugly feelings toward her, or when you just don't know how to let go of them. The first thing that usually comes to people's minds when I bring this up is the situation where the partner has had an affair. But it comes up in lots of other ways as well: a name she called you or a belittling remark, making a decision without consulting you, and so on. It's possible you may need to forgive her before you can move on. We don't hear much about forgiving these days, but I have found it to be wonderfully beneficial. Basically it means saying, "Even though I don't like what you did or said, I'm willing to let go of my hurt, my anger, and my desire to get back at you. I want our relationship to work, so I want to let bygones be bygones and get on with our lives."

Unfortunately, it may not be that simple. You may find that you can't simply forgive, that you need something from her in order to forgive her.

Take as much time as you need to consider what it would take for you to be able to forgive. Maybe you need an apology, or you need her to explain in detail why she did what she did so that you can understand it better, or maybe you need her to promise not to say or do it again. Or it may be something else entirely. Whatever it is, write it down and put it away for a few days. Then come back to what you wrote and see if it still sounds right. Next, spend a few moments imagining that she does what you want. How do you feel about that? Can you then forgive her and let go of the feelings you've been carrying? If the answer is no or you're not sure, consider again what you need to forgive her. Maybe there's something else.

Forgiving is usually easier if you can understand the action from her point of view. This exercise can help.

EXERCISE 13-1: UNDERSTANDING AND DEFENDING WHAT YOUR PARTNER DID

The idea behind this exercise is very simple. You are going to act as your partner's defense attorney. She is on trial for the behavior that bothers you (something she said or did). You are her attorney and have to persuade the jury (really you) that what she did was, if not right, at least understandable and reasonable. You are to make as strong a case for her as possible. Although it may be hard to believe right now, the stronger the case you make for her, the better it will be for you.

You will need lots of empathy to do the exercise properly. You'll have to set your own feelings aside and see the situation as much as possible from her point of view. And you can feel free to interview her to get information about how she saw the situation and how she felt.

The main mistake people make with this exercise is being cavalier about it. Doing it properly will take over a hour and perhaps several hours. You want to marshal all the evidence and put together a strong case for her. When you have all this in order, there are three options for presenting it: write or type the argument (at least a page long); speak it into a tape recorder (several minutes long); or present it orally to her or a third party such as a friend.

No one I've presented this exercise to has been enthusiastic at first. But it's a powerful technique. A number of my clients have discovered what a good deal of social-psychological research shows: It does result in changed attitudes.

CONSIDER WRITING A NOTE

Things can get to the point where discussion is impossible. Bad feelings arise whenever a certain subject is broached, and fights quickly ensue. Or perhaps you believe that you haven't been able to adequately express something important. If either of these things is happening in your relationship, writing a note may help.

The primary advantage for the writer is that you get to say exactly what you want to say. You can write as many drafts of your statement as you want, perhaps getting help from a friend or therapist, until it's just how you want it. And you don't have to be worried about getting distracted and forgetting to include something, or getting upset because of your partner's response and saying things you'll later regret. Yet another advantage is that you can anticipate your partner's objections and address them without the risk of getting into a squabble over them.

The main advantage to your partner is that she gets to read your note at her leisure and can digest the message without having to respond immediately. That can greatly cut down on defensive behavior.

There is one potential shortcoming of notes you should be aware of. When we talk, a great deal gets communicated nonverbally. Tone, inflection, facial expressions, and body posture can soften or strengthen the words. On paper, the words are all you get. What in a conversation would have been expressed by a look or a tone needs to be put into words in a note. So if you're not being critical or if you're feeling love or sadness or whatever, remember that the reader of the note won't know it unless you expressly say so.

You don't have to be a writer to write the kind of note I'm talking about. Literary elegance is not what it's about. Clarity of expression and consideration for how to best say what you want to get across are. The less fancy and eloquent you try to be, the better.

The best way I know of writing a note is to take some uninterrupted time, get a fix in your head of what you want to say, grab a pencil or sit down at the computer, and then just write without stopping to make any corrections or changes. Just get it all out. Later on, you can go over what you've written as many times as you desire, keeping in mind the principles of assertive communication on pages 153–156, and make all the changes you want. When you've pretty much gotten the note as you want it, make sure to put in an introductory comment about why you're sending a note. Here is an example of the first few lines of a note written by a client of mine to his lover:

Dear Marcy:

I love you dearly and want more than anything for our relationship to be as happy and satisfying as possible. Most aspects seem fine, but sex continues to be an issue. Since we haven't been able to talk about this without getting into fights, I'm trying writing. I'd be happy to hear your response, in person or in a note, as soon as you're ready.

It is best not to be present when your partner reads your note. Let her choose how and when to respond.

CONSIDER PROFESSIONAL HELP

Since I make my living doing therapy, it is probably self-serving for me to suggest that you seek help from me or my colleagues. Yet regardless of what it may do for me, consider that it has been estimated that less than one percent of divorced couples had ever had couples therapy. Also consider the finding of a recent study that of couples who do get therapy, it tends on the average to be six years (that's not a misprint) after they detect serious marital difficulties. The longer they wait, of course, the longer the therapy will take and the smaller the chance that it will be effective.

I hope you can use the material I have presented in this and the preceding chapters to your benefit. But if you try them and they don't help, consider getting professional assistance. Couples therapy and sex therapy need not be long or drawn-out. Sometimes just one, two, or three sessions can help. And sometimes it may take several months. But isn't your relationship worth that kind of investment?

"I liked what you said earlier about asserting yourself, but now you seem to be contradicting yourself. Understand your partner, agree with her criticisms, apologize to her, write her love notes—just give in and make nice to her. It all sounds so weak and wimpy."

I agree it can sound like that and that many men have trouble with these parts. You're not the first to see it this way. The important thing, I think, is not so much how something sounds but how well it works. There is a great deal of power in these methods. My experience is that following the ideas in this and the preceding chapters does *not* reduce assertiveness or result in men feeling weak or wimpy. On the contrary, men report feeling stronger because they have more control over conversations that they previously felt helpless to influence. They also report more harmonious and satisfying interactions with their lovers. Whatever doubts remain, I would ask you to put it to the test. Give these methods and ideas a trial for a fair period of time, say a month or two, and then come to your own conclusions.

I like the ideas in this and the preceding chapters not only because they work so well but also because of the powerful metamessage they send to your partner. You are in effect saying: "I care so much for you and what we have that I'm willing to do what's hard for me, to tell you what goes on inside of me. I'm also willing to listen to what's going on with you, even when it hurts and even when you talk in anger and exaggerate, and to try to work problems out. I'm willing to apologize when I've wronged or hurt you, and when I say I'll do or not do something, you can count on it. If doing our very best doesn't get us where we want to go, I'm willing to swallow my pride and go with you to see if professional counseling will do the trick." This is a very caring, very loving kind of message, and it can only result in better, more satisfying relationships. Such sentiments are also, I think, the mark of a civilized human being.

CHAPTER FOURTEEN

Touching

I wasn't touched much as a child, even by my mother. My father only touched when he spanked. The result is that I don't touch my wife or kids much. It upsets her, and I'm sure it's not good for the kids. I know touching is good; I like it when they touch me. But it isn't easy. I have to keep reminding myself to touch and hug them.—*Man, 41*

We still have sex sometimes, even though it's difficult because of my medical problems and hers. But touching is the main physical thing we do, touching of all sorts, and it means a lot. It makes us feel close and keeps the loving feelings alive.—*Man, 41*

ALTHOUGH THE WORD *sex* usually conjures up images of genital-to-genital contact, our hands and lips are usually more active in sex than our penises. Hand-to-skin (as well as lip-to-skin) contact usually precedes more explicitly sexual activity. If that touching does not go well, there may not be any further activity. Many women report that if they don't like how a man touches and kisses, they figure they won't like sex with him either and therefore terminate the proceedings then and there. And even during explicitly sexual acts, the hands are usually busy. Touching is crucial if you want to be a good lover. But touching is also important in other ways as well.

Unfortunately, our culture is ambivalent about both sex and touching. Since touching is an integral part of sex, and since we're confused and ambivalent about both activities, it makes sense that we would tend to confuse them. We have sexualized touching to the point where all but the most superficial types of touch (handshakes, pats on the back) are thought to be sexual invitations.

Touching is a vital human need, from infancy through old age. Studies of a wide variety of animals, including humans, have demonstrated that without touching, the animals tend to die in infancy or grow up to be quite peculiar in all respects—and this goes for humans as well.

Although it seems that America has become a more touching society in the last thirty years, it still has a long way to go. And before the last thirty years, there wasn't much touching at all. I've been amazed at how many clients can barely recall even a few instances of physical affection between their parents. As usual, the exceptions prove the point. I have a friend whose parents have always been affectionate. They often hold hands, hug, and touch each other. When other people see this, or hear my friend's report about it, they are amazed. Common reactions are: "They must really be in love," "God, I never saw my parents hug at all," and "I didn't even know if my mom and dad liked each other."

If the child does see his parents touching, it is often followed by embarrassment or by their going off to the bedroom, telling him they don't want to be disturbed. And the media, from which he learns so much, reinforce the message. People hug, then kiss, then they have sex. Slowly but surely, the child acquires the societal understanding about touching: It is sexual.

Boys fare worse in this drama than girls. Females of all ages get more touching than males. Mothers and fathers know the masculine model and fear that too much "mothering" may make sissies of their sons. And even mothers, who are much more in tune with the need for touch than fathers, may fear that their sons may interpret touching as sexual and that this may lead to psychological difficulties. So the boy is weaned early from such "childish" or feminine practices.

Fathers, having lived in a culture that is terrified of affectionate physical contact between males, don't touch their sons much after infancy. Since it is the father the boy will emulate, a powerful lesson is transmitted by this lack of touching. The boy also does not see other males touching.

Boys learn that physical contact is acceptable only in sports, in roughhousing, and in sex. There are no taboos on touching if you are playing football, wrestling, boxing, or in some other way being rough. One cause, as well as result, of this notion can be seen in the way fathers handle their sons. They often seem uncomfortable just holding or cuddling their boys, being more at ease when throwing them around or engaging in mock wrestling bouts. Since roughness is what we learned, it's no surprise that we often show affection by being rough, by wrestling with our lovers and playfully punching our friends. And it's no surprise that we're often rough in sex, less gentle than our partners would like.

The equating of touch and sex also gets in the way of physical contact between both same-sex and other-sex friends. Men who have been friends for twenty years are often afraid to touch one another because that might suggest sexual interest to someone. And to touch a woman friend might be construed as sexual by her, by you, and by God knows who else. The link between sex and physical affection even works to keep lovers from touching each other. Since touching is seen not so much as a thing in itself but as the first step toward intercourse, many people won't touch unless they feel ready and willing to "go all the way."

The taboo on touching except as a part of sex confuses us about what we want and how to get it. Ashley Montagu, author of the classic study *Touching,* says that "it is highly probable that . . . the frenetic preoccupation with sex that characterizes Western culture is in many cases not the expression of a sexual interest at all, but rather a search for the satisfaction of the need for contact."

Because girls are allowed much more freedom to express and explore their desire for physical contact, they learn to differentiate their needs for support, comfort, validation, and connection from the need for sex. In fact, given the way girls are brought up, sex is the one need they have trouble noticing and expressing. Boys, of course, go in the other direction. Wanting sex is legitimate, even encouraged, while wanting to be held or loved is unacceptable.

These needs do not disappear in boys and men. They simply go underground and get reorganized and relabeled. Wanting a hug or to feel close to another sounds too feminine, but wanting sex is the epitome of masculinity, and in sex you can get some of these other things as well. After years of practice, the man just never feels a need for closeness or comfort or support. All he wants is—sex. Whenever he feels something that might be called warm or close or loving, he reads it as indicating a desire for—sex.

While this may seem like a brilliant feat of engineering, the result too often for too many men has been a confusion about what they want and therefore an inability to meet many of their needs. One place where this is especially evident is in relations among men. Many men are realizing that they want something from other men: closeness, understanding, support, and so on. But as soon as they start getting any of these things, they often pull back in fear and sometimes come into therapy to discuss their "latent homosexual feelings." This is especially true of men who have engaged in some physical contact with other men and found it pleasurable. Because of the link between sex and touching in their thinking, they decide that what they really want from other men is sex, and because that is unacceptable to them, they should stay away from any physical contact with men.

What they fail to see is that touching need not be sexual, any more than feelings of love or closeness or caring need be sexual. One can hug or cuddle a man, woman, or child, or even an animal, for that matter, and not have sex.

But can't touching lead to sexual feelings and erections? Of course it can, but that in itself doesn't mean a lot, nor does it imply a necessary course of action. Erections can be caused by lots of things that do not necessarily indicate a desire for sex. Your erection need not run your life. For example, John frequently rode on buses as a teenager. The vibrations of the bus, sometimes combined with adolescent sex fantasies, often produced arousal and erection. Despite the sexy feelings and the erection, John somehow managed to contain himself and never became a bus-fucker!

Even if your feelings about someone are clearly sexual, you don't have to act on them. It is possible for all of us to be turned on by many different people and things. I've talked to men who became aroused and erect while stroking a child or pet, and to some who were aroused while listening to music or watching a sunset. And neither they nor you have to do anything about such events except appreciate and enjoy the good feelings.

It is becoming clear that all of us, men and women, need different things from different people. Men need men as well as women, and many feel incomplete unless they can also relate to people much older as well as those much younger than themselves. It seems a great tragedy if we separate ourselves from those we want to be with because of our fears about what being close and touching imply. They need indicate nothing more than what they obviously are, and I don't mean sex.

Men need physical affection as much as women do, but many men don't get as much as they need. This is partly the result of not knowing when they want touch and partly of not knowing how to get touched even when they know they want it.

Ask yourself if you're getting as much touching—holding, hugging, kissing, cuddling, massaging—as you'd like. Ask your partner the same question. If either of you wants more, you have some work to do.

Touch can do all sorts of things. It's one of the best sources of comfort known to human beings. When you're feeling defeated or crushed, when something terrible has happened, being held or getting a hug won't necessarily solve the problem, but it sure can make you feel better. Some men have trouble accepting a comforting touch or hug, perhaps because it reminds them of when they were small and comforted this way by their mothers. Some men even push women away when the women try to hug or hold them. If you are in this category, you might want to consider accepting a hug next time it is offered. It really can make a difference—it can make you feel you have the other person's support, understanding, and love. Touching can also be a great facilitator of conversation. When someone is talking about something difficult for them, a brief touch on the hand or arm can help them continue.

Touching between parent and child is extremely important. Children need to be touched and hugged, and so do parents. You might want to ask yourself if you're touching your children, whatever their ages, as much as you want and as much as they want. If you think more would be better, why not gradually increase the amount?

THE SECRET OF PLEASURABLE TOUCH (AND SEX AS WELL)

Much of the touching we do, even with lovers, is perfunctory and meaningless. A man kisses his wife as he leaves for work, for example, but his mind is elsewhere and he could just as well be kissing the lamp. Often in sex there's a similar situation. The man is hugging his partner or kissing her, but his mind is on what he hopes will come next, not on what he's doing now.

The only secret to pleasurable touching and sex is to be fully present, to be alive in the moment, even if the moment lasts only a few seconds. The difference is immediately noticeable. When you're really present, the touch means something, no matter how brief it may be. When you're not present . . . well, you're just not present. You can't experience something if you're not there when it happens.

Being present takes no more time than being absent. But to be fair, I need to say that it will take a bit of effort to change how you touch, at least for the first few weeks. If you want, just decide that tomorrow when you kiss your partner good morning or goodbye or whatever, you will focus on what you're doing for the few seconds it takes. Let go of your concerns about work or whatever else may be on your mind by focusing on the feel of your lips on hers or on how your bodies fit together in the hug. Focus on your body, on the sensations and feelings evoked by the touch. And do this with the ideas and exercise offered in the rest of the chapter. In the underground science-fiction classic of some years ago, *Stranger in a Strange Land*, the heroine is asked what she means about Michael's being such a great kisser. Her answer says it all: "Mike doesn't have any technique . . . but when

Mike kisses you he isn't doing *anything* else. You're his whole universe . . . and the moment is eternal because he doesn't have any plans and isn't going anywhere. Just kissing you. It's overwhelming."

SELF-SENSUALITY

Touching oneself can be an important step in becoming a more sensuous person. I know you're not supposed to do this—it's not nice—but you might want to consider it. Taking a warm bath and rubbing yourself gently (or even not so gently) with a washcloth or towel can be a nice way to treat yourself. The same is true for rubbing body lotion or oil onto your hands and arms, legs, or your whole body. You may get aroused while doing this and want to go on to stroking your penis, but it's not necessary.

Touching things can also help develop sensuousness. Many of us don't even notice or experience the objects we touch almost every day. Yet being aware of what we're doing can add to our sensual abilities and yield pleasure. An orange feels different from a peach, leather different from silk or cotton, wood different from vinyl. When you want to, pay attention to what you're touching, touch it in different ways, and allow yourself to experience the sensations.

PROFESSIONAL MASSAGE

One of the nicest things a person can do for himself is get a professional massage. It's relaxing and refreshing. In many other countries, this idea is taken for granted. Athletes and many other people routinely get massages. In America, however, we are so confused about sex and touch that *massage* is often a code word for a blow job or some other sexual activity. Needless to say, when I say *massage* I mean massage and not sex.

If you've never experienced a professional massage, you might want to treat yourself. (This is also a nice gift for someone you care about.) Find yourself a reputable nonsexual masseuse or masseur and make an appointment. If you have any qualms about this, take the shortest appointment he or she gives; for example, a half hour rather than an hour.

An added benefit to professional massages is that it can help increase your awareness of the possibilities of touch. You can transfer this knowledge to touching yourself and your partner. I'm not implying, by the way, that you need to become an expert at massage or that you should mainly be a student when you get a professional massage. The main thing to do is experience and enjoy, but you'll learn anyway, without even trying.

BEING AFFECTIONATE WITH A PARTNER

There are many ways of touching your partner. Holding hands while walking or sitting in a theater is always nice, as are a brief touch of her shoulder or arm as you pass her chair, lightly touching or holding her face during a close moment, and squeezing her thigh in the car or at the dining table. Here are some other ideas.

Hugging and Holding

If you and your partner agree there should be more hugging and holding, just get to it. Every day devote a few moments to holding one another. It will help if the two of you have a brief talk in which the ground rules are established. The most important thing is that both of you understand that touching need not lead to sex. Each of you should feel free to touch when you want without feeling that you may therefore be required to do something that you're not in the mood for.

There's nothing wrong with going on to sex if both of you agree that's what you want to do, but there's also nothing wrong with just touching.

Scratching

Scratching isn't a very sexy or sensual term, but many people enjoy having their backs and other places scratched, and this is a nice thing lovers can do for each other.

Touching Your Partner's "Things"

No, I don't mean those things! What I have in mind here are items like her clothes and her hair. Hugging or touching her when she's wearing a silk shirt or dress is different than touching when she's wearing something else or nothing. Pay attention, and you'll notice and experience the differences. And what about her hair? Have you ever really touched and stroked it, just to experience the feel of it? If not, why not give it a try? Many women have told me it's a treat when their lovers brush their hair for them. You might want to consider doing this if your partner is up for it.

Washing Your Partner

Being bathed caringly is something all of us experienced as children, and we took it as a loving act. Unfortunately, many of us never got to experience that again. What about washing your partner slowly and lovingly while you're in the shower or tub and having her do the same for you? If you want to go all out, you can do it just as it is done for children. One of you, let's say it's you, runs the bath and maybe adds bubble bath or lotion as well. Then slowly and with care you wash her. After that you dry her, maybe also applying powder or lotion. Keep in mind that getting clean is only the secondary purpose of the bath; showing care and love is the primary one.

A Slow Hand, and a Gentle One as Well

Women routinely complain that men are too hurried and too rough in their touching. If you believe this complaint might apply to you, you can consider what you want to do about it. For most people, the kinds of touch that convey love, support, closeness, and understanding are gentle and slow. This is not to say there aren't times when a quick or firm touch isn't appropriate. But most of the time, soft and slow is where it's at. You have nothing to lose by starting out this way.

Body Rubs

A body rub is simply you touching, stroking, or massaging some or all of your partner's body (except for the genitals). There are two basic formats. In one, you touch her for your own pleasure; she will intervene only to let you know she doesn't like what you're doing. In the other format, she touches you as you direct her to, but you don't touch her back. Many men have trouble with this one, because it involves a more passive role than they are accustomed to. Aside from giving oral instructions, however, you're just supposed to lie back and enjoy the stimulation. You may find that you're also touching her. Try to resist that impulse. Most of us men are already good at being active. We need to learn also to be more passive, just to accept pleasure without giving anything in return at the moment.

I have found that body rubs work best if they are not considered medicinal—that is, if they aren't the deep muscle manipulation that often goes under the name massage and is usually used for muscular aches and pains. If you want your partner to massage your sore shoulder, that's fine, but it's not a body rub.

If you have a sexual problem, body rubs are an excellent first step to take before you begin the partner exercises to resolve the problems that are described in Chapters 20 and 22. They are also an excellent first step in learning how to be comfortable in telling your partner how you like to be stimulated.

EXERCISE 14-1: NONGENITAL BODY RUBS

In both steps of this exercise, one of you gives a light, stroking body rub to the other for 15 to 20 minutes. How light depends on individual preferences, but you should avoid the heavy, kneading type of rubbing usually done for sore muscles and in some kinds of massage.

You will need a warm room, a comfortable place for the receiver to sit or lie, and a lubricant (skin lotion, massage oil, or talcum powder).

First you must decide who will give and who will receive in a given session. The receiver is not to touch or do anything else to or for the giver, except as specified in the instructions.

Since the receiver may not feel like doing anything active after the session, it's best not to plan to have two sessions back to back. Wait at least half an hour between sessions.

One goal of both steps is to allow you to experience touching and being touched without any other ends in mind. The giver should focus on touching and the receiver on the sensations produced by being touched.

The other goal is for both of you to make each experience as positive—relaxing, pleasant, pleasurable—as possible. *Sexual arousal is not the goal of this exercise.* It sometimes happens, and it's fine if it does, but that's not what we're looking for. The exercise is not a prelude to anything. It is simply what it is.

In each step there is a clearly designated giver and receiver, with different roles to play. These distinctions are important and should be adhered to. After each step, spend a few minutes talking about what the experience was like for each of you. Say what you liked most and least about it, what the main feeling was, and also indicate any difficulties you experienced. This talking is useful for learning how to communicate better about physical preferences; include it after every session, and be as specific as possible.

Step A: The receiver, the one who is going to be touched, is in complete control. He asks for the body rub and gives directions on how and where he wants to be touched. The giver simply follows the directions.

The receiver should use this opportunity to discover what kinds of touching he most enjoys. You can ask for anything at all except genital touching. Try new things and places even if you aren't sure you will enjoy them. If you've ever wondered how it would feel to have the areas between your toes touched, or the backs of your knees, or anything else, now is the time to find out. Make sure you are getting precisely what you want, no matter how many times you have to explain or demonstrate to the giver.

Since fifteen to twenty minutes isn't enough time to do a whole body, you should focus on one area, such as face or feet or perhaps your whole front, from scalp to toes. Take your time and get into the sensations. The receiver is the one who calls time.

The giver should do everything that is asked so long as it is not obnoxious or uncomfortable for her. She should feel free to ask for more specific instructions if needed.

Step B: The giver initiates the exercise and touches, strokes, and rubs his partner for his own pleasure, doing whatever he wants. The receiver should accept what is done without comment unless there is discomfort or pain, in which case she should ask the giver to do something else.

The giver should use this opportunity to explore his partner's body with different types of touch, pressure, and rhythm. Touch where and how you want to *for your own pleasure.* It's important *not* to try to give the receiver a good time or to turn her on. Give yourself a good time. I emphasize this point because many men have trouble with it, focusing their efforts on giving the partner a good time rather than themselves. Do whatever is necessary to follow the directions.

Spend no more than twenty minutes on this. The giver is the one who calls time.

When time is up, remember to face each other and give a few moments of feedback to your partner on what the experience was like for you.

After you have done the body rubs a few times as they are described, feel free to experiment. Some couples make them a regular part of their lives, a treat to be enjoyed when they have a few minutes free and want something physical but not sexual. Some couples use them as a means of stress management because they find getting a body rub is a wonderful way to relax. Some couples use them as a transition activity that takes them from work or chores to sexual activity. The body rub helps them let go of what they were doing before and helps open them up to an erotic experience. And many people find that what they learn in doing body rubs—giving directions regarding the physical stimulation they want, accepting and focusing in on physical stimulation without doing anything in return at the moment, following a partner's directions for desired stimulation, and touching a partner for one's own pleasure—transfers quite nicely and easily to more erotic activities.

I am not prescribing touching as a panacea for all your ills or as a compulsory ritual that should be followed whether you like it or not. Rather, I see touching as a very important human need, one you should be free to fulfill in ways and with people of your own choosing. It won't change the world and it won't solve all your problems, but it will probably make you feel better and bring you closer to the people you love. Men need touching as much as anyone else, and there is no good reason to deprive yourself in this area.

Get in touch with those you care for. Stay in touch. Literally.

CHAPTER FIFTEEN

Sexual Arousal

Being turned on is the best feeling in the world. It's even better than orgasm because orgasm is an ending while turn-on is a beginning. Makes me feel totally alive and awake.—*Man, 34*

I think arousal is what it's all about. I love feeling sexually excited and I love my partner feeling it. Her turn-on pushes mine even higher and mine does the same for hers. It's an incredible spiral of greater and greater passion. —*Man, 46*

WHEN PEOPLE TALK about "getting it up" in regard to sex, they usually mean the man's getting his penis up. But there is another kind of getting it up that is more important for men, and women too. I'm referring to getting your arousal up. Arousal, a feeling that is also called *excitement, passion, lust, turn-on,* and *horniness,* is what powers erections in men, lubrication in women, and orgasm in both. Arousal is also most of what makes for a sexual experience that feels really good.

EXACTLY WHAT IS AROUSAL?

Arousal is like love; even though we know what each one is, neither is easy to define. Let's start with what arousal is not. It definitely is not the same as the overwhelming excitement described in the popular media, which can make all of us feel inadequate. Even at the peak of passion, few human beings have felt that their bones were melting, or that they were floating in paradise, or that they were experiencing a tidal wave of unbearable pleasure. Arousal is also not the same as an intellectual interest in sex. For example, if you say to yourself, "Gee, it's been six weeks since I had sex," but don't feel any excitement, you're not aroused.

Although *desire for sex* and *turn-on* are often used synonymously, clarity is served by making a distinction between them. I use *desire* to mean wanting to have sex. It's easy to understand wanting sex when you're already aroused. But it doesn't have to be this way. You could also want to have sex for other reasons. Perhaps your partner gets irritable and provokes a fight unless she has sex twice a week. Since she's starting to get irritable and you want to avoid a fight, you initiate sex. But what you really desire is to avoid trouble; having sex is merely the means to this end. There are men and women who want lots of sex even though they have trouble getting aroused. One reason for their high desire is the hope that if they keep working at it, they'll figure out how to get turned on.

It also works the other way. There are people who get easily and highly aroused in sex but don't want much of it. This sounds strange but really isn't. A man in this category may feel that sex is a distraction from other things—usually work—that have a higher priority. Or he may believe that too much lovemaking makes him more committed or vulnerable than he wants to be.

I use *desire* to mean only that you have an interest in sex, whether or not you're aroused. A high level of desire simply means you want sex a lot. Arousal, on the other hand, is how high you get when you anticipate sex or engage in it.

The most important thing arousal is *not* is an erection. The two often go together—arousal is usually what makes your penis get hard—but they are best thought of as separate. You may, for instance, wake up in the morning with an erection but without any excitement. That means only that you have an erection and are not turned on. And just as it's possible to have an erection without being aroused, it's also possible to be very sexually aroused and not have an erection (because fear, anger, another feeling, or a medical condition is getting in the way). Some men with erection problems say that erections accompanied by lust feel different from those without the feelings. When there's no turn-on, the erection seems like an anomaly, not at all connected to you. When there's an erection and arousal, you feel more connected to your penis; it's part of who you are as a total person at the moment. If you want to keep sex as good as possible and prevent erection problems, don't attempt to use your penis unless you are turned on. If you are already having trouble with erections, this becomes an absolute rule.

Let's go to what arousal is. Above all, it has to do with things you sense and feel. One way of looking at it is that your body (and mind) is on, as in "all systems go." One man put it this way: "My heart was racing, my body was tingling, and I was raring to go"—not as extreme as having your bones melt, but pleasurable nonetheless. Terms frequently used to describe arousal, aside from the synonyms already given, include *warmth* or *heat* (as in "I was hot"), *tingling, blood rushing, heart pounding, wild, wanting to have her,* or *to touch her* or *to be inside her.* Arousal is almost always described in positive ways; it feels good. Think of an activity in your life that excites you: skiing, tennis, running, sex, closing an important deal, or whatever. Then recall a specific example of that activity when you were even more excited than usual. Take a moment or two to get into the details of how you felt. It's as if you're all fired up, your attention is narrowly focused, the blood is rushing through you, and you feel fully alive and terrific. That's what I mean when I say *arousal* or *turn-on,* even though we're talking about the high end. I wouldn't expect that you'd be that aroused every time you went skiing or had sex. But the extreme does offer a good way of defining the idea for yourself.

I hope you don't get upset if you discover that you get most excited by something other than sex. That's not unusual. You may never get as wild in sex as when you learned you were accepted by the college of your choice or as you do when closing a million-dollar deal. But if you feel your sexual arousal is not as high as it could be, you can do something about it.

Now recall a time when you were very sexually aroused. You were really hot for it and really into it. You could feel it in your pelvis (whether or not you had an erection) and elsewhere, maybe in your heart or stomach. This is what we're talking about.

When people are highly aroused, they are narrowly focused. Their attention is devoted to what they're doing and going to do. So one way of telling how aroused you are is by asking how distracted you are by extraneous matters. A person who's distracted in sex by common outside noises (barking dogs, backfiring cars, the normal creaking of houses, and so on) is probably not very aroused. A person who's repelled or disgusted by a partner's varicose veins, or hair in a place he doesn't think there should be hair, or similar items is probably not very aroused. When you're excited, you either don't notice these things or they don't bother you much because you're too focused on something else.

RATING YOUR DEGREE OF AROUSAL

Although not necessary, it can be helpful to learn to rate your degree of arousal. The best way I know to do this is to recall the time when you felt most excited in sex, whether it was last night, last week, or twenty years ago. Try to recall exactly how exciting that was. And assign that degree of excitement a 10. At the other end of the scale we need a 0, a time when you felt no arousal at all. Any occasion when you weren't thinking about sex or having any sexual feeling will do.

Now you have anchored your scale at both ends. You might want to assess your average degree of arousal in sex. Go over in your mind the last three or four times you had sex and rate your arousal for each. This can be a bit tricky, because your arousal probably varied during each experience. The most intense feeling was during or just before orgasm. A good way around this is *not* to include orgasm or the seconds just before it. Rate arousal based on how you felt before orgasm was imminent.

If your usual arousal is less than 7 on a scale of 10, and certainly if it's less than 6, you might want to consider following some of the suggestions in this chapter. If your arousal is generally 5 or less, you should definitely attend to them. There's an excellent chance you can increase your excitement and enjoy sex more.

One wonderful feature of arousal is that it is responsive to direct effort; it's fine to work on increasing it, to try to make it higher. I mentioned earlier that trying to get and maintain erections can lead to problems. There's too much pressure put on the penis, and its response may be the opposite of what you want. In general, however, this danger does not exist with arousal. So feel free to focus on arousal during sex and at other times and to consider what might intensify it. The more you can work on increasing and enjoying arousal during sex, and the less you try to force your penis to do anything, the more fun you'll have and the more functional you'll be.

I now turn to some ways of increasing arousal, all of which work for some men. You should read them over and experiment with those that seem relevant to you.

MAINTAINING AN ONGOING EROTIC CONNECTION

I discussed the importance of an ongoing erotic connection between you and your sweetheart in Chapter 8. If you have sex regularly, talk about it regularly, and touch in sexual ways regularly, this will do wonders for your arousal, and your partner's as well. This is a very powerful practice.

CONDITIONS

As mentioned in Chapter 6, determining and meeting your conditions is essential. Certain conditions will allow higher arousal than others, and the absence of these conditions may make arousal impossible. It will pay you to do the conditions exercise in Chapter 6 if you haven't already done so.

Randy, for example, had been badly stung by the derogatory remarks his ex-wife had made about his masculinity and sexual abilities around the time of their divorce, and so he was wary about getting serious with another woman. At the same time, however, he sought women's company and their bodies. But either he had difficulty getting an erection or he ejaculated very quickly. It soon become clear that he was very tense with these women, whom he saw only once or twice, and not the slightest bit aroused. This is not a good foundation for enjoyable or even functional sex. As we did the conditions exercise, he realized that in order to get aroused, he needed at least three things: to be less tense with a partner (which necessitated knowing her much longer than a few hours), to like and be attracted to her, and not to feel such tremendous pressure to prove that his wife was wrong about his sexual prowess. It took several months to meet these conditions, but once that happened he started enjoying sex again.

GETTING THE BEST PHYSICAL STIMULATION

One of your conditions may be getting certain types of physical stimulation. If so, it's important that you be able to express what you want.

First, however, you may need to find out what you want. Many men have little idea of what they like in sex and dismiss the question with a blanket "It all feels good." If you think it all feels the same, you can do a lot to improve your sex life by challenging that notion. The problem, I think, is that we men are so busy performing that many of us haven't taken the time to determine what pleasures us the most. If you want to find out more about what feels best to you, get your partner to do different things. You can also try touching yourself in different ways during masturbation. Focus in on the sensations and see how you feel. That's all there is to it. Doing this over a period of weeks will give you more information about what you like.

However you discover what you like, you may still need to express your desires to your partner. Even if she was there when you realized you like her to hold your balls when she strokes your penis and during intercourse, this does not mean she's going to know you want her to hold your balls right now or that she should hold them tighter. Only you can let her know. Rereading the chapter on assertiveness will help you be more forthcoming about your desires.

If you already know what kinds of stimulation you like, you might want to consider showing her. This is often more effective than simply telling her. The kissing seminar exercise (page 171) will give you some pointers. Another possibility, if you're comfortable with the idea, is to masturbate in her presence so she can see how you like to be touched.

The most important suggestion for expressing your desires is to put it positively and avoid the impression of blaming your partner for not doing it right. In other words, say what you want, not what you don't want. The following will definitely *not* work: "That's too light. I've told you I want a firmer touch. Why can't you remember?" Here's a better way: "A little harder . . . harder yet . . . that's it, just like that, feels great." This will be even more effective if you reinforce it later, after sex is over, with a comment like this: "I really enjoyed the stronger touch today. Thanks."

Try not to assume that she'll remember what you want the next time. If she doesn't, there's no need to get upset. Not doing it just right does not mean she didn't listen or doesn't care. More likely it means only that it's difficult for her to change her habitual way of touching. Just remind her by saying "harder" again. You may need to do this many, many times.

Men and women I know who are good lovers give feedback like this all the time, even to partners they've had for many years. It's no big deal to them, just an integral part of lovemaking and getting exactly what they want.

FOCUSING ON SENSATION

In talking to thousands of people over the years about what they think about during sex, it's clear that many of them are light-years away from what's going on and are thinking about work, tomorrow's schedule, or sports. In general, not focusing on what's going on will decrease arousal and make sex less enjoyable. Focusing, on the other hand, will amplify the sensations, make them feel better and more intense, and increase arousal.

Focusing on sensation means exactly that. You put your attention in your body where the action is. When you're kissing, keep your mind in your lips. This is *not* the same as thinking about your lips or the kiss; just put your attention in your lips. When your partner is touching a part of you, put your attention in that part. When your penis is being touched or when you are having intercourse, put your attention inside your penis; be aware of the fit between the penis and whatever is around it, pressure, texture, temperature, and wetness.

I have noticed that when I ask men to focus, some of them screw up their faces and grit their teeth. They're working very hard. When I ask about this, they usually say this is how they concentrate. Focusing need not and should not be hard work. The tension generated by trying too hard does not help. See if you can focus in a relaxed way, with no pushing or shoving—just gently moving your mind, your attention, to where you want it.

A problem with focusing is that our minds tend to wander. There is no cure for wandering minds—that's what minds do—but practice will help yours wander less often. What you need to do is gently bring your attention back to where it belongs as soon as you're aware that it has drifted off.

Some men find it helpful to move back and forth between focusing on sensation and focusing on a fantasy. That's fine and often very arousing. You can also shift between focusing on sensations and focusing on feelings. You may be aware of how good it feels when your partner is touching your penis and then may shift into focusing on your feelings of love for her. That's fine, too.

EXPRESSING COMPLAINTS AND CONCERNS

Sex therapist Bernard Apfelbaum makes the important point that in sex we all try to be as positive as possible and to cover up any complaints or problems. If it doesn't feel good kissing your partner because she has bad breath, we try to ignore the odor and continue with the kissing. If we feel pressured by our partners to have erections, we do almost anything to avoid telling her about this.

Apfelbaum goes on to say that expressing the negative feelings— doubts, fears, concerns, complaints—can be very liberating. It can allow you to feel more in control of your life and to get more aroused. It is important, of course, that what you say be put in a way that will be possible for your partner to hear. Blaming and accusing statements will cause trouble and decrease everyone's sexual arousal.

One man I saw with erection problems was making progress by refocusing on sensation when he started to feel anxious in sex. Then I suggested the effectiveness of this strategy could be increased if he also told his partner about the anxiety when he felt it. His report about it is instructive.

> I used to internalize the anxiety. But keeping it inside seemed to make it stronger. Tuesday I externalized it by telling her, and it was amazing. I felt free of it, and it was easy to refocus on sensation. My penis behaved like a champ. I like this idea and will continue with it. It makes me feel more in charge of what's going on.

That may seem too easy, because although he was expressing a concern, it was about his own anxiety and wasn't in any way critical of his partner. So let's take a more difficult example, your sense of pressure from her to get an erection. Whether or not the pressure is truly coming from her, what you know is that you feel some urgency coming from somewhere that you get hard, and this is making you anxious. Here's a way you might express it, in this illustration when you're not in the middle of sex: "Ever since I failed to get hard on our trip, I've felt tremendous pressure to have an erection when we're in bed. It makes me tense and I can't even pay attention to what we're doing. I know a lot of it comes from me. I feel rotten about disappointing you and not doing my part. But lately I feel that some of this pressure is coming from you. My impression is that you're as tense as I am and it's like you're demanding that I get hard. That's how it feels when you're using your hand on me. Is there anything to what I'm feeling?"

There's probably a good chance she'll agree with your impression. It makes sense that she'd be feeling anxious. She wants the problem resolved and, perhaps more important, she doesn't want to feel that you're not hard because you aren't turned on by her or that she's not stimulating you in the best way. If this is the case, the two of you are now in a position to decide what to do to relieve the tension.

EXPRESSING PLEASURE

While expressing concerns can clear the way to feeling more arousal, expressing pleasure with words, sounds, and movements can amplify the good feelings and get you more turned on. It will probably also excite your partner, and her increased passion will undoubtedly do the same for you. I discuss this issue in detail in Chapter 10, so I will do no more than under-score it here as a means of increasing arousal. The more you express your excitement and pleasure, the more turned on you will feel.

LOCATION, LOCATION, LOCATION

One of the easiest ways to increase arousal is to have sex in different loca-tions. Sure, the bed is nice and comfortable and it's also where people are supposed to make love, but it can get boring if you never take a vacation from it. What about sex on the living room or den floor, in the hallway, or in some other room? In the shower or a walk-in closet? On the desk in the den, or even at night on the desk at work? Or with one of you sitting on the washer or dryer while it's on spin cycle, or with one of you on the kitchen or bathroom counter? You could also try sex in the car or van.

Wherever you can lie, sit down, or bend over, or one of you can get a tongue or hand on the other's genitals, that's a good place to consider. Sex in different locations gives a sense of variety and adventure and is usually a huge turn-on. Sex in unusual places is worth doing even if the actual act isn't as great as it would be in a more familiar and comfortable setting. For example, although a favorite fantasy for lots of people is sex on a beach or in a meadow, the reality is often uncomfortable. You may well end up with sand or dirt in your orifices and mosquito bites all over you. But even when that happens, people fondly recall the memory years later.

SIMMERING

Virtually all of us, including many who say they aren't turned on very much, experience surges of sexual energy during the day. Unfortunately, we don't do anything with these feelings. But why let these bursts of sexual arousal disappear? Why not use them? Here is a simple but effective tech-nique that sex therapist Carol Ellison and I developed some years ago. It's a way of hanging on to and developing your spontaneous sexual urges through the day, which can result in more arousal and better sex.

EXERCISE 15-1: SIMMERING

Time Required: A few minutes a day

The next time you're aware of a sexual feeling, hang on to it for a few seconds. Get into the experience by imagining what you'd like to do with that woman you see on the street or on TV, or by recalling in greater detail that fantasy or memory of a good experience. Whatever you're imagining, get into it. Imagine the touch of her lips, hands, breasts, vagina, or whatever. Feel the texture, the temperature, the way your bodies connect. In other words, run your own X-rated movie of what you want to do. Continue this for a few seconds, or even longer if you prefer. Then let the image fade away.

An hour or two later, close your eyes and get back into the image again for a few seconds. You can imagine exactly what you did the first time or change the experience any way you like.

Continue in this way every hour or two during the day, whenever you have a few spare seconds.

One way to enhance the simmering is to do a few Kegels (see page 214) while you're imagining your scene.

The last step in the simmering exercise is to incorporate your real partner in the fantasy if she's not already included. You can do this when you're on the way to meet her—say, driving back home from work. Start the imagery with what you'd like to be doing with the person who started the simmering, then fade her out and put your partner into the fantasy. Might you enjoy doing the same things or something similar with her? Develop this idea any way you like. When you get home with your partner, you'll probably be highly aroused and ready for a good time.

Unless your partner is almost always ready for sex—which probably means she already knows about simmering—it's smart to include her in your thinking. A short phone call is all that's required. This way you'll both be ready to go when you get together, or at least you'll be aware of what obstacles may exist.

Simmering should become a regular part of your life. People who consider themselves sexy and have good sex lives do it all the time. It does not get in the way of doing your work or interfere in any way with your life. But it does make you feel good and keeps your sexual feelings flowing, ready to blossom when the time is right.

If you find that you don't have many surges of sexual energy to simmer with, carry around a small notebook or some index cards in your pocket for a week or two and write down each instance of such an impulse (rating it on a scale of 0 to 10) and the stimulus. An example would be: "10 A.M., Mon., 7, tall redhead in store." Almost every man I've worked with who has done this for a week or more discovered that he was indeed having sexual impulses. He just hadn't been paying attention before.

USING FANTASY

Simmering is one way of using fantasy to increase arousal. But there is at least one other important way: fantasizing during sex with a partner, something many people do. The fantasies can increase arousal and therefore help maintain erections and intensify orgasms.

If you haven't been fantasizing during sex, you might want to try it. Whenever it feels appropriate or useful, conjure up in your mind an especially arousing image and stay with it as long as you like. For further information about sexual fantasies and their use, read the rest of this chapter and also Chapter 5.

USING EROTIC MATERIALS

There are a number of erotic materials that can help increase arousal. These include magazines such as *Playboy* and *Penthouse*, popular and pornographic novels, and R- and X-rated videos for the VCR.

Even if your initial feeling about erotica is negative, you might want to give it a try. Many people who thought they couldn't stand reading or looking at this stuff found out that they got turned on anyway. The question of why this is so need not detain us here. The point is simply that reading, viewing, or listening to erotic materials can increase your arousal.

But, as with everything else, it's important to let common sense be your guide. If you always use these materials, they will themselves become boring. And if your partner is new to them or shy about them, you need to take her feelings into account and proceed slowly and only with her permission. You would certainly do well to start with the softest-core stuff and not with the raunchiest. A selection from a romance novel or D. H. Lawrence may do more for her, and be more acceptable, than a hard-driving pornographic account. There are now also many collections of erotica written by women, and erotic films made by women, that may be more to her taste, and perhaps yours as well.

Many women are more turned on by love than sex, so love poems and literature may be a more promising field to explore for the purpose of arousing your partner. Her greater excitement may well have the effect of turning you on more. And if you're willing to check out the kinds of things that arouse her, she may be more willing to explore those that do the same for you.

ROLE-PLAYING

One very powerful way of increasing arousal is through role-playing or the acting out of fantasies.

Many years ago I was involved with a woman who sometimes would drop into a role in the middle of sex. She would suddenly say something like, "You haven't been a good boy today, so you're not going to get any." Since what we can't have is infinitely more exciting than what we can, my passion immediately skyrocketed, even though I knew she was only acting. I fell into step and would start apologizing and begging. She would repeat her refusal and give in gradually. "Well, okay, since you apologized, you can touch my pussy, but that's it. Just a touch." This would progress through steps including "You can put it in but only halfway. Not an inch further" and "Okay, your behavior is getting better, so you can put it all the way in, but no moving at all." It seems ridiculous on the written page, but I assure you the effect was real and powerful.

There are infinite possibilities as to what roles or games to play. You can get ideas from erotic literature, movies, and your own fantasies.

There is one common kind of role-playing that deserves special mention. When one person (let's say it's your partner) pretends to resist—to not want to have sex or engage in a certain activity—it is crucial that certain rules and signals be worked out beforehand and strictly adhered to. She has to know in her gut that if she really means *no, stop,* or *not yet,* and expresses it, you will understand and immediately comply. Trust has to be taken for granted.

Don't ignore your own fantasies. I find that many men are quite creative in their own minds but don't follow up on their ideas for a number of reasons. If your mind throws you an idea that really turns you on, consider it. If it is not likely to harm you or your partner and not against either of your values, maybe there's some way you could try it out.

I recall one man who got very aroused by fantasies of having sex on an airplane on one of the frequent trips he and his lover took. He hadn't thought about putting it into practice, because he couldn't figure out how both of them, being large people, could even fit into the toilet on a 747, let alone do anything there. After he finally mentioned the fantasy to me, I asked why it had to be in the toilet. His incredulous response was, "In the aisle?" No, not in the aisle; that would get him arrested. But on the night flights they frequently took, there are usually rows of empty seats, and you can move the armrests out of the way. The session ended on that note and nothing more was said about the matter for a month. But when they returned from a cross-country flight, they happily reported that the armrests could indeed be moved. They haven't yet managed intercourse, but they did some other interesting things and were pleased.

RESISTANCE, FEAR, AND UNCERTAINTY

Some degree of resistance can heighten arousal (and desire as well). One problem in long relationships is that sex is too easy. You can pretty much have it when and how you want. Although this is convenient, it can lead to boredom. Contrast this to the situation most of us were in when we were younger and dating. There was resistance from our family and society (you're not supposed to be doing this) and maybe from a partner as well (we shouldn't be doing this yet). Most people agree that such resistance increased arousal.

This is why being sexual where you're not supposed to be (say in the bedroom next to your parents' when you and your girlfriend are visiting them, or in a public place like a parking lot or an airplane) is so exciting. This is also why role-playing where your partner pretends to be uninterested or resistant in some way can be so exciting. Violating prohibitions and overcoming obstacles make our blood boil, so to speak.

Uncertainty plays a role as well. In the role-playing example I gave above, for example, my partner was pretending to resist, one result of which was that I wasn't sure how far I would actually get. The lack of certainty helped drive my arousal up off the charts.

Anxiety can also heighten passion. Although anxiety can have serious negative consequences for sexual functioning, at least one kind of fear— the fear of being discovered—can actually make us more aroused. This plays a part when we have sex in public places. You have to be careful with this, of course. If you have sex in a bedroom or bathroom of someone else's home where a party is going on and are discovered, you will have to live with the consequences. But if you can lock the door and make sure no one knows for certain what you're doing, you may find your arousal breaks all your records.

One couple I interviewed regularly used resistance, uncertainty, and fear of discovery to enhance their lovemaking. Whenever they went to a party, for example, they'd look for a room—bathroom, bedroom, pantry, basement— where they could have a quickie. They dressed appropriately, with clothes that allowed easy access to the genitals and usually with neither of them wearing underwear. Once in the room of their choice, they'd do a role-play. A favorite scene was where they pretended they were strangers and he was trying to seduce her while she resisted (and sometimes they reversed roles; she came on to him but he was reluctant because his "wife" was in the next room). To heighten what was already a very high turn-on, either or both might say that they thought they heard someone coming, someone turning the doorknob, the door opening slightly, and so on. This may or may not be your cup of tea, but I know this couple has had a passionate sex life through their twenty-two years of marriage and neither one has had an affair.

ENHANCING ORGASM

Since orgasm is just the extreme form of arousal, everything in this chapter can help make it more intense.

If you believe your orgasms aren't as exciting as they could be, if they are significantly more intense with masturbation than in partner sex, or if a partner has mentioned that you seem unexpressive or to be holding yourself back, be aware of what you're doing the next few times you orgasm. Some men do seem to be keeping themselves in check by restricting their breathing, movements, and sounds. If this is true of you and you want to do something about it, start letting yourself be a bit more expressive. Focus on the pleasurable sensations and let your body move as it desires, let yourself breathe (very important under any circumstances), and let some sounds come out. Don't try to let go of all your controls at once. Make small changes in one area at a time. If embarrassment is an issue, you might want to start being more expressive in masturbation before you do so with a partner. Gradually relax more of your controls and see if you experience fuller orgasms.

Another method for increasing orgasm intensity (and sexual feeling in general) is by strengthening the pelvic muscles by doing Kegel exercises, named for the man who invented them. I have been using this exercise with clients for almost twenty years and have received numerous reports of greater sensation in the pelvis (including the penis), greater desire and arousal, and more powerful orgasms.

EXERCISE 15-2: KEGELS

Time Required: A few minutes a day

First you need to get in touch with your pelvic muscles. The best way of doing this is to pretend you are in danger of urinating or having a bowel movement but that you need to control this until you can reach a toilet. The muscles you squeeze to hold things in are the ones we are interested in.

The exercise itself is quite simple. Start by squeezing and releasing the muscles fifteen times, twice each day. Don't hold the contraction; just squeeze and let go. At first you may also be squeezing your stomach and thigh muscles. A few days of practice should allow you to isolate the pelvic muscles and squeeze only them. You can do the exercise unobtrusively anywhere: while driving a car, watching TV, reading the paper, during a meeting, and so on. It works best if you pair the exercise with something you do every day—for example, doing Kegels each time you get on the freeway ramp or each time you read the paper. That way you'll automatically do them whenever the event occurs.

Gradually increase the number of squeezes until you're doing about seventy-five, two times each day.

When you reach that number, you may want to do a variation: Instead of immediately releasing the contraction, hold it for a count of three, then relax and repeat. These are a bit more difficult. Work up to about fifty of these long Kegels. If you like, you can do one set of short Kegels and one set of long Kegels each day.

Continue doing Kegels for at least six weeks. Results usually aren't noticeable for a month or more. As you continue with them, they will become automatic and require no conscious attention or effort.

Squeezing your pelvic muscles when you're having an erotic fantasy, when you're being sexually stimulated, and when you're having intercourse can increase pelvic sensation and help turn you on. Some men have reported squeezing and holding the contraction just before orgasm. They say it holds off orgasm for a few seconds and makes it more powerful. Feel free to experiment as you see fit.

More than anything else, arousal is what drives good sex. It *is* the spark. It is also the cornerstone of a sexuality based on pleasure rather than on performance. If you want more exciting and more satisfying sex, go for greater arousal.

CHAPTER SIXTEEN

Sexually Stimulating a Woman

THIS CHAPTER IS my response to the requests of many clients and workshop participants and also letters and e-mails from a number of men who asked for more explicit information on sexually stimulating their partners. I can't cover everything here, but the feedback I received suggests the following ideas were helpful. In other places in the book I have talked about kissing and hugging. This chapter focuses primarily on genital stimulation.

FEMALE SEXUAL ANATOMY AND RESPONSE

First, let's check out the territory. Although male and female genitals develop from the same basic structures, they end up looking quite different. The external genitalia of a woman are illustrated in Figure 7. Of course, women's genitals, just like men's, differ in many ways—size, color, placement—but the figure will do for our purposes.

The clitoris is unique in having no function other than giving sexual pleasure. Men have nothing quite like it, since the penis also serves as an organ of elimination. Aside from that, however, the penis and clitoris are similar. Even though the exposed part of the clitoris is small, it is as richly

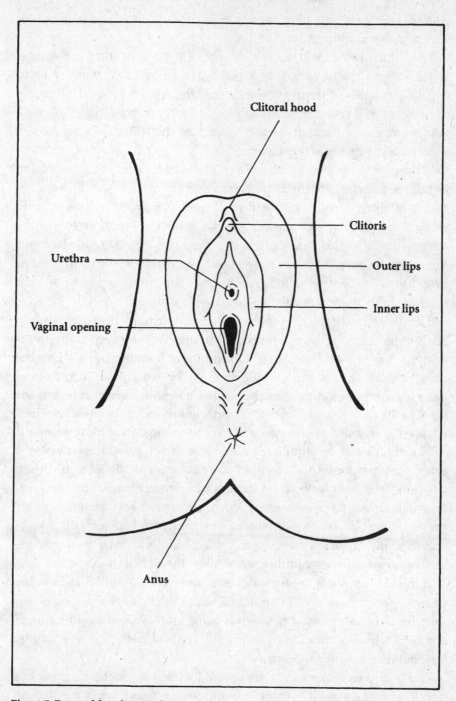

Figure 7: External female genitals

endowed with nerve endings as the head of your penis and is therefore very sensitive to stimulation.

The clitoris is for most women the site of their most intense pleasure. When women masturbate, they typically do so by rubbing the clitoris, which is so sensitive in many women that they prefer stimulation to the right or left of it rather than actually on it. Rarely do they insert anything into the vagina. By now it is widely accepted that clitoral stimulation is what leads to orgasm in most women.

Some men don't like this idea. They, like Freud, believe that the vagina should be the core of female pleasure and that women should have orgasms in intercourse, just like men. Freud thought that in a mature woman the sensitivity of the clitoris was somehow "transferred" to the vagina. Just how this magical transfer was supposed to take place was something he never bothered to spell out. But his theory was sufficient to make many women feel inadequate because this metamorphosis did not occur and they could not have so-called vaginal orgasms.

The clitoris rarely gets direct stimulation in intercourse. It is difficult for a penis to be in the vagina and touching the clitoris at the same time. To accomplish this in most positions would require an L-shaped penis, which became extinct at the same time as the dodo. As the penis moves in and out of the vagina, however, it tugs on the vaginal lips, which are attached to the hood of the clitoris, and therefore provides indirect stimulation to the clitoris. But this stimulation is insufficient to produce orgasm in most women.

The clitoris can be stimulated in a more direct fashion by rubbing it against the man's pubic bone. This can be achieved in the woman-on-top position if she leans forward far enough and also in the man-on-top position if the man positions himself high enough so that his pubic bone presses against his lover's clitoral area. However, such contact is often difficult to maintain during intercourse. Even if maintained, it does not necessarily provide sufficient stimulation to allow the woman to orgasm.

If the woman wants to orgasm in intercourse, one option is to have her or her lover stimulate her clitoral area with a finger or two during penile thrusting. No matter what position is being employed, someone's fingers are usually free for this. Doing it this way is a lot easier and usually more efficient than any other alternatives.

The outer lips of the vagina are covered with pubic hair. The inner lips are closer to the vaginal opening and are usually closed. When the woman spreads her legs, they part, exposing the urethra and vaginal opening. Both the outer and inner lips are sensitive to touch in most women, although such stimulation in itself is unlikely to produce orgasm.

Although I've already made a number of statements about what is and is not likely to lead to orgasm, I should add a qualification. Erogenous zones and orgasms vary from woman to woman. While what I've said is true of most women, there are others who are different. Some women can orgasm through stimulation of areas other than the clitoris, vagina, or breasts, a few through breast stimulation alone, and a much smaller number solely by means of fantasy. While on the subject of differences among women, it's important to add that these differences apply to breasts as well as other body parts. Although most men find touching, licking, sucking, and otherwise stimulating a female breast to be exciting, there are some women who do not derive much pleasure from having their breasts stroked or touched. They don't mind it and are happy if their men enjoy doing it, but it doesn't arouse them. And virtually every woman, no matter what her usual breast responsivity, has times during her menstrual cycle when her breasts are too sensitive to be touched.

While often thought of as a hole, the vagina is actually a potential space rather than a real space. In the unaroused state its walls are relaxed and touch each other. When sexually excited, the walls balloon out, forming a real space. The space will accommodate itself to fit snugly around whatever object is in it, from the smallest penis to a baby's head.

The outer third of the vagina, the part closest to the entrance, contains the most nerve endings and probably the only nerves in it that are sensitive to touch. The inner two-thirds are insensitive to touch but are sensitive to pressure and stretch in many women, and the thrusting and distention that occurs during intercourse can be very pleasurable for them.

Women who have no-hands orgasms in intercourse (meaning no simultaneous finger stimulation of the clitoris) seem to do it in one of two ways. One way, already discussed, involves pressing the clitoral area against some part of the man, usually his pubic bone. The other way is solely through vaginal responsivity. These women report having hot spots or particular areas of sensitivity in their vaginas. When stimulated, these spots generate orgasms. Three researchers caused a stir a few years ago when they gave a label to this sensitive area, calling it the G-spot, and suggested it was a true anatomical structure like the clitoris or nipple. Unfortunately, the evidence for an anatomical structure is shaky unless we want to say that any very responsive place is the G-spot. The vaginally sensitive women I've talked to locate the spot in different places in the vagina. Whether it makes any sense to use the term *G-spot* remains to be decided, but the important point is that some women are definitely responsive in their vaginas and do orgasm solely through the thrusting of intercourse.

Most of what was said earlier about sexual response in men also applies to women. As with men, women have many different ways of having a sexual experience.

When a sexually meaningful stimulus is present, an increased volume of blood is pumped into various parts of a woman's body—including, but not necessarily limited to, the pelvis, breasts, lips, and earlobes—increasing their size and sensitivity to stimulation. Vaginal lubrication, produced by the vaginal walls in a process similar to sweating, begins soon after blood starts flowing into the pelvic region.

There are many parallels between the assumptions we make about erections and their lack in men and vaginal lubrication or its lack in women. Profuse lubrication does not necessarily mean a woman is highly aroused, and little or no lubrication is not necessarily a sign of lack of arousal. A woman colleague who read this chapter in draft form wrote the following:

> I don't think men know enough about what lubrication does and does not mean. They assume lubrication means the woman is turned on and vice versa. This is *not true*! There are times in my menstrual cycle when I'll be wet all the time and other times when my secretions will be minimal, regardless of how turned on I am. And, to make it more confusing, sometimes I'm dry on the outside when aroused but quite moist inside.

Women also differ tremendously in how much they usually lubricate. Some women lubricate so profusely that they often have the wet panties pornographic writers love to mention. Most women lubricate somewhat less, and other women lubricate very little no matter what time of month it is or how aroused they are. To further complicate matters, lubrication can be very sparse or absent in a woman who has recently given birth or who is nursing, regardless of how turned on she is.

The best way to determine what lubrication or its lack means is talking about it. And whatever you do, don't make the common mistake of assuming that the woman is ready for intercourse just because her vagina is wet. She may be, and then again she may not be.

The flow of blood to the sexual tissues causes them to enlarge. The breasts, clitoris, and inner and outer vaginal lips puff up. The vagina starts expanding and lengthening at the same time. As stimulation continues, the outer two-thirds of the vagina narrow, creating what Masters and Johnson call the "orgasmic platform."

As blood flows into it, the clitoris expands in a process similar to penile erection. It always increases in diameter, but only in some women does it also get longer. As stimulation goes on, the clitoris retracts under its hood. This can come as a great surprise to a man who is stimulating it and now wonders where on earth it went. There's no need to look for it because you probably won't find it. Even though not visible, however, the clitoris continues to respond to stimulation of the area around it.

During a woman's sexual experience, increased muscular tension may be evident in the face, hands, thighs, abdomen, or almost any other place. There may also be involuntary contractions or spasms in the pelvis, buttocks, and elsewhere.

As with men, if the woman is distracted, gets anxious, or starts receiving less than optimal stimulation, her emotional excitement will drop, accompanied by physical changes reflecting the lesser degree of arousal. This is nothing to get concerned about. Reinstating the conditions and activities that led to the higher level of arousal will probably have the same effect again.

Orgasms in men and women are similar both physically and emotionally. In both women and men, orgasm is a reflex that releases the muscular tension and reverses the flow of blood to the erotic areas. The main physical difference is that men ejaculate and women apparently do not. The reason for the qualifier *apparently* in the last sentence is that several sexologists, the same people who brought us the G-spot, have recently claimed that at least some women do ejaculate. They base their claim on the fact that some women expel something when they orgasm, but the exact nature of that something has yet to be determined. Several studies have concluded that it is an involuntary expulsion of urine caused by the contractions of orgasm. At this point, perhaps the fairest thing that can be concluded is that while virtually all men ejaculate something that is not urine, the vast majority of women do not. Emotionally, men and women describe orgasm in similar terms. There is tremendous variation among individual men and individual women, and among different orgasms in the same person.

Not having an orgasm is not a tragedy for either sex. Emotionally, however, it can be something else, depending on the woman's perceptions. If she feels good about the relationship and believes her partner is interested in her satisfaction, it's usually no big deal if she doesn't have an orgasm on any given day. On the other hand, if she feels that the man cares only about his own satisfaction and isn't willing to do anything for her, there will be problems.

In many women orgasm is accompanied by contractions of the pelvic muscles, which you may feel if your finger or penis is in the vagina. While some sexologists feel these contractions are the defining characteristic of female orgasm, others argue that orgasms without noticeable contractions are not only possible but common. I side with the second group. Orgasms, like so much else in sex, follow no absolute pattern. There may be evident pelvic contractions or there may not. Only your partner knows if she has had an orgasm.

Men's orgasms are easier to figure out because we tend to assume that ejaculation means orgasm. If you see the white stuff, that means he came. Since most women don't expel anything, how can you know? Many men are troubled by not having definitive evidence of their partner's orgasm. In fact, it is one of their most common questions about female sexuality: How can you tell if she came? The only way to determine for certain is to ask her. But a lot depends on the circumstances and how the question is asked. Some women respond angrily or anxiously because they feel they are being tested or put in a position of having to prove themselves. In a stable relationship, of course, it should be possible to tell your partner that you're interested in her satisfaction and want to know when and how she orgasms. But in newer relationships, perhaps the best question is something like "Is there anything special you want?" or "Is there something I can do for you?" Or perhaps a simple statement that you are interested in her satisfaction and would be happy to hear about anything she wants would work.

But beware of becoming too involved with the issue of her orgasms. She didn't hire you to be her sex therapist. We all prefer to be given what we need and want, not what someone else thinks we should want. Women, more than men, tend to evaluate sex in terms of feelings rather than performance. If a woman feels good about what happened, whether or not it included a noisy orgasm or any orgasm at all, let her keep the good feeling.

The issue of how many orgasms a woman can or should have has become important since Masters and Johnson demonstrated that some women in their laboratory could have more than one orgasm in a relatively short period of time with continued stimulation. As word of this possibility spread, some men got the idea that their lovers needed to have strings of orgasms, and some women began to feel inadequate because they can't even have one orgasm or can have only one.

The fact is that while some women, and we have no idea how many, can have multiple orgasms, many cannot, and even many who can are often satisfied with just one or even none. If your partner likes to have several orgasms in one session, that's nice, but no nicer and no more proof of anything than if she has only one or none on a particular occasion. The only reason for having more than one orgasm is that it feels good and right at the time—unless you or she is training for the orgasm Olympics. If your partner desires continued stimulation to have another orgasm, you are free to decide whether or not you want to participate in the process.

The last part of a sexual experience is basically the same in men and women. It is simply a return to the unaroused state. The swelling in the genitals and other areas decreases as blood flows away from them, the muscles becomes relaxed, and the organs and tissues return to their normal positions. This process occurs more quickly if there has been an orgasm than if there has not. Sometimes, if there has been high arousal and no orgasm, a woman's return to the unaroused state can take more than a few minutes and there may be some discomfort. Masturbating to orgasm can bring relief, if it is desired.

As already indicated, men and women display somewhat divergent tendencies after sex is over. Many men either immediately go to sleep or leap into some other activity, whereas many women like to cuddle, talk, and in other ways continue being together.

PHYSICAL STIMULATION

On to physical stimulation, which leads to a caveat: **The only real expert on how and where she wants to be stimulated is your partner.** No matter what I say, no matter what you have read, no matter what worked with another partner, no matter what worked for her on another occasion, if your partner says she wants something different, try to do it without hesitation or comment.

The best way to find out what your partner likes is to get a guided tour of her genitals. I think every partner, male and female, should get such a tour early in the relationship, yet, as far as I can determine, most people never do. You might want to see if you can get one. The situation will be clinical, and it should be. She should introduce you to her sexy places and tell or show you how she likes them stimulated, and answer any questions you have. You should reciprocate then or at another time with a similar tour of your genitals.

Of course, it doesn't hurt to have some ideas of your own as long as you're willing to abide by her feedback. The important thing is to get the two of you exploring, experimenting, and talking.

There are several almost foolproof principles. You have much to gain and very little to lose by following them.

▲ **Establish an ongoing erotic connection with your partner.** Read or reread and start applying the information in Chapters 7 through 14 about talking and listening to your partner and lavishing compliments and appreciations on her, as well as affectionate touches. Unless you do this, the material in the rest of the chapter will not have as much benefit as it could.

▲ **Keep connected to the person who owns the parts you're messing with.** Looking into your partner's eyes at times and expressing yourself with words and sounds are helpful in this regard. Also helpful is kissing on the mouth. Most women adore this kind of kissing and can't get enough. Take a break now and then from her breasts and genitals and give her a passionate kiss.

Lover-to-lover connection is so important that many a woman feels lonely when a man is going down on her. He's way down there and she has no one to hold or hug and maybe can't even see him. One way to remedy the situation is to put one of your hands up to play with her breast, to hold her hand, or for her to suck on. Another way is to take a break now and then and put your head up, look at her, and say something loving or sexy. "I love you," "I love eating you," "I love your wetness," "I love the taste and smell of you"—all these comments and others like them are always welcome and appropriate.

▲ **Attend to your personal hygiene.** Make sure, for instance, that your fingernails are clean and clipped. Shave regularly (or keep your beard trimmed), and take a shower or bath daily, or as often as you need to. And brush your teeth.

▲ **Take it slow and easy.** Except in rare circumstances, go slow. You can always speed up if the situation calls for it. If you start too fast, on the other hand, it can be a turn-off to your partner. Recall the line in the Pointer Sisters' song: "I want a man with a slow hand, I want a lover with an easy touch."

▲ **Make sure she knows how much you like and enjoy the aspects of her you're attending to.** Tell her how beautiful her lips, face, breasts, buttocks, and vagina are, how satiny they feel, how much you like to gaze at them, hold, cup, and squeeze them, nuzzle, lick, and bite them. Make certain she knows that as far as you're concerned, she's got the greatest, sexiest butt or breasts in the universe.

▲ **Go from the less sensitive spots to the more sensitive spots.** In other words, don't go immediately for the hot spots. Start elsewhere and work your way to the erogenous zones.

▲ **Always use lubricant when stimulating a woman's genitals.** This is not much of a consideration during oral sex, because the tongue is self-lubricating. But with your fingers, always use a lube of some kind. Saliva is a good natural one, as are her own vaginal secretions. But it's good to have something artificial within reach at all times. Some women like unscented massage oil, and some like Astroglide, Probe, Liquid Silk, or K-Y. Whatever she likes, use it and plenty of it.

▲ **Even at the hot spot, don't go to the hottest part of it right away.** Again, go from least to most sensitive. When she puts your hand on her vulva, that does not mean you should directly focus on her clitoris, the most sensitive area. The vulva has lots of interesting aspects that can be enjoyably stimulated before getting to the clitoris.

▲ **Take off your hat and stay awhile.** If a certain type of stimulation is working, don't immediately rush off elsewhere. If your partner is enjoying the stimulation of her hair, lips, toes, belly, or breasts, stay there long enough for her to really get some pleasure from it.

▲ **Let her indicate when it's time to get more vigorous or to enter her.** This prevents a lot of ugly situations where you did what pleased you but she didn't feel ready.

What about times when your partner indicates she wants immediate attention to a hot spot or wants immediate intercourse even though there's been no preparation? Then you break the rules and do what your partner wants. If she pushes her nipple in your face, by all means attend to it. If she indicates she wants you inside of her despite the lack of foreplay, by all means feel free to comply.

There are times when a couple is so heated up, they want nothing more than to rip off their clothes and get right to it. If that is what is clearly wanted by both partners, of course you should go with it. Be aware, however, that such occasions are rarer than you might think from reading contemporary novels or watching contemporary movies. And when they do occur, they usually do so after the couple has spent considerable time flirting, provoking, and titillating one another on the couch, in the restaurant, or at the party.

BREASTS

Don't go immediately for a woman's breasts or genitals unless that's an established MO in your relationship and you're sure she likes it that way. Start with hugs and kisses first. When you do get to the breasts, don't focus exclusively on them. Take in a larger area with your tongue or hands and just casually touch the breasts as you move around. When you do focus on them, don't immediately go for the nipples. Trace your lips, tongue, or hand around the whole breast first, then perhaps try some holding or light squeezing. Breasts are sensitive, so always squeeze lightly. Don't handle a breast any more roughly than you'd want your balls handled. If she wants firmer or harder touching, let her ask for it. By the way, don't devote all your attention to one breast. The other one gets lonely. It doesn't have to be fifty-fifty, but do give some attention to each. If you have your mouth on one, use your hand on the other.

While stimulating her breasts by hand or mouth, at times continue the stimulation with your hand while you give her a kiss on the mouth. One woman reader of an early draft of this chapter wrote in the margin: "Tell them kiss, kiss, kiss, then to breasts, back to kissing, then to belly, back to kissing, then to vulva, back to kissing, then to clit, and so on." I think that pretty well sums up most women's attitudes about kissing. But of course while you're kissing her mouth, your hands can continue their play elsewhere.

Touch the nipple in passing, but don't jump on it. Tease around it a number of times. Make her anticipate the more serious stimulation of the nipple to come, make her want it. When it's time to focus on the nipple, again remember to take it easy. You can rub a nipple with a finger, flick it with a finger, or rub or squeeze it between two fingers. You can rub and flick with a tongue. You can also suck it or even bite it lightly. In one lovemaking session you can do all of these things. And while you're doing one of them with one nipple, you can be doing the same or something different with the other. If you don't get instructions to the contrary, change what you're doing now and then, but not every second.

A very enjoyable position for breast stimulation is from the rear. That is, when the man is standing or sitting behind the woman or having rear-entry intercourse. From this position, you can hold the breasts from underneath, cup them, and do most of the other things we've already mentioned.

Don't entirely forget the breasts when the action moves south. A woman with sensitive breasts will enjoy stimulation on them when you're going down on her, using your finger on her genitals, or having intercourse.

BUTTS AND WHAT TO DO WITH THEM

Behinds are fun. Stimulating them doesn't lead to orgasm, but touching, squeezing, massaging, fondling, licking, and sucking produce wonderful sensations.

Although butts are less sensitive to gentle stimulation than most other body parts, light touching can be nice. And firm pressure and handling are quite acceptable. You can really grab your partner's butt without causing discomfort. A man can clasp or knead his partner's butt cheeks while having rear-entry intercourse or variations of the missionary position that allow one or both of his hands to be free. This can feel wonderful to both of you. Some men and women also find that having their butts tapped or slapped is very arousing. There are even little whips made especially for those who like a spanking now and then.

A sexy kind of stimulation for many women is for the partner to squeeze and knead the butt while at the same time licking or sucking her breasts or playing with her clitoris or vagina. Light biting of the buttocks is also enjoyed by many couples.

Yet another kind of stimulation enjoyed by many women is a light exploration of the crease between the cheeks, basically just slowly running a finger or two back and forth. The finger(s) may or may not touch the anus itself, depending on what the partners like. If a finger does touch the anus, it is important that it not be inserted into the vagina until after it has been washed.

Behinds are fun to play with and have played with, so if you haven't given your partner's backside much attention, try it next time.

STIMULATING WOMEN'S GENITALS

Before getting to actual stimulation, we need to consider positions to stimulate from, an important but neglected issue.

Positions to Stimulate From

The usual position for hand stimulation is for you to be hugging or holding or kissing her and reaching down to her genitals with one hand. An option is to sit facing her between her open legs while she's either sitting or lying. A much-overlooked position for both manual and oral stimulation is with her sitting on something—bed, sofa, kitchen counter, table, stairs, or stool—and you kneeling or sitting between her legs.

The most common position for the man doing the woman orally is for him to lie on his belly facing her genitals, but this creates a huge problem: you have to lift your head up, which quickly tires and strains the neck. This is a big reason why men don't like to do oral stimulation for long periods. One solution already noted is for her to be sitting on something with you kneeling between her legs so that your mouth is, shall we say, exactly where it ought to be. Another option if you want to do it lying in bed is to raise her up with a pillow under her buttocks and raise you up with a pillow under your upper chest. Yet another option is for her to sit on your face; that's what it's called, but actually it's her kneeling over it. You need a pillow under your head for support, but that's a great way to be face-to-face with her vulva and give really great oral sex. Whatever positions you try, it is crucial that both of you be as comfortable as possible. The strategic placement of pillows can be a big help.

Now to the actual stimulation. Before getting to her vulva, attend to the surrounding territory, the abdomen and thighs. The inner thighs are especially sensitive to light stimulation, so run your hands and fingers over them. Pressure on and above the pubic bone can be quite stimulating at the beginning. With the belly and thighs, rub, stroke, lick, nip, and lightly bite. Then move on to the crotch.

Before we get to rubbing and stroking, consider that it can be very friendly and also stimulating just to put your hand over her vulva, kind of cupping it. This can be done at almost any time your partner is open to it, and certainly before and after more direct stimulation. Just a nice way to say hello. You can also lightly vibrate the hand back and forth quickly. Lightly playing with her pubic hair is a friendly thing to do, too.

The whole vulva is as sensitive to stimulation as the area encompassing a man's penis and scrotum. Since that's the case, it's a good idea to reconnoiter the whole vulva before going to the clitoris. First run a finger or two over the outer and inner lips—which very much like to be touched—and between the outer and inner lips. You can touch around the clitoris and take a little side trip into the vagina if you like, but don't get stuck there.

Going back to the vaginal lips, pat lightly with your fingers all over and press some flesh lightly. With your thumb and forefinger, take hold of the outer lips and gently pull them and stretch them. See how your partner reacts to these touches. Gradually work your way up to the clitoris.

Another kind of stimulation is touching and rubbing the shaft of the clitoris, the part behind the clitoral hood. You can get a finger on each side, or thumb and finger, and do a little rubbing (with copious lubrication, needless to say). If you've never done this before, you might want to check it out.

What you want to do with your hand or mouth is basically what your partner does to herself when she masturbates. As already indicated, getting a demonstration is the best way to find out what this is. For most women, the action is around the clitoris, although not directly on its head. Women do not usually masturbate by thrusting a finger in and out of the vagina, so you probably shouldn't do much of that either unless you're asked to. The motion on the clitoris that works best for most women is a light rubbing or rocking motion on the side of the clitoris itself. The lighter and more lubricated the touch, the better. She'll let you know when she wants a firmer touch. This often happens as she gets more excited. Circular motions around the clitoris are also welcomed by many women.

There is an interesting alternative to the moving finger. This is to press down lightly on the top of her vulva with several fingers, one of which is on or just to the side of the clitoris. Your hand stays fairly still and she moves against it to get exactly what she wants. Obviously she has to be willing to be active. If she is, try this out. It's pretty fantastic.

EATING IT

I'll be talking mainly about licking, but don't take that too literally. Licking is only part of the picture. Don't forget to use your lips to kiss, grasp, and pull. The mouth is very adaptable and resourceful. Use all its abilities.

It can be a loving gesture as well as a practical aid if the woman uses her fingers to spread her lips apart so that her clitoris and vagina are most accessible. If she doesn't, you can do it.

A friendly thing you can do and that many women like at the beginning of oral sex play or afterward is to lightly blow on the vulva and clitoris. It doesn't generate an orgasm, but it can be fun and arousing. **Warning: Do not blow directly into the vagina.** This could cause a fatal air embolism.

Here's some things you can do with your tongue. You can also do most of them with a finger as well.

▲ Give relatively light, relatively quick thrusts or licks of the tongue on her clitoral area. With all tongue movements, get some help from your head by moving it up and down. Your tongue will quickly tire if it does all or most of the work.

▲ Try long and usually slower strokes with tongue and mouth. This type of licking covers more of her lips and vulva than the shorter licks. In this case, you're moving your head more than your tongue. In fact, your tongue can remain stationary.

▲ With your tongue on her clitoral area, move your head to the right and to the left a number of times. This is not something you would do for a long time, but doing it now and then can be a nice change.

▲ Move your head in circular motions, keeping your tongue out. Some women absolutely adore this one. The circular and back-and-forth movements are even easier to do with a finger, so try them when you're stimulating her by hand.

Just as with blow jobs, a lot of the work of oral sex for women is done with the hands. Here are some things you can do with your hands and fingers at the same time as you're doing any of the techniques above with your mouth.

▲ Put one or two fingers into her vagina, usually thrusting in time with your licks. When inserting into the vagina, start small and slow. One finger inserted slowly and only partway, one or two knuckles in. If you put your finger all the way in, do it slowly and gently. Angle the finger up, toward her pubic hair, if you want to stimulate the G-spot, more about which in a moment.

▲ Use one hand to play with her breasts.

▲ Reach out with one hand to hold her hand.

▲ Reach up to her mouth with one hand so she can suck a finger. Many couples find this sexy and fun. You're licking her clit and she's giving a blow job to your finger.

▲ Use a finger to rub her perineum, press it against her anus, or insert it into her anus. Not all women like something inserted into their anus, but many of them enjoy some pressure against the anal opening. If you're going to insert the finger, use lots of lubricant. And always wash the finger before inserting it into the vagina or touching the area around the urethral opening.

▲ Use one or both hands to cup and massage her buttocks.

▲ Try thrusting into or exploring the vagina with your tongue. Although there are few if any women who get an orgasm this way, it can be a nice thing to do. You can use your tongue in her vagina while she stimulates her clitoris with her finger. Or you can use your finger on her clitoris while licking her vagina with your tongue.

So far I've been talking about licking with a little thrusting thrown in. But there are other possibilities to check out. For example, suck the clitoris as you would a nipple. Little nips and even bites (small ones, of course, with lips over your teeth) are also worth exploring. Anything you can do with a nipple can be done with a clitoris. Just keep in mind that the clitoris is ever so sensitive. Always start with light stimulation.

THE SCENT OF A WOMAN

Although the vagina is designed to be self-cleansing as well as self-lubricating, more than a few men (and many women as well) have voiced concerns about vaginal odor. A scent does exist, but it varies greatly from woman to woman and from time to time. Some men like the smell, some don't. It may help to keep in mind that unless your partner has a vaginal infection or poor hygienic practices, her odor shouldn't be so strong as to offend you. This is especially true when you consider that your mouth isn't usually in or on the vagina and your nose is an inch or more away. If you have your tongue on her clitoris, your nose will be above it, probably in her pubic hair. Of course, pubic hair has its own fragrance (in men as well), but many men find it less objectionable than vaginal odor.

If there are concerns about odor or anything else regarding oral sex, why not talk to your partner about them? Washing before sex, or maybe a fun shower or bath together—which many couples consider essential if oral sex is on the menu—will help.

Keep in mind that women are very sensitive about your reactions to their genitals. Even if they have their own issues about their genitals, they hope you're not displeased or offended. So approach this whole issue with tact and discretion. If you suggest a bath before sex, suggest it for both of you, not just her.

THE G-SPOT

Interest in the G-spot runs very high. While I was hosting a sex chat forum for America Online, for example, questions about the G-spot were more common than any other. The area on the upper inner surface of the vagina (toward the belly) an inch or two in has been known for several thousand years, at least to practitioners of Tantric sex, as a very interesting place; they called it the sacred spot. Whether or not the G-spot is a true anatomical entity is not known at this point, and it really doesn't make any difference. I encourage you to explore this area—or any area inside or outside your partner's body—as long as you and your partner are not going to make yourself crazy if you don't get the results you think you should.

Assuming you want to check out the sacred spot, the best way is with a finger rather than a tongue or penis. The woman needs to urinate, completely emptying her bladder, before this activity. Stimulation of this area presses on the bladder and gives the woman the feeling of having to urinate. If she's just gone, she can remind herself that although it feels like she needs to pee, she really doesn't.

What you want to do after the necessary preliminaries is, with her sitting or lying on her back, insert one finger and then angle it upward just past a ridge you should feel on the top side of the vagina. Your finger will be inside of her only about to the second finger joint, not all the way. It's probably best to just let your finger rest there for a moment or two, simply pressing lightly, so that your partner can bring her consciousness down to that area. This is especially important if she doesn't have much experience with stimulation of that area. Then use the "come hither" motion. (This is where having clean and trimmed fingernails becomes important.) How fast and hard is, of course, up to your partner. Some women like a light coaxing motion; others like it more direct and firmer. The urge to urinate usually subsides in a moment or two, and then she can focus more on her arousal. Anything new usually takes some getting used to, so don't give up after ten minutes or one session. Check out this kind of stimulation a number of times and see how she feels about it.

Some women report a sensitive internal area in a different place than where the G-spot is supposed to be. Feel free to explore that one in any way she desires. Some women also report that their sensitive spot shifts depending on where they are in their menstrual cycle.

ORGASM CONSIDERATIONS

Two more things about orgasm require comment. Men should know that some women become very still and quiet just before their orgasm, as if they're listening or waiting for it. If your partner does this, it's crucial that you be accepting of it. Unless you're told otherwise, just keep doing what you've been doing.

The other thing about women's orgasm is that you should not stop stimulation when she begins to come. No matter how much moving and thrashing she's doing, do your best to continue stimulation until she asks you to stop. Men and women are very different on this. Once a man reaches the point of ejaculatory inevitability, really the beginning of his orgasm, he will orgasm completely even if all stimulation ceases. Not so a woman. She needs consistent and continued stimulation until she's done. If stimulation stops before her orgasm is complete, it may well abort the rest of it. The clear message to us men is: When she starts coming, don't stop what you're doing, and don't change it. Just keep on truckin'.

There can be a difficulty with this, however. In the advanced stage of excitement—that is, when she's nearing orgasm—a woman's clitoris retracts under its hood and may seem to have disappeared altogether. *Do not go looking for it.* Just keep stimulating the general vicinity in which it was last seen.

Sometimes the woman will seem to draw away from you. That can mean that she doesn't want any more stimulation there, or that she does but wants it to be gentler, or something else altogether. Unless you're told to stop stimulating, just move with her and keep on doing what you've been doing.

AFTERWARD

When the manual or oral sex is over and you're being loving together, don't forget to mention how much you love to touch and lick her genitals and taste and smell her juices. If you've been doing primarily stimulation with your finger, putting that finger in your mouth and licking her juices off it with appreciative sounds can be very meaningful and loving to your partner. The same is true if you've given her oral sex and happily lick the juices off your lips with your tongue. Whatever you say or do, by all means stay connected.

CHAPTER SEVENTEEN

Sex and the Single Man

I'm the guy all girls' parents warn them against. I know someday I'll get married, have children, and be faithful. But what I want now is sex with every attractive woman I meet. I just want to get my fill and move on. It's fun and it's also an ego thing. My problem is that I've met only a few women who feel the same. Most of them want some kind of relationship, some hope for the future. I don't like to hurt them, but the situation is set up so that someone has to lose. If I'm honest, I won't get as much sex as I want. If I pretend I'm more interested in a relationship than I really am and then disappear, she gets hurt. I wish there was a way to be honest and still get what I want.—*Man, 33*

While I was married, I didn't think much about the singles world. It seemed like it was on another planet. Now that I'm divorced, I feel like a babe in the woods. Women are much more sophisticated than they used to be. They talk about sex easily and all of them come off as experts in oral sex and anal sex—who would have imagined!—and five hundred positions of intercourse. And I'm so scared of AIDS and all the other bugs that I'm not sure I really want sex.—*Man, 46*

IN SOME WAYS, the dating scene has changed dramatically in recent years. There are new ways of meeting Ms. or Mr. Right. Singles organizations, dating services complete with videos and other high-tech accoutrements, and personal ads have become popular alternatives or supplements to the old ways.

Since the sexual revolution, there's also a new attitude about sex. It is no longer the let's-do-it-even-though-we-don't-know-each-other's-name-yet notion of the 1960s and '70s, but there is a strong sense of entitlement about sexual activity and pleasure. The vast majority of dating men and women expect sex to be part of their activity within a few dates. The sense of freedom and entitlement about sex, however, has now been complemented by a new sense of fear about it. We're finally getting the message that sex isn't risk free. There's also a feeling among many people, men as well as women, that sex ought to make sense, that it ought to fit into one's life and values in a reasonable and positive way. What that way is, however, isn't always easy to determine and is bound to be different for different people.

It's now far more acceptable for dating couples to talk about sex before having it, especially about protection against disease and pregnancy. It's not that everyone is doing it, or even a majority of couples, only that it's no longer unusual. It's also more acceptable than, say fifteen years ago, for dating couples to put off getting into sex for a time. No longer do you have to have sex by the third or fourth date to feel okay about yourself. I see all these trends as positive and hope they continue.

There are changes in our views not only of sex, but also of relationships. There is a kind of wariness about getting involved that didn't exist a generation or so ago. More and more young men (and women) come from homes where it was apparent that their parents' marriages, whether or not they ended in divorce, left a great deal to be desired. And there are large numbers of men (and women) dating who themselves have suffered through unhappy marriages and divorce. Although surveys indicate that most men and women do want to commit themselves to a relationship, and although the marriage statistics clearly indicate that the institution of marriage is flourishing, there exists a kind of jadedness and caution that is new.

Despite the changes regarding how and where to meet people and the new concerns about sex and relationships, there is a great deal of continuity. Males and females still dream of finding Ms. or Mr. Right; they still wonder where to meet that special person and if they can offer enough to attract and keep him or her; and, sexual revolution or not, they still wonder when to get sexual and what that means.

THE IDEA OF GRADUAL INVOLVEMENT, OR TAKING IT SLOWLY

There's no question that a great many problems that plague daters result from rushing into things and not taking the time to reflect on how you feel and what you want. A simple example is when you ask out a woman you've never met and don't know (you've gotten her name from a friend) for an extended date, say for Saturday night or an all-day outing. If the two of you don't hit it off, you're both going to be miserable. There's all that time looming in front of you, and you don't want to be there. This is also a convenient and destructive way of getting into sex. You don't know what to do with all that time available, so you resort to something you're comfortable with, your sexual routine. The problem is that you're likely to feel worse afterward rather than better.

The whole process of dating can and should be one in which you take your time getting to know someone, reflecting after each encounter what you feel about her and what you want from her. This allows you to stay within your zone of comfort and to make the best choices for yourself. I know it doesn't sound half as romantic as love or lust at first sight, but it makes a lot more sense for people who've gotten beyond letting their eyes, hearts, or penises run their lives. By the way, what I'm saying is relevant not only if you're looking for your one and only, but even when you're just looking for someone to spend a few nights with.

I've been a voyeur at the many professional conferences I've attended over the years, taking a lively interest in who shacks up with whom and with what results. One thing that's always amazed me is how often a man hits on a woman, makes an immediate decision to spend the night with her if he can, succeeds in his quest, and then can't stand the sight of her the next day, nor she of him.

I'm not a prude and I have nothing against a night or two of pleasure with someone new, provided you both understand what the rules are. But if you feel like hell when you wake up next to her the following morning and wish you were elsewhere, what's the point? It's better, I think, to put a little more time and effort into getting to know her before getting into bed.

I very much like the idea of "coffee dates," or gradual involvement, which is just a structured way of taking your time. At a conference or on a vacation, this means only that even if you are smitten by a woman, don't try to rush her into bed or let her rush you. Better just to have a cup of coffee together, a meal, or a walk, then separate for a while so you can consider how you feel about her. If all the thoughts and feelings are good, then by all means arrange to see her again. But then back off once again for reflection.

A first date should be time-limited, no more than an hour or two. If you like her, it will be easy to arrange a longer get-together for the next time. If the two of you don't hit it off, you haven't lost much and you don't have to worry about how to fill up endless hours.

Needless to say, the gradual-involvement idea implies that you should take your time becoming sexual with a new partner. As I hope will become clear in the rest of this chapter, there's a great deal to be gained from this approach and almost nothing to lose.

THE QUESTION OF HONESTY IN DATING

A huge problem in the singles life is that many people get hurt because of different expectations about what being together or having sex means. Men often feel that they have to lie to get sex. They think they can't simply say, "You turn me on and I'd like to spend the night with you." So they have to concoct stories about wanting a relationship even when they don't.

It can help to realize that not every woman is looking for a big-time relationship. There are many women who would be happy to spend a weekend or a week with you without any promises of more to come.

If you're honest about your desires, you will certainly be rejected some of the time. Some women you're interested in will not have sex with you if that's all you want. But you'll also get what you want some of the time and you won't have to feel bad afterward. I suggest honesty.

If you're at a conference or at Club Med and you only want company for the night or week, why not say so? "I get lonely at these meetings. It's much nicer if I can find someone to spend my free time with." Or, "I'm just taking a week to get away from it all. And I'm looking for someone who wants to enjoy the time with me."

The same kind of honesty can be used in more common dating situations. If you're not looking for a big-time relationship but want some company, why not just say so? "I've only been divorced six months and that whole business has taken a lot out of me. I'm not ready to settle down again, but I enjoy company and want to have a good time." Suppose she asks if you think you'll ever want to get married again. An honest answer might be: "I really don't know. It's going to take me some time to sort out the whole business about love and marriage."

HONESTY AND SEXUALLY TRANSMITTED DISEASES (STDs)

What to do and say about STDs is a big issue. If you know you're disease free, you might want to find out if she is. If you know you've got something, what are you going to do about that?

Surveys show that many men, and women as well, don't tell new partners about their diseases and don't do anything to prevent infection. For what it's worth, I think this is immoral, immature, irresponsible, and probably illegal as well. How would you feel if you had sex with a woman and it turned out that you had contracted herpes, genital warts, or some other disease from her? I'll bet you'd be furious, and you'd have every right to be. So how do you think she'd feel if the tables were turned and she got something from you?

I think partners owe it to themselves and each other to (1) use condoms and spermicide every single time they have intercourse and (2) be completely honest about any diseases they have. This is simply basic human decency.

Once again, of course, rejection rears its head. Yes, it's true that if you tell a new friend you have a disease, she may not want to have sex with you even with a condom or even though you know that you're not infectious right now. That's just the way it is. It's her right to make the decision, just as it's your right to decide what you want to do if she has a disease.

"But why do I have to tell her I have herpes or genital warts, or whatever? Wearing a condom will protect her."

But condoms are not 100 percent effective. Nothing is. Even with a condom, she might get what you've got. She's the one who needs to make the decision, not you. By not giving her the relevant information, you're robbing her of a basic human right, the right of informed consent.

If you have something to tell your friend, just tell her. There is no best time, place, or method, which is another way of saying that any time (before sex), place, or way is acceptable. Here is an example: "This is difficult, but there's something I need to tell you before we go away for the weekend. I have genital herpes. It's not active now and I wouldn't have sex when it was, and I always use a condom, but I wanted you to know."

What about the situation where you're disease free but want to know about her? This can be a bit difficult, too, and I disagree with a lot of the advice from experts in recent years regarding this question. Many of them suggest interrogating your about-to-be sex partner. I have nothing against asking, but I'm convinced that you can't have total faith in the answers. First of all, some people will say they're disease free when they're not. Second, some people aren't aware they have a disease. So even if she tells the truth as she knows it, it may not be accurate.

Feel free to ask if you want, but use protection in any case. Condoms aren't perfect, but they're a lot better than nothing. Condoms used with generous amounts of spermicide aren't perfect either, but they are even safer than condoms without spermicide.

Speaking of condoms, you should consider in detail ahead of time exactly how you're going to get a condom into the act. How are you going to bring up the subject, what are you going to say, and what are you going to do? Working out a routine and rehearsing it a number of times in your mind will help ensure that you actually do what you want to do. Having condoms available in a number of places will also help. You can always carry some in a shirt or jacket pocket (but *not* in a wallet or glove compartment, please, because the heat there can weaken latex), and have a few in your usual place for lovemaking, say a bedside nightstand.

Suppose you're asked how many women you've had sex with. A recent survey indicates that some men and women lie by underreporting. Women feel pressured to do this because they fear being thought loose. And these days some men feel pressured to underreport for the same reason and also because a large number of partners implies the possibility of disease.

So what to do? Here again I believe honesty is the best policy. There's little point to pretending to be someone you're not, because sooner or later your friend is probably going to find out who you really are. If she isn't going to like that person, it's best to find out as soon as possible. And it doesn't help the development of trust, a crucial component in any decent relationship, when people start lying to each other.

DON'T SAY YOU'LL CALL HER IF YOU AREN'T SURE YOU WILL

Speaking of honesty, women are confused and enraged by men who say they'll call and don't. My understanding of the man's position is this: He's either sure he will call (or won't call), or he's not sure. If he thinks he will, he's just being honest. If he's not sure or knows he won't, he's using the promise that he'll call as a solution to a potentially unpleasant situation. He doesn't quite know how to say goodbye or good night. "I'll call you" offers an easy way out.

The problem arises when she wants you to call and takes your promise seriously. She's looking forward to hearing from you and seeing you again. When you don't call, she feels disappointed and upset, and then angry: "Why did he lie to me?"

Once again, I believe some kind of honesty is a better policy. I don't think it's necessary to say anything unkind or to get into a hassle. At the very least, though, if you're not positive you're going to call her, don't say you will. If you don't promise to call and then you do, that might be a nice surprise for her.

If you find yourself in the awkward position of having said you'll call and then realizing you don't want to, it is probably a good idea to call or, better yet, write a short note. For instance: "I enjoyed our date last week, but after thinking about what you said, I don't think we should get together again. You said you wouldn't be ready to settle down for a long time, and I'm looking for a steady relationship now." If it's something potentially more embarrassing or hurtful—you just don't care that much for her, or she's not as ambitious, smart, or pretty as you want—a little white lie can be used: "I enjoyed out time together but realized later that the chemistry just isn't there" or "I think we're just too different to make it as a couple." This way, you're doing what you want, not seeing her again, but you haven't left any loose ends or bad feelings.

Not saying you'll call when you aren't sure you will is just one example of being honest and not making false promises. Although honesty isn't always the best policy—there are some circumstances where it's best to keep one's mouth shut—it should be the first policy we consider.

SUPPOSE YOU'RE A VIRGIN

Despite the common myth that all males over the age of eighteen or nineteen are sexually experienced, there are in fact many men in their twenties and some in their thirties, forties, and even older who have never had sex with a partner. Although the reasons vary—shyness, fear of women, fear of sex, fear of closeness, not feeling a need to have an intimate relationship or sex, being preoccupied with work or other things—one thing these men have in common is a sense of inadequacy because they haven't had sex with a partner. When they decide they'd like to become sexually intimate with a woman, they often feel conflicted about a number of things, one of them being what they should say about their situation. They feel women will be turned off by their lack of experience, but at the same time they don't want to lie; even those who have considered the possibility of lying fear their lack of experience will show.

Yet again, I think honesty is the first thing to consider. It's not necessary to announce, "Hi, I'm a virgin," but if it becomes appropriate or if you're asked a relevant question—such as "What have your past lovers been like?"—why not tell the truth? It's doubtful that your new friend is going to be horrified by your response. And if she is, you don't need her anyway. Although I can't guarantee it will happen to you, some women find a male virgin interesting.

Some men are virgins because their attempts at intercourse haven't worked out (ejaculation before insertion or inability to get or maintain an erection) and they've given up. If this is true for you, the material in the rest of this chapter and in Chapters 20 to 23 may help.

For some men, the problem is that they are very shy and find it extremely difficult to meet women or to ask them out. Although dealing with this issue is beyond the scope of this book, there are several good works on shyness and developing social skills available. A therapist can also help.

If the reason for your virginity is a fear of women or the closeness that sex might bring, you should consider professional therapy. Most of the time these problems can be worked out and you can learn to enjoy a close relationship.

Whatever the reason for your virginity, try to remember that it's not a disease or something you have to be ashamed of. It's just a fact, and if that fact bothers you, there are a number of options that can help you get what you want.

SEX FOR THE FIRST TIME WITH A NEW PARTNER

The first time a couple has sex is a poignant moment. Two people come together to share an experience and themselves, often in conflict or confusion within themselves, and perhaps with differing goals and expectations. Each hopes for at least a tolerable experience and fears a humiliating one; each yearns for acceptance and fears something less. Both are concerned that they will be found wanting in some way: that their bodies, behaviors, or personality will be compared to some superior standard and be found inadequate.

Men usually feel responsible for how the lovemaking goes. They wonder if they can do all they believe they should do: get the partner interested and aroused, get and maintain lasting erections, and provide the kind of ecstasy they assume their partners desire. They hope their performance will be, if not fantastic, at least passable.

Their partners often go through very similar types of questioning and agonizing. The woman wonders if the man will find her body attractive, if she'll be able to please him, and if he will find sufficient interest and pleasure to want to return.

It's totally understandable that people should be uneasy when they have sex with someone new. Even in these so-called liberated times, sex still means something special. It's not something you do with just anyone. In sex you allow a unique access to yourself—to your nudity, to the feel and smell and taste of your body and its fluids. And it can go even further. You may allow access to your emotions, at least to your interest and excitement. In doing so, you run the risk that this may be the start of real contact with the other person, a kind of intimacy, with all the possibilities and dangers that intimacy implies.

Because of the tension that accompanies first-time experiences, they are often unsatisfactory. Many men do not get or maintain erections, or they come quickly and then feel bad about these "failures." Other men function adequately but don't derive much pleasure. A great many women do not have orgasms the first time they have sex with a partner, a fact for which many men blame themselves. A woman I know says that the first few sexual encounters with a new partner are so bad she considers them "throwaways." The only reason she engages in them, she says, is that she can't figure out how to get to the fifth or sixth time—and good sex—without going through the first and second times.

It doesn't have to be this way. Although there is no way of dissipating all the strangeness and tension involved in first-time experiences, there are ways of making them better and more satisfying, with far fewer "failures" and bad feelings.

No Sex Before Its Time

The single most important point is this: **Don't rush into sex. Go slowly and get into sex only when you're comfortable with your partner and your conditions are met.** This is the notion of gradual involvement applied to sex. There's no good reason to rush into sex on the first or second date, or even on the fifth or ninth date. Sex should occur only when you and your partner feel comfortable with each other and really want to engage in physical intimacy. This is especially true for men who've had problems in sex.

In case you're wondering how women feel about this idea, I'm happy to tell you that the vast majority of women I've talked to over the years have agreed that taking one's time getting to sex is what they prefer.

If you've read Chapter 3, you know there are lots of things you and your new friend can do besides the old foreplay-intercourse routine. As your comfort with each other develops, you could, for example, engage in more intimate forms of touching (hugs, kisses, massages, necking, petting, sleeping together, dry humping, hand jobs, and so forth). There's certainly no shortage of activities.

It's clear from everything we know that sex goes best if it's done when both partners feel it's what they want. If one or both feel pressured into the activity, it will be something less than wonderful. It's well known that women often feel pressured into having sex. What's not so well known is that so do men. Men feel pressured by their notions of manhood: that a man should make sexual advances very quickly in a relationship, and that a man should never rebuff the sexual advances of his partner.

Of particular relevance here is what you can do if your new partner pushes for sex before you feel ready. This situation is no longer unusual. A woman may make a sexual advance because she truly wants sex with you or because she's trying to deal with the insecurity generated in her because you haven't made one. Regardless of her motives, you're going to have to do something.

Probably the most common choice is to go along regardless of how you feel. I don't recommend this, because it can easily lead to bad sex and bad feelings. It is far better to get into your assertive and expressive mode and let her know how you feel. Here's one example of what you might say: "I'm flattered you want me to stay the night. I've enjoyed our times together and am very turned on to you. But getting into sex this fast doesn't work well for me. I'd like us to take our time, getting to know each other better, and get to sex when it feels right for both of us. Can you understand what I'm saying?"

Here's another: "I'm a little shy and it takes me a while to be comfortable enough to have sex. But I really enjoy you and want to spend more time with you. Does the idea of [insert activities you want to do, such as trading back rubs, doing more kissing and petting, and so on] tonight do anything for you?"

Suggestions for Sex with a New Partner

▲ Get to know her and give her the opportunity to know you. Give yourself time to determine if you really want sex with her.

▲ Be sensual with her before being sexual. Hold hands, hug, kiss, snuggle, or do anything else that feels good. Always stop when you want to, when you feel anxious, or when you get a signal from her that she wants you to stop.

▲ Do whatever is necessary to feel comfortable with her and get your conditions met. You might want to talk with her about both your expectations and hers. You might also want to talk about the kinds of physical contact you enjoy. Establish a habit of discussing your preferences and try to get her to do the same. This will serve you well when you become sexual with her.

▲ Always stay within your comfort zone. Refrain from activities that make you tense.

▲ Consider a session or two of massage or body rubs before you get to sex.

▲ You might also want to consider actually *sleeping* or taking a nap with her, which can be a nice and cozy way of getting more comfortable. It's possible that sleeping together might lead to sex, which is fine if that's what feels right at the time. But make sure your conditions are met and that sex is what you want. If not, just sleep.

▲ Have a talk with her about protection against conception and disease before you get anywhere near genital contact. It's a mistake to assume that this is the woman's responsibility. Since both of you will have to deal with any consequences that occur, it's the responsibility of both partners.

▲ When your conditions are met, when you are aroused, and when you want to, feel free to engage in the sexual activities you like (as long as she also likes them). Keep in mind what was said about sexual choices. Intercourse isn't required. If you have had erection or ejaculation problems in the past, it is best not to have intercourse the first few times you are sexual with her. Do other things that feel good to both of you.

▲ Give feedback about your experiences with her. Tell her—during and after sensual and sexual activity—what you like and don't like, and encourage her to do the same.

▲ Express your feelings. If you have feelings that get in the way of your sexual responsiveness or your ability to relate to her in any way, you would do well to discuss them with her. It will help her to know you, and it may totally or partially resolve the problems.

▲ Don't do anything you don't want to do. If she suggests sex before you feel ready for it, let her know how you feel, no matter how difficult this may be. If she suggests activities that aren't your style, let her know immediately: "I'm sorry, but I really don't want your dog in bed with us." Take care of yourself.

▲ Keep intake of alcohol and other drugs to the absolute minimum you can tolerate. The last thing you need is some chemical screwing up your mind and nervous system.

IF YOU'RE HAVING ERECTION OR
EJACULATION PROBLEMS

No one envies a single man with a sex problem. It's a difficult situation to be in. Different men react in different ways. Some don't date at all, thinking it's better to go without love and without sex than to be humiliated. Others date lots of women, but only for brief periods—as soon as they think sex might come up, they find someone else to go out with. Still others try to have sex. Sometimes everything works out and the problem is solved, but this isn't typical. More often than not, the problem recurs and the man is devastated (whether or not his partner is). And there are still other men who try to fix the problem before dating by using self-help books or going to therapy.

There are several things a single man with a sex problem needs to keep in mind. Perhaps the most important is that having a sex problem doesn't make you an undesirable person. It just means you have something that needs work, no different from any other problem. Because men with sex problems tend to do a lot of negative and destructive self-talk, it's important to read and master the information in Chapter 19. It also does you no good to keep away from women. Believe it or not, this will tend to make the problem worse.

There are several options. One is to have surrogate therapy for the problem (see Chapter 23). Another option, probably the one most frequently chosen, is just to date and see what happens. Some men with erection problems find that getting into sex slowly with a partner who really turns them on is helpful. After a few times with her, the problem often disappears. These men can benefit from following the suggestions I give in this chapter. Unfortunately, this method is not likely to help a man with a long-standing inability to control the timing of his ejaculations or a long-standing erection problem.

Still other men won't go out, at least not beyond a second or third date, until they believe they've done something to resolve their problem. The twelve suggestions given earlier in this chapter on sex with a new partner will help, as will doing the appropriate masturbation exercises in Chapters 20 and 22. And so will the following suggestion.

Consider Telling Your New Friend About the Problem

If you're like most of the men I've seen in therapy, this idea will make you uncomfortable. Despite that, there are a number of good reasons for thinking about it. Before I get into them, however, let's dispense with one piece of silliness. I'm *not* at all suggesting you introduce yourself like this: "Hi, I'm Fred, and I have an erection problem." That's not the way to do it. But somewhere on an early date (not the first one, though), when it looks like the two of you are moving toward becoming sexual, you can find an opportunity to tell her.

One advantage to telling her is that you'll eliminate the women whom you fear the most and whom you shouldn't be with in the first place: those who, for whatever reasons, can't handle the problem. The last thing you need is to be with someone who's unsympathetic or even hostile to your situation. Telling her before you get anywhere near a bed will ensure that you don't end up with such a person. Of course, it may feel very bad that this woman you're so attracted to says she doesn't want to see you again. Just keep telling yourself that there are plenty of other women you'll be attracted to and who will not be put off by your problem.

The other advantage of telling is that you'll feel a lot better. You won't have to try to hide the problem if she already knows about it, and you'll know you're with someone who can deal with it. The men I've worked with who have told women they're dating about their sexual problems have felt incredibly relieved. For example:

> I feel wonderful! I was scared to death before I told Jane about my situation. I was sure she was going to tell me to get lost. But she was wonderful. Said there were plenty of things we could do without an erection and she was looking forward to doing them. I can't tell you how good I feel!

It's understandable that men are very uncomfortable with the idea of telling a woman they're attracted to and don't know very well that they have a sex problem. The main reason is fear of rejection. As one man put it: "Oh, that's just terrific. Here we are just getting to know each other, just starting to think what sex together might be like, and I'm supposed to say, 'By the way, I can't get it up.' It makes perfect sense that she'll tell me to get lost."

It is possible that she will tell you to get lost. The chances are probably small—most women I talked with would not react like that—yet they are real. But you have to realize that none of the options is good. To tell her is difficult, and you may end up rejected. But not to tell her isn't exactly a bed of roses. You'll be worried about her finding out—and how is it possible that she won't?—and about her reaction to the discovery. This worry will make it harder for you to enjoy sex and to function as you'd like. And if you get rejected in bed, it may be much more difficult to deal with than if you got rejected before you had sex.

It's important to realize that getting rejected doesn't decrease your worth as a human being, a man, and a lover one bit. You do have a problem, but it's resolvable under the right circumstances. If she decides she can't deal with it, that's because of something in her. A common reason why a woman might not be able to deal with this sort of problem has to do with her own insecurity. In talking with women over the years, I've often raised the question of what they would do if a man they were attracted to mentioned a sex problem before they had sex. The vast majority of the women said it wouldn't be an issue as long as he took responsibility for the problem and would be willing to get help if it didn't clear up on its own.

But a few said they wouldn't be able to see him again. One articulate woman put it like this:

I know it isn't fair. But to me, him not getting hard would mean I wasn't sexy or skillful enough. I know that's my own button, but it would be too much for me to handle. I'm sure I could cope if he developed an erection problem after we'd been together awhile. But at the start, when I'm so insecure anyway and so worried about my effect on him, I just don't think I could deal with it.

It's clear that she has the same fear of rejection you do. Your not getting erect seems to her like you are rejecting her.

Although I reported earlier that no man has reacted positively to my idea of telling potential partners about the problem, a great many of them ended up doing so. After considering the options, they realized this was the one that made the most sense.

So how did they go about this? The story of one client, Charles, offers some ideas. Charles dated lots of women in the months after his divorce, but only once or twice each, because of his fear that sex might come up and he would be humiliated. Finally, feeling he couldn't go on this way, he came to see me. When I brought up the idea of telling a woman about his problem, he tenaciously resisted. There was no way, he said, he was going to announce to a woman he barely knew that he was impotent. The idea of telling Janet, a woman he had been out with once and who he was quite interested in, was frightening.

I suggested that since none of the options open to him was terrific, the only question was which of them was the least bad. He said he'd think about it. The next time he saw Janet, he told her. Here's his report:

> I realized that I had to tell her. I couldn't go on dropping women after only one or two dates. It was only making my fears worse. So I thought about how to bring it up. I realized we'd both been recently divorced and had talked a little about that during our first get-together. Since I see my problem as a consequence of a failing marriage and then the divorce, I realized that I could bring it up during another discussion about divorce.
>
> I had planned to steer the conversation toward the subject of divorce the next time I saw Janet, but I didn't have to. She did by mentioning that one outcome of the divorce is that she's more guarded around men. I saw my chance and dove in. Told her I'm also more guarded and I've also got another consequence to deal with. With great difficulty I explained my erection problem. I was almost afraid to look at her while I was talking. But I did look at the end and she was smiling. Said she didn't see it as a big problem. People who care about each other can do lots of fun things that don't require erections.

If you think the problem is transient, here's something you can say: "It takes me a few times with a new woman to get comfortable enough so my penis feels it can do its stuff."

The same kinds of things can be said if your problem is rapid ejaculation, depending on whether the difficulty is transient or long-term. If you know from experience that your control will get better after a few more times, you can say: "I usually can last a lot longer after I've been with someone a few times." If the problem is chronic, you need to say something different.

Using Chemical Aids

Some men these days are using chemical aids to help their erections, and others are using antidepressants to help them last longer on their sexual encounters with new partners. No doubt this practice will expand now that Viagra is with us.

If your problem is transient and you are able to function without the drug after a few times, there may not be much for you to say to your partner or for me to say to you. It is another story, however, if you continue to need the aid over time.

Sooner or later, something needs to be said, as she will discover that you are taking pills or shots. One young man who was taking Paxil to help him last longer was surprised when his girlfriend asked him why he hadn't told her he was taking drugs for depression. While he was sleeping at her place, she decided to include his shirt in a load of laundry she was doing, and the vial of pills fell out of the shirt pocket. "I wasn't prepared to tell her," he reported, "but I had no choice. So I had to explain that I wasn't depressed and why I was taking the pills. She wasn't thrilled that I hadn't told her sooner."

At some point—which could be four weeks or three months into the relationship, depending on the woman and the situation—not telling her becomes withholding important information. A woman broke off the relationship with her boyfriend of eight months when she found out he had been taking penile injections the whole time without telling her. For her, this was a betrayal. "I had the right to know he had an erection problem. His not telling me means I can't trust him. I wonder what else he hasn't told me. I can't be with a man like that."

I know a number of men who used injections or pills to help them function with a new partner and then, after a bond had been formed, told their partners what was going on. In each situation the partner responded positively. In some cases the man kept using the aid. In other cases they had sex therapy to find a better solution.

What to Do When a Problem Occurs

When a problem occurs—whether or not you've spoken to your new partner about it and whether or not you've ever had this problem before—you should probably say something. Suppose you come fast in intercourse. Try saying something like this: "I was so excited, I couldn't control myself. I'd like you to feel as good as I did. Tell me what you like."

Let's take the same scenario but make one change. Instead of coming fast, you don't get an erection. Your partner uses her hand and her mouth on you, but to no avail. Chances are good that her efforts, as well-intentioned as they are, will only make things worse, because you'll feel under even greater pressure to get hard.

There are several ways to handle this situation, but perhaps the best might go like this. You recognize you're tense and probably won't get hard. So you stop her from trying to stimulate you and say something like this: "He's [referring to your penis] shy the first time, and I don't think he'll come out to play tonight. How can I make you feel good?" An alternative is: "I just realized I'm a little tense. I don't think I can get hard. Let's do something else."

Suppose she says: "That's so disappointing. I was looking forward to having you inside me." You could respond like this: "I was looking forward to it, too. But look, I've still got a hand and a pretty wicked tongue. Wanna play?"

But suppose she says no and tells you she's no longer in the mood. If that happens, it's not a tragedy—just another fact to consider. Here's a way to deal with it: "I'm sorry you're so disappointed. Here, let me rub your back. That often helps me when I feel disappointed." Or (as you put your arms around her): "Maybe holding each other will help relieve the disappointment."

Do Not Apologize for the Problem or for Yourself

Although I think it's smart to tell a partner ahead of time about a problem and to acknowledge the problem when it occurs, it is *not* wise to apologize for it or for yourself. Men with sex problems feel bad because they "can't deliver" and tend to feel guilty and apologetic about everything. Continuing to apologize for the problem may help relieve their guilt for the moment, but it does nothing to endear them to their partners. It's difficult to be with someone or find him attractive if he seems to be apologizing for his existence.

My best advice is: Do not apologize for your physical appearance, your mental abilities, your personality, or your sexual history or performance. It's bad enough if you don't like any or all of these things. Apologizing will only call attention to them and get her to dislike them, too. No one likes to be with a wet blanket. If you're terrible and life is terrible and everything is terrible, and that's all you can say, you should consider sitting home alone and not inflicting your misery on others.

Better yet, consider changing your perspective and feeling and acting more positively. Yes, you have a problem, but it is solvable. Explain it, acknowledge it when it occurs, have a good time in spite of it, and get on with resolving it.

RESOLVING PROBLEMS

CHAPTER EIGHTEEN

Getting the Most from
Your Self-Help Program

Everything has gone to pot. The tension about sex has infected every part of our lives. We don't touch anymore, we don't have fun, and both of us blow up at the slightest pretext. I feel bad all the time, and I'm sure she does too.
—*Man, 42*

LET'S FACE IT. It's no fun to have a sex problem, and the prospect of having to follow my suggestions isn't the most exciting idea you've ever heard of. You have my sympathy. Over the years I've followed various athletic, dietary, medical, and therapeutic regimens myself, and I think I know what you're feeling. I did very well with some of my programs, fared less well with others, and failed completely with a few. But I learned something important: I did best when I made the programs fun. When I had to rely on willpower alone and grit my teeth every time I had to do something, I didn't do very well. In fact, it didn't take long before I was off that program altogether. I also did best when I clearly understood what I was doing and stuck to a schedule.

I'm surprised at how many people plunge into a self-help program without doing the proper thinking and planning ahead of time and then just as quickly drop the program. This is why most people who join health clubs show up only a few times and are never heard from again.

To work productively on a sex problem and maximize the chances of a successful outcome, three general requirements must be met: (1) if you're in a relationship, you need to get it in as good a shape as possible; (2) you need to understand what will be asked of you and to make the necessary arrangements; and (3) you need to get your mind working with you instead of against you. These three topics are covered in this and the following chapter.

THE RELATIONSHIP THING AGAIN

Estrangement is frequent in couples who are having sex problems. Sometimes the sex problem is the cause. Partners blame themselves and each other, they stop touching and feeling close, and frequently the woman is angry at the man for not being willing to get help sooner. In other cases the estrangement predates the sex problem or is independent of it; the couple is angry and distant for reasons other than sex.

Regardless of what is causing the distance and hostility, closeness and cooperation must be reestablished before productive work on sex can be undertaken. A great deal of the time I spend with couples in sex therapy, especially at the start, is not devoted to sex. Rather, it involves getting them to stop blaming themselves and their partner and to repair the damage caused by the blaming, the withdrawing, and the fighting. Below I give some pointers about what you can do for yourself and your partner before you start to work on sex per se. You should also read or reread Chapters 7 through 14 as soon as possible and start applying the relevant ideas and suggestions.

1. Have a talk with your partner in which you acknowledge the problem and what you are going to do about it—for instance, use the exercises in this book or see a therapist. If your partner believes that you have been dragging your feet about resolving the sex problem, this belief needs your immediate attention. You should let her know that her perception was accurate, and you should apologize for not realizing this sooner. You should also tell her that you want to get your relationship on a better footing before working directly on sex. For example: "You were right all along—this problem really needs attention. I'm sorry I didn't see it sooner. But I'm ready to deal with it now. There are exercises in this book I think would help, but before doing them maybe we should start having some good times again."

2. Start being more positive about yourself. The worse you feel about yourself and your situation, the harder it is to make your partner happy and have a good relationship with her. So it's crucial to keep self-criticism down to the absolute minimum. I address this issue in detail in the next chapter.

3. If you've been staying away from physical affection, get back into it—assuming, of course, that this is acceptable to your partner. Touch, hold, massage, hug, and kiss your partner when the spirit moves you, and be responsive to her touches and hugs. Depending on what has been going on with the two of you, it may be advisable to first have a talk about touching, so that she doesn't construe a hug or kiss as meaning you want sex. If she's too angry to engage in physical affection now, try to be understanding of her position and keep on with the other ideas and exercises that are acceptable.

4. If you've been withholding compliments and words of love, now's the time to start expressing them. Let her know all the things about her that you like and love.

5. If you haven't been having sex, you should consider starting again if both of you are willing. If you've been making love but also having fights about it, it's time to start on a new path. After you've started expressing compliments and words of love, and after you've started touching again and had some good times, talk with your partner about sex. Is it okay with her to do something other than intercourse if you lose your erection or come fast? If either one of you isn't sure what the options are, read and talk about the section on sexual options in Chapter 3. Can the two of you agree to use some of the options and not get upset or get into arguments about what's happening? If the answer is yes, then go to it.

6. Do your best to see that each sexual encounter ends positively for both of you. For example, if you come fast in intercourse or lose your erection and you know she isn't yet satisfied, you could say something like "I'd like to make you feel good" as you start to stimulate her by hand or mouth. Another possibility is to say nothing but just start stimulating her in a way you know she likes. Yet another way is to say, "Roger [or whatever name the two of you use to refer to your penis] is out to lunch, but I'd love to go down on you." Since I assume you've already talked about options, still another way would be to say: "I don't think I'm going to get hard. Would this be a good time for me to hold you while you use your vibrator?"

7. Make a firm pledge that there will be no more sulking, name-calling, or apologies about the problem. You know about it, she knows about it, and there's no need to belabor the obvious. And try not to blame her when the problem recurs. Even if it's true that she's somehow contributing to or even causing the problem, blaming and accusing will only make her defensive and make matters worse. The more the two of you can have good times together, sexually and otherwise, and be kind and caring in your interactions, the better the chances that the problem will be resolved.

Another way of saying what I've covered so far in this chapter is this: Don't make the problem worse. The more you withdraw from sex and your partner, the more tension that's generated, the more blaming that goes on, and the greater the sense of failure, the harder it will be to make positive changes. The worse things get, both in your mind and between you and your partner, the more difficult it will be to resolve the problem. So seriously consider putting the seven ideas into practice as soon as you can.

If you think all is well in your relationship and that nothing extra is required, check this out with your partner. Make sure she agrees that you're ready to do the exercises. If she doesn't, start applying the suggestions given above. And feel free to use any other ideas you have for making your relationship better.

"It doesn't work. We can have good times sometimes but my partner is so angry with me for not taking care of the problem before that she goes into rages whenever I mention doing something without a long-lasting erection."

This situation is common. You should make sure you've acknowledged the problem, apologized for not wanting to deal with it sooner, and assured her that you're going to get help now. If she needs to vent, let her express herself, agree as much as you can with what she says (for example, "I can see why you're so furious. I didn't take you seriously and it's caused you a lot of pain"), and then renew your offer to get help. If that doesn't work, suggest the two of you see a therapist before any further damage is done to your relationship.

"Nothing works. We've been in a horrible place for months. We can't be civil, can't have a good time, can't have a reasonable conversation."

If nothing in this chapter can be applied, then you need a therapist who works with both relationship and sex problems. Get that help now. The longer you wait, the more difficult it will be. Ask your partner if she'll join you, but if she says no, go by yourself. I've been involved in a number of cases where the woman refused to go to therapy until after her partner went himself for several sessions. Once she believed that he was serious about trying to improve their relationship, she became willing to participate.

THE DETAILS OF SELF-HELP

> I never thought "working on sex" could be fun, and it sure wasn't the first few weeks. But after I finally admitted to myself that I had a problem and had to work to overcome it, April and I settled in and made the best of it. It wasn't half as bad as I imagined. We made fun and games of it whenever we could, and the result is that the problem is largely resolved, we both learned a lot, and we're closer as a couple.   —*Man, 45*

One thing to do early on is set one or more goals. Read this whole book first, or at least the chapters that seem relevant. Then set a specific goal for yourself; for example, improving your ejaculatory control to the point where you can usually decide when to come in intercourse, or keeping your erection in intercourse at least 70 percent of the time. If you have a regular sex partner, setting goals should be a joint endeavor. Make sure the two of you agree on what you want to achieve.

Then go over the sections in the book that are most directly relevant to reaching that goal. If you have a partner who's working with you, she should also read the same material. Discuss it together. Are there any differences of opinion about what you're going to do that need to be worked out now?

If you're working with a partner, I cannot emphasize enough the importance of getting and keeping her cooperation. It's crucial that you and your partner agree about what you're going to do and that disagreements and conflicts that arise over the program or over anything else be resolved as quickly as possible.

A great deal is being asked of your partner, and she has a critical role to play. Her attitude and behavior can make the difference between reaching and not reaching your goals. A supportive, cooperative partner is a blessing, and you need to do everything in your power to help her be this way.

It's crucial that she allow you to satisfy her with nonintercourse sex (sex without an erection) until you reach a point where you are able to have good, long-lasting erections. This is necessary because virtually every man I've worked with needed to believe that he could give his partner a good time in bed without a hard penis. Without that belief, it's almost impossible to reduce the pressure he feels to have long-lasting erections. That pressure, of course, is at least a part of what's causing his problem. If he knows he can satisfy her in other ways, having an erection, or one that lasts a long time, becomes less important to him, thus reducing his anxiety.

Unfortunately, some women find this difficult to accept. These women are usually orgasmic in intercourse, and either they haven't learned to be orgasmic with other kinds of stimulation or they have but find these other ways not quite good enough. And often these partners convey—sometimes subtly, sometimes almost brutally—that they won't be happy until the man has good erections and can engage in intercourse. One of the subtle ways is by refusing to allow him to sexually pleasure her. This usually makes the man feel guilty. She's doing all this work for him and giving him pleasure, but he can't reciprocate. This is not a good setup. The man invariably picks up on his partner's frustration and impatience. Under these circumstances, the chances of resolving his problem are close to zero.

These issues can often be worked out in therapy, but they can be difficult for some couples to resolve on their own. So make sure to discuss them with your partner before undertaking a program. If they can't be settled with good feelings, do not try the exercises. Instead, have a consultation with a sex therapist.

Whether you're working with a partner or on your own, you should determine if now is a good time to undertake the program. Make sure you don't have events on your calendar, such as an extended visit from relatives or an especially busy time at work, that will make staying on the program difficult. It's fine to put off starting the program until a more propitious time. Once you do start, pull out all the stops and go for it.

Plan for systematic effort over a period of two to five months. In general, you'll need to devote two to three hours a week to the program, usually in segments of twenty to thirty minutes. This is an average, of course, and it's certainly fine to take a brief vacation from the program. What doesn't work at all is to skip weeks altogether or do the exercises on an occasional basis. Learning new skills or habits requires consistency and frequency.

Set up a definite schedule for doing the exercises, such as Monday, Wednesday, and Friday at 8:00 P.M., and stick to it. If either one of you is not in the proper mood and can't get in one when the appointed time arrives, skip the sexual exercise but do something else that's relevant. For example, review your progress, read or reread a chapter in this book, be close and loving in some way, and so on. I guarantee you that regular schedules work better than relying on willpower or doing the exercises when the urge strikes you.

The biggest mistake people make is not doing the exercises often enough until the goal is reached. One reason that isn't immediately apparent is that although the exercises are fairly simple and easy to do, they can begin to feel like a burden over a long period of time. The people who do best with them are those who find ways of making and keeping them interesting. They keep the goal in mind and how good they'll feel when they reach it, and they approach the exercises in a positive and lighthearted way. They also stay disciplined and get through the program as soon as possible. The more you stick to your schedule and the more quickly you move through the program, the better the results will be.

Please understand that you need prime, unhurried time for the exercises. It doesn't help to do them when you're fatigued or when time is short. You've got to be relatively relaxed and alert to benefit. The time given for each exercise is only for the exercise itself, but you shouldn't just jump into an exercise; rather, start by spending a few minutes talking or touching, to feel close and get into the proper mood. Then do the exercise.

It will help you keep to your program if you make all the necessary arrangements in advance. If you're going to do exercises in your bedroom, as most people do, you may want to make sure the room is clean and exactly as you want it. Have anything you might need for that particular exercise—for example, a clock or a lubricant—in place. Since you may need to refer to this book, it's also a good idea to have it on the nightstand and turned to the appropriate page.

One question that comes up a lot is how much flexibility is allowed. Do you have to do every single exercise, and do each one exactly as it's written? The answer is, that there is room for selection and creativity; just take care not to lose sight of what you're doing. When I see a man in therapy for erection problems, for example, I don't necessarily ask him to do every one of the exercises in Chapter 22. Everything depends on his situation and the results of the exercises he's already done. Doing all the exercises I give in any chapter would represent the safest, most conservative route.

Some individuals and couples skip some of the exercises, doing only those they feel are most relevant to them. Others make changes in the procedures to better suit their situations. For example, an older man with an erection problem may realize that in doing the exercises three times a week, his own body is working against him; after an ejaculation his body isn't ready to produce another erection for two or three days. If that's the case, it makes sense to do the exercises only twice a week. On the other hand, many men wanting to develop ejaculatory control learn that progress is swiftest when they do the exercises four or five times a week instead of the three times I recommend.

There is nothing wrong with changing the routine to better suit your needs provided you are willing to readjust if things don't work out. If, for example, you skip an exercise and then have difficulty doing the next one, you should consider doing the one you skipped. Similarly, if you change an exercise and it doesn't produce the intended results, you should consider doing it in a manner closer to what I've written.

Before doing any of the partner exercises, both you and your partner should read it over together so that you'll both know what is being asked of you. Discuss her feelings, your feelings, and what is to come, and work out any disagreements.

Since how long you'll need to continue doing the exercises is largely a function of how often they are done, you need to reach an agreement about frequency. Your partner should also understand that in the majority of the exercises, you are in total control—of the type of stimulation, of when to stop and resume, and when to end the exercise. You should make clear your willingness to satisfy her manually or orally before or after doing an exercise. Difficulties will arise if she feels she is doing all the work and getting nothing in return. Do whatever is necessary to prevent this from becoming a problem.

One way for you to prevent problems is to take total responsibility for initiating the exercises. Even if the two of you have already planned to get together at 9 P.M. on Tuesday, it's up to you to initiate the process at that time. This point is crucial. I've witnessed many arguments because the woman thought the man wasn't initiating the exercises; this fed into her fears that he was putting the whole burden of the program on her. The way to avoid this, and it must be avoided, is to be very disciplined about initiating the exercises.

Another way to maximize harmony and effectiveness is to schedule a regular meeting with your partner—say once a week—to discuss how the program is going for each of you. This is similar to what you'd be doing if you were seeing a therapist. During this meeting, each of you should be able to talk without interruption for a few minutes about anything that is relevant. It will pay to listen with full attention when your partner gives her point of view.

If you're doing exercises without a partner, a weekly meeting with yourself is helpful. Use the time to think about how things are going, what needs to be changed, and so on.

Some people object that all this scheduling seems rigid and unspontaneous. They're right. It's supposed to be that way (although I prefer the words *disciplined* and *systematic*) because that's what works best when you're learning new skills. If you were serious about learning new skills in sports or business, you wouldn't just go to class or practice when the spirit moved you; you'd probably have some kind of regular schedule. And that's exactly what's needed here as well.

But scheduling time in advance for being together does not rule out spontaneity. There's nothing wrong with doing an exercise when the spirit moves you even though your schedule doesn't call for it that day. There's also nothing wrong with occasionally taking a day off from the program and doing whatever the two of you want to do.

It's important not to restrict physical activities with your partner to the exercises. Make sure you do some holding, hugging, kissing, and any other mutually enjoyable expressions of physical affection. Have fun together in other ways as well.

And learn to be a little patient. Most of the men I've seen with sex problems want the problem resolved yesterday! They wish for a pill, shot, or some magic words that will straighten things out instantaneously. One man I saw with his wife beautifully exemplified this attitude. He had been having erection problems for ten years, with all the usual complications— sex had become almost nonexistent, touching had diminished, she had almost given up on ever having good sex again, and he had become increasingly depressed. I gave them a few assignments to do at home. When they came in for the next session, he said this: "We're talking more and we feel closer. And we're doing more touching. But it didn't work. Nothing has changed." What he meant was that he hadn't gotten an erection with her. After a decade of no erections, he expected to get one after only a week of work.

Even though sex therapy is brief and highly effective, it takes a little longer than a week or two. See if you can accept this fact. Talk to yourself when you feel impatient and are starting to think that nothing will help: "I know I'm being impatient, and I have to realize that the process takes longer than a few days. Look, in some ways things *are* better. We're having more fun, and she's being more cooperative and supportive than before. Things are improving, and I'm sure the problem will be resolved. I just have to be a little more patient."

Talking to your partner can also help.

YOU: I feel so impatient. I'd like this to be over.
HER: I know exactly how that feels.
YOU: I know this has been hard on you, and I feel guilty for putting you through it. The sooner it's over, the sooner you'll feel okay and the sooner I can stop feeling so guilty. I don't know if it's

possible, but I would feel better if you could reassure me in some way. Maybe you could tell me that you're okay about going through this with me. Is that possible?

Above all, find ways to make the program enjoyable. Some of my clients inject a bit of humor into their activities by saying, "I wonder if all this hand stuff will make us go blind." Others talk about the hows, whens, and wheres of the sex they'll have once the problem is resolved. Yet others remind themselves of all the benefits of undertaking the program, such as an increased ability to talk about sex, an increased ability to talk about other things as well, a new knowledge of sex and intimacy, feeling closer, and so on.

I know you wish you didn't have to be doing exercises and that you didn't have the problem. But since you do have the problem and are going to do the program, why not make the best of it?

CHAPTER NINETEEN

Getting Your Mind on Your Side

For the first month, these positive statements were just words. I said them, I heard them, but although they made me feel a lot better than the negative statements I had been making, it's like I didn't really connect with them. And then, about two weeks ago, I started believing. Yes, I really would be a great lover. Yes, I really would show my partner a good time whenever we made love and have a good time myself. Now these statements are part of me.—*Man, 38*

IT MAY BE going too far to say that the mind is everything when it comes to sex. But if it's not everything, it's certainly far ahead of whatever is in second place.

Let's look at two men who both had a problem the last time they had sex—say they didn't get erections. The first one, Bud, was disappointed but not greatly upset. He had a good time anyway. He's eagerly looking forward to making love with his partner again today. He tells himself it's going to be another great experience and imagines kissing and fondling her breasts, which gives him great pleasure. Because he's feeling so good about the prospects, his mind conjures up a picture of her taking his penis in her mouth, which gives him even greater pleasure. When he and his partner get together in bed, his mind will focus on the pleasurable sensations he's feeling, thus maximizing the chances that he will get aroused and that the arousal is translated into an erection.

Art, on the other hand, keeps thinking about what he calls his "failure." He tells himself he may be impotent, that he may not get it up the next time. He too has images, but they're different from Bud's. He imagines his wife indicating she's ready for intercourse but himself being totally soft, which makes him feel terrible and hopeless. He's working up a nice stew of defeat and failure. As he gets caught in this muck and mire, he has more depressing thoughts and pictures. Finally he imagines his wife getting furious and telling him he's not a real man. He gets into such a state of anxiety and despair that he almost jumps out of his skin when she tries to hug him. If he does try to make love, his mind will be busy focusing on the possibility of failure and its consequences rather than on what's happening at the moment, thus helping to ensure that failure is what he gets.

Two men, two minds. One is headed for pleasure and a good time, the other for anxiety and a miserable time. The difference is not in their penises but in their heads. This fact deserves your attention. The reality is the same for both men: no erection the last time they had sex. But they deal differently with that reality. As psychologist Albert Ellis, the father of what is now called cognitive therapy, has been demonstrating for five decades, it's not reality itself but rather how you construe or interpret it that makes all the difference.

Your mind can make for beautiful, functional, and satisfying sex, but it can also make sex an agony. Perhaps most important for our purposes, it can create and maintain sex problems and make resolving the problems difficult or even impossible. With your mind on your side, however, it's much easier to solve any problems.

To get the most from your self-help program, it's essential to make sure your mind is working with you rather than against you. In a number of places earlier in the book, I have given examples of using your mind to your advantage, such as mentally rehearsing things you want to say and do, and using fantasies to increase arousal. But now we need to get into more detail.

The mind operates in basically two ways: through thoughts (ideas) and through pictures (images). It's constantly talking to itself with words and images about you. Because these messages are to and about yourself, they are called self-statements. You may or may not be aware of these internal communications, but take it as an article of faith that you spend a good part of every day talking to yourself about you. If you're not aware of what you're saying, you soon will be.

Thoughts and images can be mainly positive or mainly negative. In what may be a sad commentary about the state of humanity, a very large proportion of the population goes around making negative statements and showing itself negative pictures. The result is what is called low self-esteem. People who tell and show themselves negative things feel bad much of the time. The bad feelings affect their relationships, behavior, sex life, and everything else.

Men who have had sex problems or who for some other reason don't feel good about themselves sexually do a lot of what Albert Ellis calls "catastrophizing" and "awfulizing." Any disappointment or frustration, any less-than-perfect event—such as a sexual activity that doesn't live up to every single standard in the man's mind—is made into catastrophe. Lack of erection becomes "I'm impotent" or "I'm over the hill" or "My wife will leave me."

Self-statements have a kind of magnetic quality. They attract other statements of the same kind and build on one another. If you regard your latest sexual activity as positive, your mind will tend to call up supporting positive ideas and images. It may recall another very satisfying sexual event from the past, or some sexual compliments you've received. This will reinforce and heighten your good feelings. Unfortunately, it works the other way as well. Negative thoughts and feelings tend to conjure up other bad experiences, thoughts, and feelings. One bad experience recalls another and another, until you're feeling totally discouraged.

If you're having a sex problem of any kind, it's probable that you are helping to maintain that problem by the activity of your mind. Such negative thinking makes it difficult for the problem to fix itself and for therapy or self-help materials to work.

You need to get your mind out of your way and on your side. Put differently, you need to think more positively. A negative thought (or image) is anything that leads to negative or bad results for you. A positive thought (or image) is anything that leads to better feelings and helps you do what you want. More positive and helpful thoughts, and fewer negative thoughts, is what you need.

It's crucial to understand that what's important are the effects of telling yourself certain things or having certain images. Whether or not these ideas and images are true is entirely beside the point. People tend to say, "That's not negative thinking, that's reality!" My response is that *it doesn't make any difference if it's true or not; what counts is the effect it has on you.*

In 1989, as he approached the last day of the Tour de France, the world's most prestigious bicycle race, American cyclist Greg LeMond knew he had to accomplish something that most experts considered impossible. He was fifty seconds behind and would have to make up more than that on a very short ride. LeMond didn't deny the difficulty of the task; he simply didn't bother with it. Focusing on how difficult the task was would only make him feel bad. Instead, he focused on riding the race of his life. He would focus only on his position on the bike and his pedaling technique, and what would be would be. Greg LeMond won the race by eight seconds, the closest Tour ever run.

I'm not suggesting you deny reality—facts must be faced—but only that you don't dwell on its depressing and discouraging aspects. Focus instead on the positive aspects of the situation—things that make you feel good, increase your confidence, maintain your ability to think clearly and to take appropriate action—or get away from all evaluations, whether positive or negative, and simply focus on the task at hand. That's what positive thinking is all about, and it's what Greg LeMond did so well in the Tour de France.

There are several questions you can use to judge what's going on in your head. All of them have to do with how helpful or unhelpful the idea or picture is. I'll use a made-up example to illustrate the use of the questions. The example goes like this: You have the smallest penis in the world. Scientific measurements demonstrate that no one anywhere has a smaller penis than you. To make the example more interesting, let's throw in two more things. One is true, that medical science has no way of providing you with a larger penis. The second is made up, that no woman in the world could have an orgasm in intercourse with your little penis. When you find yourself thinking about your penis, ask yourself these questions:

1. **Does this thought or image make me feel better?** If telling yourself that you have the smallest penis in the world makes you feel bad, as it almost certainly will, it's not helping you. Without denying the size of your organ, you need to move on. Focus on the assets you have that make you a desirable lover—for example, your genuine liking of women and sex, your sensitivity to the feelings and desires of others, your ability to listen and learn, your ability to satisfy women with your hands and mouth. Focusing on these matters will make you feel better.

2. **Does this thought or image help me behave the way I want?** If telling yourself that you have a small penis makes you fearful of approaching women for sex, or even of dating, it's not helpful. It's preventing you from behaving the way you want.

3. **Does this thought or image help me think productively about the situation?** If telling yourself you have a small penis puts you in a funk where you can't think productively, it's not helping you. Negative thoughts often have the effect of stopping all constructive thinking.

4. **Does the thought or image reinforce positive images I have about myself?** If focusing on your small penis reinforces a larger, more destructive idea—for example, that no one will want to have sex with you or that you'll never have a relationship—it's not helpful.

5. **Does the thought or image improve my relationship?** If imagining

your partner joking with her friends about your small penis makes you want to get back at her or withdraw, it's not helpful to your relationship. You need to change the idea or image to help you feel better about the relationship.

No matter what your problem or situation, there are always two ways to go with it. The negative way leads to discouragement, despair, and self-hate. The more positive way leads to useful thinking, good feelings, and solutions.

Some people think the idea of positive thinking is simpleminded and a denial of reality. To be sure, some advocates of positive thinking are simpleminded and do deny reality. But what I'm suggesting is something different. If your sex life is boring, if your ejaculations are very quick, if you and your partner don't agree on how often or what kind of sex to have—if any of these things are true, they are facts and need to be acknowledged. But acknowledging something does not mean dwelling on it; you need to move on. Just because your penis hasn't been working lately doesn't mean it will never work. You can make changes.

Changing the thoughts and pictures in your head isn't difficult in principle. You simply argue with and change unhelpful thoughts when they occur to make them more positive and constructive, and show yourself positive images as often as possible. I said this process isn't difficult in principle, and it isn't, but there is a catch: It requires consistent effort over a period of time. We're not talking about changing a negative thought to a positive one once or twice or even a hundred times. We're talking about doing this dozens of times a day, every day, for months. It's simply a matter of repetition and perseverance. There are no brilliant insights to be had and no magical shortcuts. It's by sheer repetition that you change your negative ways to more positive ones.

Consider if you've ever made any of these comments to yourself:

My penis is too small.
I'm not a good lover.
Other men are better at sex than I.
I don't know how to satisfy my partner [or women in general].
Sue and I will never have an exciting sex life.
I'll never overcome this problem.

If you've said one or more of these things to yourself every now and then, it probably doesn't mean much. But if you habitually tell yourself things like this, you're going to feel bad about yourself sexually. And that needs to be changed.

The following exercise will help you get started.

EXERCISE 19-1: TRACKING NEGATIVE THOUGHTS

For the next week or two, carry a small notebook or some index cards in your shirt or jacket pocket wherever you go. Whenever you're aware of having a negative or unhelpful sexual thought or image, jot it down. Obviously, there will be times when you're aware of something but can't write it down; this may happen when you're with others or when you're driving. Jot it down later if you still remember.

If you're unsure if a thought or image is negative or not, use the five questions on pages 266–267, to help you decide.

At the end of a week or two, go over all your negative self-statements and pictures. These are the things that you need to change that we'll get to in the next exercise.

Here is what one man who had erection problems wrote in his notebook on one day:

I'm a failure in sex.
An image of not getting it up and a woman making fun of me.
My dick is defective.
Sex just isn't my thing.
Recalling Marge [his wife] saying I wasn't a real man.
I wish sex didn't exist.
An image of Marge passionately fucking another man and afterward telling me that I'm just a limp dick.

These thoughts and pictures are enough to depress anyone. Constantly replaying them is a great example of awfulizing and catastrophizing. It will make you feel terrible, as with this man, and will probably doom any efforts to solve the problem. You have to change such thoughts.

How can you change self-statements? Just change them. Here are some examples. The self-statement comes first. The italicized response that follows is an example of what you could say to yourself. My comments are in brackets. You don't need to use my words exactly, but do something to make those statements more positive.

My penis is too small. *Hey, wait a minute. I measured it and it's the usual six inches, about what most other guys have. It's big enough to give pleasure to me and to Marge.* [If it's true that you really do have a small erect penis, then you need to acknowledge that fact but then focus on your strengths, like this: *Okay, so my penis is on the small side, but it's also true that my fingers and tongue are very sensitive and have given orgasms to many women. And don't forget that Kit and Wendy didn't have any problems having orgasms in intercourse with me.*]

I'm not a good lover. *Let's change that. It's true I've been having some problems keeping an erection, but other than that I'm a good lover. Marge frequently mentions how sensitive I am to her needs. I'm going to take care of the erection problem by using this book and I'll be even better.* [This man isn't lying to himself. He acknowledges the problem, then commits himself to changing it. If, on the other hand, the man had reason to believe that he really wasn't a good lover—maybe his partner had said something to that effect—then he would want to say something like this to himself: *I have more to deal with than just the erection problem. Marge has commented that I don't seem to be aware of where she is or what she needs. I think that's because I'm so focused on how my cock is doing that I forget about her. Okay, I have two things to work on. And work on them I will. First I need to pay more attention to Marge. If I do, she'll probably become less critical and that will help take some pressure off of me to get hard. But I also need to start working on getting my penis to function better.*]

Image of Marge passionately fucking another man. *That hurts, but it's my fantasy, not Marge's. She'd like to fuck like that, but with me, not someone else. I'm going to get some help to make that possible. And right now I'm going to do that movie again, but this time with me and Marge going at it.* [This is a simple technique where you take a negative image and make a more positive one of it. In this case, he runs a series of images, a movie, in his mind of him and Marge making passionate love. Then he tells himself: *That's how it will be.*]

EXERCISE 19-2: CHANGING NEGATIVE THOUGHTS

This exercise is based on the results of Exercise 19-1. Now the task is to take issue with and change your negative sexual thoughts and images into more positive ones, as in the examples above. Whenever you are aware of having a negative thought or image, make the positive changes. If you're too busy at the moment, come back to it later when you have time. It might be hours or even a day later. That's fine. For example: "When driving home yesterday I kept telling myself Marge and I would never work this out. That comes out of my despair, but I don't think it's true. We're going to do the exercises in this book and we're going to make it better."

The words and images you use must be acceptable and believable. Some men have no problem saying "I will be a great lover" or "I will overcome this problem." For other men, however, such statements are too strong. They might do better with "I will be a better lover" or "I'm working on this issue." Use the kinds of words and pictures that work best for you.

Even with acceptable and believable statements, it takes a while, usually months, for them to really sink in. Of course, the more often you talk positively to yourself and the more often you combat negative thoughts and images, the sooner the positive ideas will sink in.

Do this exercise as frequently as possible for as long as necessary, which may well be months, until it becomes your natural way of using your mind.

The previous exercise involves modifying negative thoughts and images of yourself. The next is not dependent on responding to negative mental activity, but simply involves having more positive thoughts and images.

EXERCISE 19-3: HAVING MORE POSITIVE SEXUAL THOUGHTS AND PICTURES

Several times a day, take a moment or two to say something positive to yourself about sex and to show yourself a positive picture (or two, or more). You'll be more likely to continue doing this if you do it at regular times—as soon as you are awake, while brushing your teeth or shaving, or when you get into the shower or sit down on the bus.

Exactly what to say and what images to have are up to you, as long as they're positive. Some examples:

▲ Imagining yourself having long-lasting intercourse (if you've been having problems with ejaculatory control or erections).

▲ Saying to yourself, "I know this program will work and I'll have longer-lasting (or firmer or more frequent) erections."

▲ Saying to yourself, "Next time Sue and I have sex, I'm going to focus on the pleasurable sensations and have a grand time."

▲ Imagining yourself experiencing the problem you have (say losing your erection in intercourse), but feeling calm about it, hugging or pleasuring your partner, getting aroused again, and getting more sexual stimulation. This is an extremely important image, because the better you feel about setbacks and difficulties, the more easily your problem will be resolved.

▲ Recalling an experience where you didn't have the problem that's now bothering you. For instance, if you're losing your erection before intercourse, recall in detail a time when you kept your erection and had great intercourse; as you imagine that time, tell yourself, "It will be like that again."

Best of all is to combine an image or fantasy with a statement that reinforces it, as in the last example. Imagining yourself having long-lasting sex and telling yourself at the same time or afterward that "I will learn to last longer" is another example.

There is a group of men, a much larger group than many people would think, who are constantly down on themselves. Women aren't the only ones with low self-esteem. Many of these men aren't able to do Exercise 19-3, or they do it but the words aren't believable. A different version of that exercise can help.

EXERCISE 19-4: FOCUSING ON YOUR VIRTUES

This exercise requires that you dwell on your good points (strengths, assets) several times a day. The first step consists of making a list of these points, preferably on index cards, one item per card. One of my clients dubbed these items his "virtues list." Over a period of several days or longer, jot down your virtues on the cards. If you can't think of anything positive, use compliments you've received; if someone thanked you for your generosity, use "generous." One or two words is usually sufficient for each characteristic. A sample list might look like this: "decisive, loyal, good provider, intelligent, understanding, gentle, willing to help, good listener." Try to come up with at least seven to ten items.

Beware of being perfectionistic. No one is always kind, always a good listener, always decisive, or 100 percent creative or intelligent. If you often exhibit the quality or virtue, or if others have complimented you on it, that's sufficient.

The second step consists of going through your list at least twice each day and focusing on one of the items. It should go like this: You read each item and say to yourself "Yes, I'm quite intelligent" or "It's true, I'm a good listener." Then take a few more seconds to recall an example of one of them ("I remember when Marge told her friends that it wasn't true men couldn't listen, that I was a great listener. This was after I had spent several hours with her, listening to her feelings about her father's death. It's true. I am a good listener"). The next time you go through the list, focus on a different virtue or recall a different example of the same one.

The entire exercise usually takes less than a minute. Twice a day is a minimum; the more often you do it, the better you'll feel. After a week or two of practice, you should also repeat some of your positive points whenever you have a spare moment: while stopped at a red light, or waiting in line someplace.

With a little effort, you'll make this exercise a regular part of your life from now on. You'll find it's a lot easier and more rewarding to focus on positive thoughts than negative ones.

HAVING A TALK WITH YOURSELF

While we've just been discussing how to talk to yourself, here I mean something a bit different. Having a chat with yourself is usually longer than the kinds of self-statements we've been dealing with; whereas a self-statement might take only a few seconds, a chat with yourself might take a minute or longer. It's a gentle, reassuring, supportive talk, even with some cheerleading, designed to calm you down, support your efforts, and keep you on the right track and doing the right things. These are the kinds of talks we often get from friends and therapists. I give them to my clients all the time.

One good time to use these talks is during time-outs (see pages 178–180). Calm yourself and then talk to yourself about what needs to be done. For example: "Take it easy, take it easy. Take a few deep breaths to get more relaxed. . . . Good. Now let's look at this. You're acting as if Ronnie is your enemy, trying to hurt you. You know that's not the case. It's just that you pushed her button when you mentioned the business with her mother. She tends to lose it when that comes up. What she said doesn't mean anything. She was just very upset. You know she loves you. So what to do? How about apologizing for bringing up her mother? That might help. Fine, let's start with that and then ask if this is a good time to continue talking about our plans for Labor Day. That's the plan. And relax. She loves you. It will be fine."

It's extremely important to have a talk with yourself when you feel discouraged about solving your problem or about how an exercise has gone. I can almost guarantee you will have such feelings sometimes. The more quickly you can recover from feelings of failure and discouragement, the better you and your partner will feel and the faster you'll make the changes you desire.

EXERCISE 19-5: SELF–PEP TALK

Whenever you feel discouraged about your progress or your chances of success, sit down in a private place for a few moments and give yourself a supportive, reassuring talking-to. Do this as many times as necessary over a period of hours or longer to help yourself feel more positive. Several examples follow, but you of course need to make changes in the wording to better suit your personality and situation.

Here's an example of what a man who is feeling discouraged about fixing his problem could say to himself (in a calm, reassuring voice):

Hey, take it easy. You're letting yourself get carried away. I know you're feeling discouraged, but I don't think there's reason to be. Let's look at the facts. It is true that you've had trouble controlling your ejaculations with all your partners. But it's also true that you're a good lover; everyone you've been with says so. And it's also true that there are ways to fix the ejaculation thing. You've already got this guy's book; why not do what he suggests? If worse comes to worst and it doesn't help, you can get a referral to a sex therapist here. This problem is solvable, so let's just be calm and get on with it.

This man's self–pep talk is based on looking at the facts of his situation, but these talks don't always have to focus on the current facts. You might want to remind yourself of another time in your life when you successfully overcame a problem. Focusing on a past success will almost certainly make you feel better about what's facing you now. Here's an illustration:

This is one of the toughest situations you've ever faced. It seems like you have so little control. But maybe you can take comfort from the fact that tough situations have always brought out the best in you. Remember the Johnson deal? Now, that was a mess. No one thought you could swing it, and you had plenty of doubts as well. Everything seemed out of control. But you found things you could do something about and you worked on them.

And you did it. What you're facing now is similar. You can't directly control your penis, but you know what you can do. Focus on things you can control, the same way you did with the Johnson deal. Yes, this is a toughie, but hang in there. You'll get where you want to be.

One other function that can be served by these talks with yourself is self-commiseration, expressing compassion for yourself. This is kind of a verbal hug you give to yourself. Men aren't used to doing this. If we get compassion, it's usually from our partners. But you can learn to supply some of it yourself and make yourself feel a lot better. Here's an example of how it could go:

This is so hard for you. Not being able to solve a problem on your own strikes at everything you hold dear. Makes you feel like less of a man, less of a person. And even though Ann is supportive and understanding, sometimes it feels like you're all alone. It hurts real bad, and you feel so down. It's hard to feel this way, hard to have the problem. You want to deny it, to run away. But there's no place to go, no way of denying it. Try to be kind to yourself, and understanding. It's rough, but—problem or not, difficult or not—you're a good person and will get through it. Just be good to yourself; be as generous as you would be if someone else had the same problem and told you about it.

This last example may seem corny as you read it, but many of us receive such expressions of compassion from the women in our lives. And many of us—if we were lucky—got something like it when we were children. Expressing compassion for yourself is healthy and constructive. Why not give it a shot when you're in need?

And try not to get discouraged if these self-chats don't have immediate results. You may have to do a number of them, over a period of hours, days, or weeks, before you notice changes.

This completes your introduction to getting your mind on your side. But we are far from done with the subject. In later chapters I'll suggest other relevant exercises. You'll be far ahead of the game if you've already started doing the exercises in this chapter.

Developing Ejaculatory Control

I've had dozens of women, and only now do I learn that I've been coming quickly all along. I didn't realize it. I thought what I was doing was normal. I feel bad about all those women I shortchanged.—Man, 26

Having better control is something I treasure. It's made for better sex and a big difference in how I feel about myself, not only sexually but in all areas. —Man, 37

LACK OF EJACULATORY control is probably the most common male sexual problem. The main manifestation of this difficulty is that the men consistently come more quickly than they or their partners want in intercourse; hence the terms "premature" and "rapid ejaculation." Although the complaint is usually stated in terms of time—he comes, say, within thirty seconds of starting intercourse—the issue is really about voluntary control of the ejaculatory process rather than time. The man lacks a vote or influence over when he comes. It happens when it happens, usually quickly and often seeming to sneak up on him.

It has been estimated that about one-third of American men suffer from an inability to control the timing of their ejaculations; that is many millions of men. Though the problem generally affects younger men and tends to improve with age, there are some men in their forties, fifties, and even older who have it. I worked with one man who had very little control over his ejaculations his whole life and still had the problem even though he was seventy. I hope you won't wait as long as he did to develop better control.

WHAT IS EJACULATORY CONTROL?

While ejaculation is a reflex and can't be controlled perfectly, a man who has developed control can enjoy high levels of sexual arousal, whether

275

from oral or manual stimulation or intercourse, without coming, and he usually has a choice when to ejaculate. He can allow his arousal to rise to a high level and then more or less level off until he wants to come, as shown in Figure 8. Don't take the leveling off too literally, however. In reality, his arousal fluctuates, increasing and decreasing, according to his desires and what's going on, until he wants to come. He can also decide to come quickly if that seems appropriate.

In contrast, a man without control tends to go from zero excitement to orgasm without leveling off (Figure 9). He has to come quickly; he has no other choice. He doesn't get to enjoy high levels of arousal for long. He may try various methods of lessening his excitement—thinking of things other than sex is a popular one—but they work neither well nor consistently. And his partner is always in a quandary. She's fearful of stimulating him, because that may bring instant ejaculation. She's fearful of allowing herself to get turned on in intercourse, because it will probably be over before she's derived as much enjoyment from it as she desires. If she has the ability to be orgasmic in intercourse, she at first will try desperately to reach orgasm before he comes, usually a futile endeavor. After repeated failures, she may stop getting turned on. What's the point of getting excited, she wonders, if the only result is to be left hanging and feeling frustrated? Even if she does manage to achieve orgasm in intercourse before he

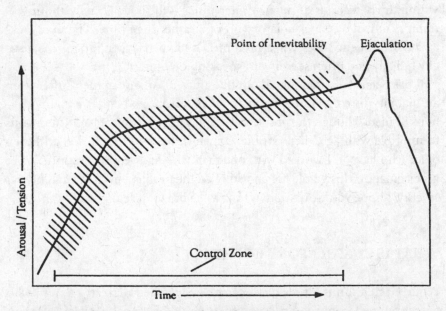

Figure 8: Male sexual experience with ejaculatory control

does, it's a hurried and anxious business and often doesn't seem worth the effort.

Lack of ejaculatory control isn't a bad problem to have, because sex therapists have been very successful in resolving it. According to a number of studies and clinical impressions, 80 to 90 percent of men learn better control in therapy, provided they are willing to devote the necessary time and energy. Ejaculatory control is a skill or habit that can be learned in eight to twenty weeks by following the exercises given in this chapter.

Many men without good ejaculatory control have a fantasy, which one of them put this way: "I'd like to be able to screw for an hour—no, make that two or three hours—without coming. I think that would feel great and my wife would love me for it." It's easy to understand how someone who usually can't have intercourse for more than a minute or two would fantasize about the effects of lasting longer. But, as usual, it's important not to get carried away. I've talked with men who do have intercourse for up to an hour, and even longer, and they are not a happy group. They have the problem of not being able to come inside a woman no matter how long they thrust, and their regular bouts of thirty-, forty- or sixty-minute intercourse really don't feel all that great.

It may seem to you that their partners would be ecstatic, but the reality is somewhat different. Their partners complain about unceasing thrusting

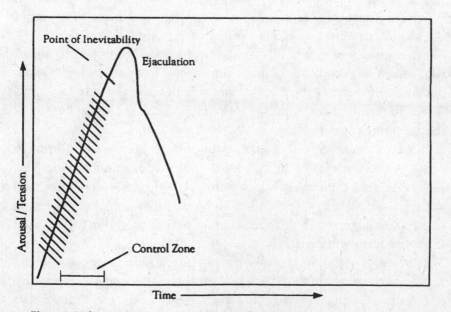

Figure 9: Male sexual experience without ejaculatory control

and pounding, sore vaginas, and a sense of incompleteness because, although intercourse seems to go on forever, the man never finishes in "a normal way." This problem, called "retarded ejaculation" by sex therapists, is far less common and more difficult to treat than rapid ejaculation.

Lack of ejaculatory control manifests itself in various ways. Some men have very little control regardless of the sexual activity. They come as quickly in masturbation as they do with partner stimulation. Others are okay when they're by themselves but not when they're with a partner. Still others, probably the largest group, are fine except for intercourse. There is yet another distinction. Most men without ejaculatory control have had the problem all their lives. But there are some who once had control but no longer do.

Most men without ejaculatory control do not also experience difficulty getting erections. But some men have both problems: Erections are difficult to get and ejaculations are usually quick. **Since many of the exercises for developing better control require an erection, men with both problems should not attempt to work on gaining ejaculatory control until the erection problem is resolved.** First things first.

Sex therapists aren't as knowledgeable about the causes of lack of control as I would like. We aren't sure why millions of males have little or no ejaculatory control, while millions of others do. We aren't sure why control gets better with age and experience for many men, but not for others.

One thing we do know, however, is that unlike erection problems, which are often caused or maintained by physical factors and drugs, rapid ejaculation is almost always due to a lack of knowledge, attention, or skill. Another thing we know is that abstinence hampers control. Even a man who usually has good control may come quickly after several weeks without sex. It also seems to be true that anxiety can cause loss of control. This is seen in men who come quickly with new partners but regain control as they get more comfortable.

In general, men without control simply don't make the adjustments in behavior necessary to stay at high levels of arousal without coming. This may be because these men are not focusing on their own sensations and therefore can't take appropriate action, because they don't know when to make the adjustments in their behavior, or because they don't know what kinds of adjustments should be made.

The benefits of gaining control are many. Better control means longer and usually more-enjoyable sex, especially intercourse. Men who've achieved this feel more confident and better about themselves as lovers, and their partners are appreciative. Also, many men report that their own orgasms feel better: "Fuller" or "more complete" is how they describe them.

It's important, however, not to confuse having better control with the woman having so-called vaginal orgasms (orgasms solely through intercourse without simultaneous clitoral stimulation). There are, of course, some women who can have such orgasms. If your partner is one of these women and you learn to last longer, she may again have such orgasms. But the clear conclusion of a number of surveys is that many, probably a majority, of women are not orgasmic in this way. They require direct clitoral stimulation (by her hand, your hand, your mouth, or a vibrator) to have orgasm, a task for which a thrusting penis is not well suited. Lasting longer will not help these women reach orgasm in intercourse.

It's also important not to assume that lack of control is always a problem. Whether it is or not depends on the couple and the circumstances. There are some couples, for instance, in which the man usually comes quickly but it troubles neither him nor his partner. If they're content, they shouldn't bother to change. There are also many men who have little control with a new partner. The first few times they're together sexually, he comes quickly. But then his control reappears. With a transitory phenomenon like this, there doesn't seem to be much point in doing exercises. The man can explain to his partner that his control will get better over time, or he might want to delay having intercourse with her until he's more comfortable.

As I mentioned earlier, some men have had good ejaculatory control in the past but have lost it. They've lost the control they once had with the same woman, or they no longer have control now that they are separated from their partner. It is difficult to say if these men should do the exercises in this chapter. The exercises certainly won't hurt, and I've seen some cases in which they've done a lot of good. But even there they seemed like supplements. For these men, the main issue is something else. Usually there's something about the current situation (the man is nervous with a new partner, for instance, or he's angry or feels guilty) that needs work before his control can reassert itself. So feel free to do the exercises, but also devote some time to figuring out what's getting in your way. The best way I know to do this is doing the conditions exercise in Chapter 6.

One man I worked with had never had great control, but it had gotten much worse in the last two years of his deteriorating marriage. Doing ejaculatory-control exercises hadn't helped at all. After his divorce, he came for therapy because he wanted to be a better lover for new partners.

It turned out that one of his main conditions for good control was feeling accepted and loved by his partner. This condition had clearly not been met as his marriage fell apart. Even when he and his wife weren't in open conflict, he'd sensed her anger and resentment. Now that she was no longer in the picture, he was able to make rapid progress with the masturbation exercises described later in this chapter. As this happened, he became involved with a woman he had known for years. He felt truly accepted by her and, after two or three sessions in which he came quickly, his control was better than ever before.

TWO APPROACHES TO EJACULATORY CONTROL

For many years the only proven way of improving ejaculatory control was the program of exercises detailed in the rest of this chapter. But recently a pharmaceutical option has been added. There are a number of medications used to treat depression that have a side effect of making orgasm harder to get to. For men who come more quickly than they want, the drugs can help them last longer. It isn't quite appropriate to use the term "ejaculatory control" for the effect of these drugs. They don't actually give you greater control. They just have the result of making you last longer than before. The control belongs to the drug, not you.

Among the drugs used are Prozac, Zoloft, Paxil, Luvox, and Anafranil. So far there haven't been enough good studies done to know which drug is best for which person. It's mainly a process of trial and error.

As you might expect, there are some problems associated with taking these drugs. Although the doses used to treat rapid ejaculation are usually lower than those used to treat depression, there still can be side effects, and these side effects tend to increase in number and severity as the dose gets higher. Among the possible side effects are anxiety, dizziness, dry mouth, headache, insomnia, and, in some cases of high doses, a significant decrease in sexual desire and even erection problems. Another downside to using the drugs exclusively to deal with rapid ejaculation is that there is no lasting effect; that is, you don't learn anything about lasting longer and you have to keep taking the drugs to last longer. When men stop taking the pills, the vast majority return to rapid ejaculation.

Which drug you should try and in what dose are things you need to work out with your physician. Individual response to these drugs varies considerably. For some men they work wonderfully well, for others the effect is more modest, and for some men they don't help at all. Some men need to take a pill every day, whether they're going to have sex or not. Other men do fine just taking a pill only on the days they have sex.

If you're willing to take these pills for the rest of your life, you need only discuss the subject with your physician. If you would rather develop your own skills at ejaculatory control, you should explore the program in the rest of this chapter. For many men, a combination of the pills and the exercises works best. Taking a drug can be helpful in demonstrating that it's actually possible to last longer. This makes you and your partner feel good. Being able to have longer-lasting sex at least sometimes (by taking a pill) gives a break from the regular menu of quick orgasms. And for some men, the increased time to orgasm also makes the ejaculatory control exercises work more effectively. In the situations where you're using a drug and the exercises, as you develop ejaculatory control by doing the exercises you can phase out the pills.

Bo had been a severe rapid ejaculator his whole life but hadn't been willing to seek treatment until his wife, Sara, threatened divorce. By the time they came to see me, Sara's anger had been stewing for years. I started Bo on some of the exercises later in the chapter, but they didn't work because Sara got so angry while doing them. Because of this, I suggested they give Anafranil a chance. Only a few days after taking the first pill, Bo and Sara had their longest-lasting intercourse ever. A day later they repeated their success. Sara was so pleasantly surprised she forgot to be angry the next time they did an ejaculatory control exercise. By alternating long-lasting intercourse (their "pill days") with the exercises, this couple was able to complete the program in three and a half months, toward the end of which Bo gradually stopped using the Anafranil. Given the intensity of Sara's anger, none of us thought we would have achieved this success without the drug. This is a good example of how a medicine that makes a man last longer can help in a situation in which the drug is not wanted as the long-term solution.

If you and your partner agree you should try one of the drugs either alone or in combination with sex therapy exercises, all you need to do is talk to your doctor.

Don't be too disappointed if you try one or more of the drugs and they don't work for you. They work for many men, but not all. And for some, the drugs make for greater ejaculatory latency but the side effects are intolerable. If the drugs don't do what you need them to, you can still benefit from the program that follows.

A SEX THERAPY PROGRAM FOR
DEVELOPING EJACULATORY CONTROL

My approach for developing ejaculatory control stems from the work of Dr. James Semans in the 1950s. Semans's stop-start technique is the foundation of all the successful procedures used by sex therapists today. Many of them have added variations of their own. I've experimented with most of them and also with some I've developed myself. What follows is the best program of suggestions and exercises for improving ejaculatory control I've come up with in twenty-seven years of dealing with the problem.

Developing better ejaculatory control involves learning two skills. One is the ability to attend more fully to your own sensations of arousal and tension. The other is the ability to make changes in your behavior that will prevent or delay ejaculation.

Let's go back to Figures 8 and 9 to understand in more detail what ejaculatory control means. The shaded area represents the time from the beginning of penile stimulation to just before the point where ejaculation becomes inevitable. I call this area the control zone, because this is where the man can make changes in his behavior to influence when he ejaculates.

The man whose experience is represented in Figure 8—we'll call him Fred—wants to enjoy a long session with his partner. He wants to get to and savor high levels of arousal without coming right away. As he nears the middle and upper ranges of his control zone, he may change his thrusting from faster to slower, and maybe he'll even stop moving altogether for a few seconds or longer. Or perhaps he'll move his hips slightly to change the angle of the thrusts, or maybe he'll do some circular movements for a few minutes. He may monitor his breathing and take some slow, deep breaths. If he knows that holding her hips or looking at her face is orgasm-producing, he won't do that until he wants to come. By making these adjustments and avoiding orgasm-producing activities until he's ready, he's able to stay in the shaded area, having a good time and enjoying the sensations. When he wants to come, he'll act differently.

Although Figure 9 represents the experience of a man without much ejaculatory control, it could also be Fred's experience under certain circumstances. Let's say that just as he begins intercourse he recalls that he and his partner have only a few minutes before they have to dress and leave the house. So he wants to come as quickly as possible. His past experiences will guide his behavior to do just that. He will do the kind of thrusting that's most arousing to him, and he may do other things as well: kiss his partner in his favorite way, touch her breasts or hips, look at her face, and perhaps call up his most arousing fantasy. Although Fred's experience in this situation seems similar to that of a man without control, there is a critical difference. Fred is choosing to have a quick orgasm. The other man has no choice. He goes pretty much directly from nothing to orgasm without leveling out. He may be aware of when he's going to come, but he's not aware of the shaded area and what he could do there. Since he's not in the shaded area very long, it's hard to be aware of it. Nonetheless, it exists and can be used. The more it's used, the larger it grows, until this man's experience is similar to that of Fred.

Fred's behavior, whether in trying to lengthen or shorten his sexual encounter, comprises a number of habits carried out automatically and largely outside of conscious awareness. He probably can't tell you what he does to control ejaculation, and he might not believe that what I've written has anything to do with him. I once interviewed a number of men with good ejaculatory control and asked how they did it. They not only didn't know, but at first denied that they did anything. Only after they carried out my suggestion to observe themselves during sex did they agree that they were actually doing things to influence when they came. This shouldn't be surprising. Although I've been an avid bicycle rider for many years, I can't begin to describe how I manage to keep my balance on the fool thing. Yet I must be doing something (actually a number of things), because a bike won't stand up alone and neither will one with an inexperienced rider on it.

At the extreme upper end of the control zone is what Masters and Johnson called the point of ejaculatory inevitability. This is the point at which the man feels he's starting to come. And that's exactly what's happening. The sensations he feels are the contractions of the prostate gland and seminal vesicles; once they contract, the ejaculation is on its way and nothing can stop it. No control can be exercised once the point of inevitability is reached.

The control zone represents either sexual arousal or tension (anxiety). For most men without good control, it's usually a combination of both. Many men have trouble distinguishing between arousal and tension, but it really doesn't make much difference for those who want to develop better control. Both can make you come quickly. When you're having sex, something in you is increasing or rising, whether you call it passion, tension, or something else. That is what you need to be aware of. The best way to increase awareness is to focus on the part or parts of your body where you most strongly feel the rise in arousal/tension. For most men, this is either the penis or the scrotum. You need to know at what level this anxiety/

arousal becomes the point of inevitability. It's before this point is reached that you need to do something to control ejaculation.

Men who have good control have learned that control, usually without knowing they learned anything. And all of us, whether we have ejaculatory control or not, have learned to control other reflexes. Urination is perhaps the closest parallel. At some point when you were very young, your parents let you know that it was no longer acceptable to urinate in your pants. You gradually learned to recognize the sensations in your body signaling that you were about to urinate, and you could tell someone that you had to get to a toilet. You could tell something was about to happen, but you couldn't delay its occurrence.

As time went on, you completed your training. You not only knew when urination was imminent, but you could also exert some control to delay it. If you were in the middle of a game or watching a TV program and had to urinate, you could squeeze some muscles, wiggle around, or literally grab your crotch to hold it back, at least for a while.

All this is many years behind you, of course, and you probably have no memory of it. The processes of control have been under automatic pilot for so long that you may not be aware that you are actually doing anything to control urination, just as many men with ejaculatory control don't realize that they are doing anything to delay ejaculation. If you have any doubts about what I'm saying, just focus your attention on your pelvis the next time you have to urinate but are in a situation that requires you to wait. If you want to see the control mechanisms in vivid detail, watch what you do when you're caught in a long and unexpected traffic jam after leaving work without urinating.

Before getting to the exercises, I need to give some definitions and principles. All of the physical exercises have a similar structure: **While your penis is being stimulated by you or your partner, you will do two things—attend to your arousal/tension level and either stop or do something else to maintain ejaculatory control.** By doing this repeatedly, you will learn more about your control area and expand it. In doing so, you will achieve control over your ejaculations. And you'll be able to act exactly like Fred.

How Often to Do the Exercises

Therapists differ on how often they ask clients to do the following exercises, from daily to two or three times a week. My experience is that three or even more times a week is best, provided this is comfortable for you and your partner and you don't have difficulty getting erections. It is crucial that you not try to force erections during the program; if your penis doesn't easily get hard, just stop and do whatever you and your partner want. Return to the exercise another day. If three or more times a week is too much, or if you sometimes have trouble getting erections, twice a week will be fine. Two or three times, however, is an average. If you do an exercise only once during a week, you might want to see if you can do it three or four times the next week. If you can't, you'll probably still be okay if you get back on track in the following weeks. Less than twice a week does not work. You will never develop better control on such a schedule.

Which Exercises You Should Do

Every reader who wants to improve ejaculatory control should do the mind-power exercises and the two masturbation exercises later in this chapter. If you think you don't need to do the masturbation exercises, it's a good idea to do each of them once just to make sure you can easily and comfortably handle them. If you don't want to masturbate, you can skip those exercises and start with the first partner exercise. After the description of the mind-power and masturbation exercises, I discuss exercises you can do with a partner and what to do if you don't have a regular sex partner.

What You Should Focus On

As your penis is being stroked, you need to be aware of your arousal/ tension level. For most men, this means focusing attention in their penis or scrotum, the places where they can feel increases in fullness, tingling, or other sensations that mean arousal/tension to them. I guarantee you will get distracted by all sorts of things: fear of coming fast, concern about disappointing your partner, concern about reaching your goals, wondering if your partner really wants to be doing the exercise, and so on. You can't stop yourself from being distracted, but what you can and must do is bring your mind back to where it belongs as soon as you're aware it's elsewhere—what I call refocusing. Just imagine your attention is like a searchlight on a swivel. When it's not where you want it, imagine gently pushing the swivel and the light back where it should be, on your arousal/ tension level. Refocusing gets easier and more effective with practice, and you'll be getting a lot of practice with it. Don't get discouraged that your attention wanders: That's natural and expected. Just keep bringing it back, over and over.

When You Should Stop During an Exercise

Many questions come up regarding exactly when during an exercise you should stop stimulation. Anytime you're in the control zone is fine—that is, anytime after stimulation has begun and you're feeling aroused. But you don't want to play brinkmanship, trying to stop just before the point of inevitability is reached. If you do this consistently, you'll find that you often ejaculate before you want. So stop sooner.

If you want something more specific, here's an option. Rate your arousal/tension on a scale of 0 to 10, where 0 represents a total lack of arousal and 10 represents orgasm. As you do the exercises, you'll be able to rate yourself at any time ("I'm about 4 right now, going to 5"). To start, choose a number you're comfortable with in the middle range—say 4 or 5—and always try to stop when you reach it. But do not choose 9. That's either the point of inevitability or very close to it, and will result in too many accidents. As you proceed through the exercise and feel more comfortable and confident, you can choose higher numbers.

How Long Do You Need to Stop?

When sex therapists were first assigning these exercises in the early 1970s, most of us told men to stop for about a minute, until the urge to ejaculate had completely subsided. This worked well for most men, but an accompanying problem was that without stimulation for a minute or more, many lost all or part of their erections. In order to prevent erection loss, some of my own clients made the stops briefer, anywhere from ten to forty seconds (these are estimates, by the way; you don't need to use a stopwatch). This worked out well for some men, not so well for others. So the answer of how long to stop is this: experiment and find out. You want the stop to be long enough for the arousal/tension level to subside to an appreciable extent, but not so long that you get bored and lose your erection. Stop for different lengths of time between ten seconds and a minute and a half and see what works best. If you need to stop again within a minute or two of resuming stimulation, you need longer stops. If, on the other hand, you're losing most of your erection, try shorter pauses.

What to Do During a Stop

I have found it helps if you do one or more of the following during most stops: (1) talk briefly to your partner just to keep in touch, (2) relax and enjoy the pleasant feelings of decreasing arousal, or (3) take several deep breaths to help you relax (see page 289). It may not feel very powerful to be just lying there doing nothing, but it is. You're doing exactly what you need to do to gain control over a reflex that's been giving you trouble for a long time. See if you can experience it that way and remind yourself that you're taking charge of your sex life.

What About Ejaculating While Doing the Program?

You can ejaculate as much as you want when you're not doing the exercises, as long as this does not interfere with your ability to get an erection when it's time to do an exercise. But be careful not to do anything that makes you feel bad about yourself. Some men want to have intercourse at every opportunity, even if this means they come quickly and feel bad. Feeling bad won't help your progress, so think about what is best for you. Of course, it is fine to come quickly when not doing the exercises if there are no negative consequences. Taking a day off from the program now and then can be fun. But keep in mind what you're trying to accomplish and stick to the program most of the time.

If you want to ejaculate at the end of an exercise, you can do so, but keep your mind focused on your arousal/tension level and maintain the stimulation at a moderate pace—that is, don't do fast, hard stimulation. Be aware of reaching the upper reaches of the control region and passing the point of inevitability.

It's important to understand that you will sometimes ejaculate without meaning to, especially the first time or two you do a new exercise. Such accidents are common and nothing to be concerned about. If you didn't have any, you probably don't need to be following the program in the first place. As New York sex therapist Michael Perelman points out, these accidents are even helpful, because they help you to define the boundaries of the control zone. They let you know unequivocally where 9 and 10 are on the rating scale. If, however, you continue ejaculating unintentionally, something is wrong. Perhaps you need to return to the previous exercise and gain greater comfort and control with it.

MIND POWER FOR DEVELOPING BETTER CONTROL

To derive maximum benefit from the physical exercises described below, you need to get your mind on your side, as we discussed in Chapter 19. A man who hasn't had ejaculatory control tends to think of himself as quick on the trigger. This is, for sure, a reflection of reality, but it also becomes a predictor of future behavior and a reinforcer of a self-image you want to change. It will be easier to change your behavior if you also change your view of yourself.

Start right away to apply the material contained in Chapter 19. Imagine yourself as you'd like to be; spend as little time as possible imagining how you've been. If you haven't read that chapter and digested its contents, now would be a good time to do so.

Mind Power A: Whenever you're aware of telling yourself that you come fast, or having an image that embodies that idea, argue with it and change it. For example: "It's true, I've always come fast. But I'm going to do this program and change that. I'm going to have good control." When you picture yourself coming quickly, say, "That was then," and follow this with an image of having long-lasting sex accompanied by words like "That's the way it's going to be."

Mind Power B: This is an image, really more like a movie, that you should spend thirty to ninety seconds on every day; doing it several times a day is even better. Imagine yourself having long-lasting intercourse with good control, which includes several components. Imagine entering your partner, feeling relaxed and comfortable, and just being still inside her for a moment or two. You're not moving, just enjoying the feel of being in her. Then imagine slow movements, just taking it easy, still enjoying the feeling of being in her. Then gradually increase the pace of your thrusts. Now slow down again. Now again increase the pace gradually, until you're moving almost as much as you want, still feeling calm and easy. Now imagine slowing down and stopping all movement. Stop thrusting and just experience the pleasure. Then gradually increase the movements, slowly building up until you're moving with abandon, letting your body do what it wants. When you want, and only when you want, imagine a wonderful ejaculation. When you're done with the movie, be sure to end with a statement to yourself of this kind: "As it is in my mind, so it shall be in reality" or "This is how it's going to be."

Mind Power C: Before you do any of the physical exercises, spend a few seconds imagining yourself doing it perfectly, exactly as it is supposed to be done. Be sure to imagine all the parts: for example, asking your partner to do it with you, attending to your arousal/tension level, asking her to stop, asking her to resume stimulation, and so on.

This mental rehearsal takes only a few seconds and can be very helpful. You can do it anyplace. For example, if you and your partner are getting ready to do an exercise, you can close your eyes and do your mental rehearsal right there, or you can go into another room—for some reason, the bathroom has been popular with my clients—and take a few seconds to do it there.

Mind Power D: Every day, preferably just after awakening or just before retiring for the night, take a few seconds to imagine how good you're going to feel once you've achieved ejaculatory control.

Mind Power E: This is the pep-talk exercise given in Chapter 19. Remember to use it whenever you feel discouraged or think you failed in an exercise.

SOME DEEP BREATHS, PLEASE

Proper breathing can help develop ejaculatory control. Put simply, taking a few deep breaths can help dissipate the arousal/tension that leads to quick ejaculations. The kind of breathing that's needed is deep, easy, and relaxing. Unfortunately, many of us don't breathe this way. When I ask clients to take some deep breaths, I notice that many of them actually get more tense. They tense their chest or shoulder muscles, and sometimes their neck and even arm muscles as well.

The best kind of relaxing breathing I know is the kind taught in most schools of meditation. There is no obvious tensing of muscles, and while inhaling, the belly (*not* the chest) swells and protrudes. That is, if you lay one hand on your belly while doing this kind of breathing, you'll notice your stomach pushing out a bit on each inhalation and going down a bit on each exhalation. If you're not used to breathing this way, it will take a little practice to learn it. Keep in mind that the purpose is relaxation, keep a hand on your belly to make sure it's protruding slightly with each inhalation, and try not to tense any muscles. If you have trouble with this, it can help to imagine that your belly is an empty balloon, being gently filled with each inhalation, then being gently emptied with each exhalation. This is a fiction, of course, since the air is always going to the same place, your lungs. Nonetheless, the image is usually helpful.

Once you can do this, it's a good idea to practice it as often as possible. A few deep breaths of this kind are perhaps the quickest way for most people to relax. Experiment with taking a few deep breaths when you stop stimulation in both the masturbation and partner exercises. You can also experiment with taking deep breaths when you're being stimulated or having intercourse. This takes a bit of getting used to, because you'll be going against the grain. The more excited you are, the more likely you'll want to take short, superficial breaths and even pant. But with some practice, most men can overcome that tendency and take deep, relaxing breaths.

If you want to go further with using relaxation to help gain ejaculatory control, you can imagine that the air you take in goes down into your pelvis, relaxing the muscles and the whole region. The more relaxed your pelvis is, the less the chance of ejaculating.

MASTURBATION EXERCISES

As mentioned above, everyone who's willing to masturbate should do these exercises even if you don't think you need them. If you really don't, you only need to do each one once.

These masturbation exercises assume that you masturbate the way most men do, by stroking your penis with one hand moving up and down over the shaft and head. Some men pleasure themselves in other ways—for example, by lying facedown and rubbing themselves against the bed, pillow, floor, or sofa. Unfortunately, these other methods are not well-suited to developing ejaculatory control. You probably should learn to do it the typical way.

EXERCISE 20-1: STOP-START MASTURBATION

Step A: With a dry hand (no lotion or other lubrication), masturbate for fifteen minutes without ejaculating. Focus on your penis or pelvic area, as discussed above, so you will know how aroused or tense you are. When you feel you are in the control area, stop all stimulation and (1) attend to the sensations of arousal or tension and (2) take a few deep breaths. When the arousal/tension level has dropped significantly (which can be anywhere from ten seconds to over a minute), resume stimulation. Stop time, the time when you are waiting for your excitement/tension to abate, is included in the fifteen minutes.

You may have to stop a number of times when you first do the exercise. As you continue doing it, you will better learn when to stop and how long to wait, and the number of times you need to stop will decrease.

When you need only one or two stops during the fifteen minutes, proceed to Step B.

Step B: Exactly the same as Step A, except that you now use a lubricant such as K-Y jelly, Astroglide, or massage oil on your hand. When you need only one or two stops during the fifteen minutes, you are ready to move on to Exercise 20-2.

POSSIBLE PROBLEMS

1. You need to stop again as soon as you resume masturbating. This probably means that you're stopping too late and that your stops are too brief. Try stopping sooner and waiting longer before resuming stimulation.

2. You lose all or most of your erection while stopping. This is not a serious problem, but it probably means you are stopping for too long. Try briefer stops.

We now move on to the idea of subtle adjustments, changes in stimulation more subtle than stopping. There is nothing wrong with stopping stimulation in masturbation, partner stimulation, or intercourse. But there are other alternatives. Years ago I discovered that men with good control don't just bang away with fast in-and-out thrusts for long periods of time. They vary their thrusts to help control ejaculation. They move in certain ways when they want to come and in other ways when they want to delay ejaculation, just like Fred. You will learn these other ways. You can use these subtle adjustments when you want, and of course you can always stop if a stop is required.

EXERCISE 20-2: MASTURBATING WITH SUBTLE ADJUSTMENTS

Step A: Masturbate with a dry hand for fifteen minutes without ejaculating and without stopping. When your arousal/tension is anywhere in the control zone, make changes in the stimulation to control your ejaculatory process. Kinds of changes you can make are: slowing down the pace; varying the site of maximum stimulation—for example, by stimulating only the shaft of your penis rather than the head; changing the type of stroke—for instance, going from longer strokes to shorter ones or using circular motions. Try one change at a time. Find out what works for you and then stick with it.

These more subtle adjustments need to be made a bit sooner than stopping. If you make them too late, you can always stop to prevent ejaculation. When your arousal/tension level has decreased, you can resume the more arousing type of stimulation if you want.

When you can comfortably masturbate for fifteen minutes without ejaculating by using only subtle adjustments, go to Step B.

Step B: Exactly the same as Step A, but now you use a lubricant on your hand.

When you can comfortably masturbate for fifteen minutes using a lubricated hand and only subtle adjustments, go to the next exercise.

WHAT NEXT?

Readers who have partners willing to do exercises with them to help develop better control should read the section immediately following, and follow the exercises and suggestions that constitute most of the rest of the chapter.

If you don't have a partner, you can continue to develop your ejaculatory control with the help of erotic videos. The plan is to go through the masturbation exercises again—dry hand with stops, lubricated hand with stops, subtle adjustments while dry and then while lubricated—while watching movies that turn you on. The videos will increase your arousal, thus making control more difficult; this is exactly what we want. Now you get to take more control of when you ejaculate in the face of higher arousal, which is the situation you'll face with a partner. These exercises have been wonderfully beneficial to a number of my clients. When you start being sexual with a new partner, take your time and realize that your new control won't be as evident the first few times as it will be after you are more comfortable with her. If it seems required, you can do some of the following partner exercises with her.

If you think you need more help before you meet a new partner, you may want to work with a team consisting of a therapist and a surrogate partner. See Chapter 23 for a discussion of surrogate partner therapy.

PARTNER EXERCISES

The following guidelines apply to all the remaining exercises in this chapter unless otherwise noted:

1. Both of you should read and discuss each exercise before you do it for the first time.

2. Both of you should agree what words you'll use to tell her when to stop and start stimulation. Words are necessary because nonverbal signals are easily misunderstood. "Stop," "hold it," "start," and "more" are fine, as is anything else that's short, clear, and mutually acceptable.

3. Do whatever is necessary for both of you to feel relaxed and comfortable before beginning an exercise. Some couples like to start right in with penile stimulation. Others prefer to begin with hugging, holding, or massage. And in still others, the man sexually stimulates his partner before she returns the favor. There is no rule to fit all couples. Do what is right for the two of you.

4. It's essential that your partner take her comfort into consideration in deciding what positions to employ. She's got to last fifteen minutes, too. If she's stimulating you with her hand, does she want to sit next to you or between your legs? These details can make a big difference.

5. During the exercise, keep focused on your arousal/tension level, not on your partner. This is crucial.

6. Unless stated otherwise, the goal of each exercise is to last for fifteen minutes without ejaculating. You can come after the fifteen minutes are up if you wish, but go slowly, be aware of your arousal/tension and the point of inevitability, and enjoy.

7. When you are using stops, you should feel confident of your control and need no more than two stops during a fifteen-minute period before going on to the next exercise. If you have a lot of problems with that next exercise and it doesn't get better after a few trials, return to the one before it and practice it until you have further developed your skills.

8. Remember, two or three times a week on average tends to work well for most couples. More is better, provided it's not an effort to get erections or to get your partner to participate.

EXERCISE 20-3: PARTNER STIMULATION OF PENIS

Step A: She stimulates your penis with her unlubricated hand in ways that are arousing to you; feel free to give her instructions on how to stroke you. Keep focused on your arousal/tension level and tell her when to stop. When the arousal/tension level has decreased, tell her to resume.

When you can last for fifteen minutes with no more than two stops and feel confident of your ability to do this again, do Step B.

Step B: Exactly the same as Step A, except that your partner now uses lotion, oil, or another lubricant on her hand.

POSSIBLE PROBLEM

You aren't stopping in time because you're focusing on your partner rather than on your arousal/tension. You may be wondering if she is enjoying herself, if she's getting bored or tired. You need to swing your attention back to where it belongs as quickly as possible. You might also want to talk to your lover about your concerns. Maybe she *is* bored some of the time. Can it be okay with you that she is willing to cooperate in this endeavor even though it's not exciting for her? However you work it out, the important thing is that you be able to put your attention on your arousal/tension level.

Now that you're comfortable using stops to delay ejaculation, you're ready for more subtle changes.

EXERCISE 20-4: PARTNER STIMULATION OF PENIS WITH SUBTLE ADJUSTMENTS

Step A: This is exactly the same as Step A of Exercise 20-3, except that this time you'll use changes in behavior other than stopping to control ejaculation. She stimulates your penis with a dry hand and you delay ejaculation by telling her to slow down the pace or change the kind of stroking. Experiment and find out what works best for you, or show her what you learned from the masturbation exercise involving subtle adjustments.

Should there be problems with this exercise that don't resolve themselves after a few sessions, consider spending some time mastering the subtle adjustments by yourself, Exercise 20-2.

When you're confident and comfortable using adjustments other than stopping to delay ejaculation for fifteen minutes, do Step B.

Step B: The same as Step A, except that your lover now uses lubricant on her hand.

Step C (optional): The same as Step B except that your partner uses her mouth instead of her hand. Do this step only if both of you enjoy oral sex.

Now you're almost ready to enjoy being inside her without ejaculating. But first you should do the next exercise. It's especially helpful for those men who come before insertion in the vagina or immediately thereafter.

EXERCISE 20-5: PENIS NEAR VAGINA

Lie on your back and have your lover sit on your thighs.

Step A: After you have an erection, rub it gently for a few seconds on her inner thighs and see how that feels. Take a few seconds' rest and then do the same in her pubic hair. Take another brief rest. Now rub it gently on the outer lips of her vagina and see what that's like. Take a pause and then put the head of your penis between her vaginal lips and enjoy that for a moment. And that's the whole exercise.

If you felt any anxiety or any urge to ejaculate, take your time and do the exercise again and again until there is no anxiety and no urge to ejaculate. Remember to take some deep, relaxing breaths before starting it and between each step. When you can comfortably do the whole exercise, move on to Step B.

Step B: Exactly the same as Step A, except now it's her hand that guides your penis.

Starting with the next exercise, your partner's vagina needs to be lubricated before following my suggestions. Natural and artificial lubrication are both acceptable, but the two of you need to agree on what's to be done.

Exercise 20-6 will probably strike you as strange. You're working on developing your ejaculatory control, and here I am telling you to come as quickly as possible in intercourse. I really do want you to do this. The reason is simple. In the exercises that follow, there will be times when you come quickly by accident, and it's crucial that you and your partner deal with these incidents relatively calmly and harmoniously. By deliberately reenacting the original problem now and handling it in a way that feels good to both of you, you prepare yourselves to deal with the situation the same way when it happens accidentally.

A word of warning. You and your partner need to read the exercise together carefully before attempting it. Some women feel so hurt and angry by the many quick ejaculations they had to endure in the past that they may not be able to do the exercise or they may need to discharge some angry feelings first. It's crucial that you listen with all the empathy you can muster to what your partner says. If she can't do the exercise, skip it. If she can, but first needs to get some feelings off her chest, see if you can just listen to her.

EXERCISE 20-6: COMING QUICKLY IN INTERCOURSE

When the two of you feel like it, engage in as much sex play as you like and proceed to intercourse. Your job is to come as quickly as possible and to make sure the experience ends up a happy one. You should use what you've learned about your mind to fight any negative thoughts and pictures, and instead to feel positive about what's happening. And the two of you should go on to do whatever you want and have a good experience. Some possibilities are you stimulating her to orgasm if she so desires, one or both of you getting a massage, cuddling, and talking. When the experience is over, talk and commit yourselves to handle future quick ejaculations (and I guarantee they will happen) in the same constructive way.

How many times you can do this exercise depends on how many times you need to, which can be anywhere from once to four or five times. But you shouldn't go on to Exercise 20-7 until both of you are confident that you can handle quick ejaculations with no problems.

Now you're ready to begin a new relationship with your partner's vagina, one that allows more satisfaction for both of you.

EXERCISE 20-7: GRADUAL INSERTION INTO VAGINA

The goal is to insert your penis, gradually and in stages, into your partner's vagina so you can develop greater comfort in being there. She needs to understand that this is not intercourse and that she needs to stay relatively still.

Using a position that will be comfortable for both of you, one of you should place your erect penis just at the opening of her vagina. Take a few seconds to get used to having it there. When that feels comfortable, move the penis in a little bit, about an inch. Again, take a few seconds to get used to the feeling. Continue in this fashion until your whole penis is inside of her. Then stay that way for a few minutes and attend to your arousal/tension. See how it feels to have your penis surrounded by her vagina. Be aware of the texture, temperature, and wetness of the vagina. Get used to being there; it's a nice place.

If at any time you feel you are losing control, slow down your breathing by taking several slow, deep breaths.

If you want to ejaculate afterward and it's okay with her, do so, but move slowly and be aware of what's happening to you.

You can proceed to the next exercise when you are comfortable being inside your partner without any urge to ejaculate.

EXERCISE 20-8: PENIS IN VAGINA WITH NO MOVEMENT

Really a continuation of the previous exercise, this one also requires your partner to be still. The goal is to have your penis in her vagina with little or no movement for fifteen minutes. Either of you can insert your penis. You don't have to do it in stages, but do go slowly. Once you're fully inside, just be there. It's important that your partner feel comfortable with you doing nothing. Of course, it's fine if the two of you want to talk about what's going on. With no movement at all, you may find your erection waning. If that happens, you can ask her to contract her pelvic muscles a few times or you can move slightly, just enough to keep you hard.

POSSIBLE PROBLEM
The first time or two you do the exercise, you get very excited and come. This is not a problem unless it continues to occur. The solution that works best is to return to the previous exercise and spend several sessions without fully entering her. That is, insert only as far as is comfortable and then spend a few moments there. The next time you do it, see if you can insert a little farther, still feeling comfortable. Continue in this way until you're fully ensconced in her. Then extend the time you can stay in her.

Now we're going to extend your ability to be inside of her with movement. The position usually recommended for these exercises is you lying on your back and her sitting on top of you; this allows you to fully relax, letting the bed support your weight so you don't have to flex any muscles, and works well for many couples. But others prefer something else. So use any position that works best for you; just remember that it has to be sufficiently comfortable for both of you so that changes in it aren't necessary during the fifteen minutes.

EXERCISE 20-9: PENIS IN VAGINA WITH MOVEMENT

Step A: This is similar to the previous exercise, except that now one of you should thrust slowly. Which one moves largely depends on the position you're using. If she's on top, she'll do the moving. If you're on top, it will be you. Regardless of what position is used and who moves, you have to be in charge of how much movement and when to stop and resume thrusting. Use subtle adjustments or stops to delay ejaculation for fifteen minutes. It's important your partner *not* start thrusting to satisfy herself. That will come later.

Start with a very slow pace. Make sure you're comfortable with it before increasing movement. Then go a little faster. When that feels fine, with no danger of losing control, increase it again. Don't forget to take some deep breaths before increasing the pace.

Continue with this step until the active one is moving at a pretty good pace but not all out, say about 80 percent of abandoned movement. This will probably not be achieved in one fifteen-minute session. Use as many sessions as you need. Then do Step B.

Step B: The same as Step A, with the other one moving. This may well require a different position.

Step C: The same as the two previous steps, except both of you move. Start with very slow movements and only increase the pace as you feel comfortable and in control. Use as many sessions as required until you are both moving as fast as you desire.

POSSIBLE PROBLEM WITH ANY OF THE STEPS
You lose control when the movements get faster. This means you are speeding up too much or before you're fully comfortable with a slower pace. Go slower and make sure you're fully comfortable and totally in control before picking up the tempo, and pick it up only slightly. Take your time and some deep breaths.

Now you are ready to experiment with intercourse positions different from the one you've been using.

EXERCISE 20-10: DIFFERENT INTERCOURSE POSITIONS

Agree with your partner on which new position to try—for example, man or woman on top, side by side, or rear entry. Your control will almost certainly not be as good in the new position as it was in the old until you have more experience with it. Use the pattern you're now used to: Start with only one of you moving very slowly. Gradually increase the pace. Then let the other one move, gradually picking up the tempo as you're comfortable. Then both of you move. Keep in mind that you'll need a number of sessions to feel in good control in each new position.

For many men, no further exercises will be needed. Their control has significantly improved. They and their partners are enjoying sex a lot more and perhaps having more of it as well. But for other couples, there's still a problem.

CONTROL IS GOOD, BUT NOT WHEN SHE MOVES WITH ABANDON IN INTERCOURSE

In couples where the woman is capable of vaginal orgasms, it sometimes happens that the man's improved control does not extend to when the partner moves with abandon in intercourse, that is, when she starts her drive toward orgasm. These men tend to focus too much on their partner's arousal, and it's as if they get sucked into it. Her arousal becomes his arousal. At first reading, this may sound fine: Her excitement fuels his excitement, and they reach orgasm at the same time. Obviously, there would be no problem if that is what happened. And it does work that way for some couples.

For others, however, what happens is not so pleasing. To make up some numbers, let's say she needs to move forcefully for twenty seconds to reach orgasm. But he either gets very excited by her excitement or gets nervous for fear of not lasting long enough, and he comes ten seconds after she starts her drive to orgasm. If he can't continue thrusting or allow her to continue for another ten seconds, she doesn't have an orgasm. (It's no problem, of course, if he can continue thrusting for a few seconds after his orgasm, until she has hers). She gets frustrated because she was so close. This may feel even worse to the woman than the old situation, where he came before she was anywhere near orgasm. Now she's so close but still can't get there.

One option is to experiment with positions and movements that are more arousing to her than to you. It may be that circular movements of your pelvis or any kind of movement that pushes your pelvis against hers may help her reach orgasm without pushing you over the edge before you want.

Another possibility is simply an extension of Exercise 20-9. That is, in any intercourse position the two of you like, she gradually increases the speed and forcefulness of her movements, always stopping when you feel you are getting too aroused. She, of course, may have to simulate driving toward orgasm. It is important that you use whatever methods have proven successful to calm your excitement—for example, deep breaths (or as deep as possible under the circumstances) or repeating a slogan to yourself such as "Her excitement is not my excitement, her passion is not my passion, I have to do my own thing." You don't need all these words, but I threw them in so you can get the message. Feel free to use whatever words work for you. After stopping and feeling more relaxed, have her resume her movements. If you do this exercise a number of times— sometimes twenty to thirty repetitions are needed—you should substantially change the threshold of your ejaculations. After you feel comfortable with this in one position, start again with another.

If you've done the exercises given, by now you have attained good control and are enjoying a more confident, relaxed, and more satisfying sex life.

You will undoubtedly have noticed that results come gradually and that it takes a while for the training to sink in and become automatic. Your learning will continue for many months. All you need do to facilitate the process is to stay aware of your arousal/tension and take deep breaths and make other adjustments as needed.

Follow these guidelines whenever you have intercourse. They have been part of the exercises you've already done. Enter your partner slowly; don't rush it. When you are fully inside her, be still for a moment or two and just savor the feelings. When you're ready to move, start slow and easy and only gradually build your way up to more abandoned movement. Following these rules will counter the tendency to move too quickly and come too quickly.

Remember that there is absolutely no way to avoid losing control some of the time. Whether because you haven't had sex for a long time, are extremely excited, are tense or angry, or maybe for some other reason, quick ejaculations will occasionally occur. As time goes on, they will decrease in frequency, but they will probably never disappear. This is simply part of normal male functioning. There is nothing you can do about it, and there's no reason for concern.

When you do come quickly, don't fight it. Let it happen, and enjoy it. There's no need for apology. And there's no need to think that all your training has been in vain. It hasn't. Just go a bit more slowly the next time, stay focused, and make your adjustments a little earlier than usual.

Keep in mind the effects of tension. Anything that tenses you up or gets you upset—whether trouble at work, conflict at home, money problems, or anything else—will tend to have a negative effect on your control. So be especially aware and careful during tense times. Anything you can do to alleviate the tension will be very helpful.

If you notice yourself slipping back into your old, quick ways, take some time, both alone and with your partner, to determine what's the cause. A brief refresher course with the relevant exercises in this chapter can be helpful. Couples who don't have intercourse during the woman's period find this a good time to practice manual and oral stimulation.

Now that you have better control, please don't assume that every sex act has to last a long time. Exercise your control when and as often as you want, but remember that good sex is not determined by the clock. You can make great love in two hours, in twenty minutes, and even in twenty seconds. The key is not how long it took but how good you both feel about yourselves, each other, and what you did.

CHAPTER TWENTY-ONE

Resolving Erection Problems: Medical Options

You want to know how I feel, I'll tell you. I feel like an absolute nothing. I know I can satisfy her in other ways and I do, but that's not the point. I feel like shit, like the center has been taken out of me.—*Man, 51*

I'm the one who feels impotent. I feel unattractive and undesirable because I can't arouse the man I love. If this isn't fixed soon, I'm the one who's going to need pills . . . maybe Prozac.—*Woman, 55*

I feel like a new man, better than I have in years. Being able to function again sexually has given me a new outlook on life and made my marriage 100 percent better.—*Man, 46*

IF YOU HAVE complaints about erections, you belong to a very large group of men. It is estimated that twenty million to thirty million Americans suffer from some kind of erection difficulty. Although erection difficulties are found at all ages, they become more common with age. A recent study found that 52 percent of men between the ages of forty and seventy had some degree of erection problem. Knowing these statistics won't fix your problem, but you may feel better knowing you have lots of company.

While any problem with sex is upsetting to a man, nothing generates as much concern, anxiety, shame, and even terror as an inability to get or maintain erections. Nothing except the loss of his job can make a man feel less of a man. The primary meaning of *impotence,* the term traditionally applied to erection difficulties, is "a lack of power, strength and vigor"— the negation of all that we consider masculine. Men have been taught to tie their self-respect to the upward mobility of their penises, and when their penises do not rise to the occasion, they no longer feel like men.

A man in therapy said it like this: "I've never felt like this before. I just don't feel like a whole person, and certainly not like a man." Other men have used terms such as "useless," "hopeless," "fraud," "lost my manhood," and "can't cut it anymore" to describe how they felt when their penises weren't functioning.

Women are often baffled by the agony a man goes through when he fails to get or keep an erection, but they have no parallel experience with which to compare it. A woman can participate in intercourse or any other sexual act without being aroused or even interested. If she does not lubricate sufficiently, artificial lubrication can be brought to the rescue. She may not have an orgasm, of course, but at least she can go through with the act and give her partner pleasure. A man is in a more difficult situation. Because of the incorrect belief that sex demands a rigid penis, he feels that nothing can rescue him. His "failure" is obvious, dangling in full view. There is no way to fake an erection, and it is difficult (though not impossible) to have intercourse without at least a partial erection.

His partner may be sympathetic and supportive, but he may be so consumed with self-loathing that he can't accept what she offers. Many men distance themselves from their partners after such "failures" and engage in orgies of self-flagellation. The result is usually a miserable time for all concerned.

Over time erection problems typically bring about a horrible equality of feelings for the man and his partner. She feels as powerless to remedy the situation as he does and often blames herself, thinking she's not attractive or skillful enough to arouse him. She starts feeling unattractive, undesirable, and unloved. The way out of this mess is for the partners to turn toward each other: to talk about what's going on, to understand and empathize with what the other is going through, and to look together for a solution. But often the partners turn away from one another, alternately blaming themselves and the other. This, of course, tends to make the situation worse instead of better.

Given all the feelings men with erection problems have, clear thinking becomes difficult. Yet such thinking is exactly what's necessary, because you have to make some decisions about how to deal with your situation. It may help you to feel better to realize that **given the various treatment options available, there is almost certainly a solution for you**. You can further improve your state of mind by using the material in Chapter 19 to focus on your virtues as a lover and a human being and by reminding yourself that you are still a worthwhile man regardless of how your penis has been acting.

There are a number of ways in which penises disappoint men. Almost all men have had at least a few experiences when they wanted an erection and didn't get one or when they lost an erection at some embarrassing point. Some men have problems with getting or maintaining erections at the beginning of a relationship. Then, after they become more comfortable with their new partners, erections become more reliable. Because these kinds of difficulties are common and transient, it's best to view them as a part of life rather than as problems. A man can explain to a new partner that it takes him a few times to get comfortable enough for his penis to join in the fun or, perhaps better yet, he can put off getting into sex until he feels more comfortable with her. And some men are now taking Viagra to help break the ice with a new partner.

There are also more chronic difficulties. Some men usually have difficulty attaining erections, while others have trouble maintaining them. For still other men, the problem is that their erections aren't as hard as they would like. And there are men who don't get erections at all, regardless of the kind of stimulation.

There are basically three ways to resolve erection problems. One consists of various medical, pharmaceutical, or mechanical interventions (which are the focus of this chapter), the most recent and best-known of which is Viagra. The second is sex therapy, the kinds of exercises I present in the next chapter. The third is a combination of the first two.

Before getting to these options, however, you need to know more about the nature of the problem. Some erection problems are primarily physical or drug-related in nature, some are primarily psychological, and a majority have both physical and emotional components. The cause does not necessarily dictate the treatment—you can try any treatment you want—but this information can be very helpful. For instance, if your problem is due to a medicine you're taking or to not having enough testosterone, going through sex therapy would be a waste of time. So please attend to the following questions.

WHAT CHEMICALS ARE YOU PUTTING INTO YOUR BODY?

This includes any and all chemicals, including prescription and recreational drugs, alcohol, and nicotine. There are a host of drugs that contribute to erection problems. For more information, check the Appendix at the back of the book. If you are taking any of the suspected drugs, the first thing you should do is talk to the physician who prescribed them. See if adjusting the dose or switching to another drug is possible. If you're taking a recreational drug on the list, you should consider getting off it and at the same time look at the available medical and therapy interventions.

Don't forget to consider your intake of alcohol. Social drinking or having "just a few drinks to relax" may inflame desire but kill erections. And long-term alcoholism—which can destroy testicular cells, lower testosterone production, and increase the production of female hormones—has serious negative effects on penises and sexual desire.

Smoking tobacco is another risk factor to consider. Studies show that smoking contributes to the hardening and clogging of arteries, including the ones that supply blood to the penis. Smokers have far more potency problems than nonsmokers.

DO YOU DESIRE SEX WITH YOUR PARTNER, YOURSELF, OR ANYONE?

If your appetite for sex is intact, we can assume your hormones are in working order and there is no need to get tested. But if your desire is low or nonexistent—if you don't notice attractive women, don't fantasize about sex, don't want to masturbate or have sex with a partner—it may well be that your testosterone level is deficient. Testosterone is the desire hormone in both men and women. When its level goes below normal, as it can for a number of reasons, desire significantly decreases or disappears. It's difficult to have a functioning penis in the absence of desire.

If your desire and penis are both in the doldrums, you should schedule an appointment with your regular doctor or a urologist to get a blood test to determine your testosterone level.

Unfortunately, different doctors and different laboratories have different criteria for what they consider normal testosterone levels. And because of the risk that supplemental testosterone can hasten the growth of already existing prostate cancer, some doctors are hesitant to give it. You need to talk openly with your doctor about the test results; if you think you're getting a runaround, seek a second opinion. Supplemental testosterone is usually given by injection, typically every two weeks. But patches are now also available. Although testosterone can be taken orally, this is not recommended because it is less effective than shots and patches and carries a risk of inducing liver problems.

Although hormonal deficiencies account for only about 5 percent of erection difficulties, they are often overlooked. I once worked with a seventeen-year-old boy with erection problems, and nothing made sense until I thought to have him get a testosterone test. I should have spotted this earlier, but who would have thought a seventeen-year-old would be deficient in testosterone? It turned out his levels were very low.

When hormone injections or patches are used, the results are often quick and dramatic. "The difference between day and night" was how the wife of a client who previously had no interest or erections put it after he got his first testosterone injection. "In the past I couldn't get him to have sex no matter what I did," she continued. "Now he's the one who says we can be late to work because we have better things to do first. I love it."

Advantage:

▲ If low testosterone production is the cause of your desire and erection difficulties, testosterone is exactly what you need and will probably resolve the problem.

Disadvantage:

▲ Although there is no evidence that testosterone injections cause prostate cancer, they can speed the growth of a cancer that's already present, especially in men who do not suffer from testosterone deficiency.

A relative lack of desire and trouble with erections can also be the result of depression. By *depression* I mean a definite sense over a period of at least several weeks that life isn't worth living and things aren't going to get any better (other possible signs are increased irritability, diminished pleasure in activities that once were fun, increased or decreased appetite, decreased ability to concentrate on what you are doing, and any kind of sleep problem). One of the signature attributes of depression is a loss of interest in sex and usually other things as well. If you or your partner think you are depressed, you should get yourself to a physician or therapist as quickly as possible. When the depression is treated with therapy or drugs, chances are good your sexual desire and erections will return.

ARE YOU GETTING AND KEEPING ERECTIONS UNDER SOME CONDITIONS BUT NOT OTHERS?

If you have erections (firm enough for vaginal insertion but not necessarily hard as a rock) by yourself but not with a partner, or with one partner but not another, or on vacation but not at home, this strongly suggests that the problem is not primarily physical in nature but instead has more to do with your feelings about one or all partners or your level of stress. This means you can choose any treatment option that you, your partner, and your physician or therapist agree on.

DO YOU NEVER GET OR KEEP ERECTIONS UNDER ANY CIRCUMSTANCES?

If you don't get erections at all—while you sleep or on awakening, with your own or a partner's stimulation—this strongly suggests a physical cause or medication side effect. It would probably be a waste of time to try the exercises in the next chapter. As soon as possible, set up an appointment for you and your partner with your regular physician or a urologist.

A man I saw over two decades ago had a strong bias against medicine. Although his penis didn't get hard under any circumstances, he refused to believe the reason might be physical. Every time he got involved with a woman, the two of them would go to a sex therapist. I was the fourth therapist he tried and, sure enough, he failed with me as well. Only after continued badgering from me was he willing to visit a urologist. A few tests revealed that the problem was indeed medically based. Soon thereafter he had a penile implant inserted, and his sex life and self-esteem improved considerably. What is sad is that he could have had a functioning penis five years earlier and saved himself considerable time, money, and energy.

If you have already tried one or more self-help programs or courses of sex therapy without substantial improvement, you should also see a urologist.

DO YOU GET ERECTIONS BUT USUALLY CAN'T MAINTAIN THEM?

This could mean the problem is either psychological or physical. One of my clients started losing erections in his early sixties. No matter what the activity, he would get an erection and lose it within a few moments. He and his wife of thirty-five years were both puzzled because nothing else had changed in their relationship or sex life. Medical tests demonstrated that although blood was getting into his penis—hence the erections—it was leaking out faster than it could be replenished. He needed a medical solution.

Another client, Larry, had a different situation. With masturbation or hand or mouth stimulation from his girlfriend, maintaining an erection was easy. It was only when they attempted vaginal insertion that his erection would disappear. This clearly was not a physical or drug-related problem. The real issue, it turned out, was that Larry had serious concerns about commitment, and for him intercourse was the defining act. As long as he didn't have intercourse with Joan, he didn't feel trapped. But deep down he believed that if he had intercourse with her, he would have to marry her. It took several months of therapy before we resolved his fears of commitment. After that, erections were no longer a problem.

BE A WISE CONSUMER

If you're going to see a physician or a therapist, it's important to be a smart consumer. Among other things, this means that you should see the right kind of person. Sad to say, many physicians and therapists have little or no training in sexuality and not much skill with sexual and relationship problems. You want to find someone who is comfortable dealing with sexuality and knows what he or she is doing. Your family physician may or may not be that person; the psychotherapist you're seeing or have seen for another matter may or may not be that person.

Whoever you see, you should review your sexual history, or at least the history of the problem, before seeing the doctor so you can present an accurate and comprehensive picture. And make a list of questions you want answered. Don't let your fear of looking stupid prevent you from asking all the questions you want. The only stupid questions are the ones you don't ask. If the doctor doesn't seem comfortable dealing with you and your situation, isn't willing to take the time you want to discuss your case with you, won't talk to you in language you can understand, or won't answer your questions, go elsewhere.

Whether you see a physician or a sex therapist, I strongly suggest bringing your partner with you. Even though it's your penis, your partner is an integral part of your sex life, has important information to contribute, and should be there to hear the pros and cons of various treatments and to ask any questions she has. Another advantage to having her with you is that she can later help you evaluate the doctor's competence and suggestions.

While you should listen carefully to the doctor's recommendations, remember they are only suggestions. Every treatment costs money and most require time and effort; some also involve pain and risk. You're the one

who will have to live with the consequences. You should get the best therapeutic and medical advice you can, and then determine with your partner
what course of action makes the most sense.

It's a good idea to get copies of your test results from your doctor. These
can then be shown to any other doctors or therapists you consult. This can
save time and sometimes money as well.

DIAGNOSTIC TESTS

If you see a physician, there are a number of procedures that may be employed to determine the exact nature of your problem. First a complete
history of the problem should be taken. Some of the important questions
are: Exactly what is the problem (don't get erections, get them but lose
them quickly, penis is full but not rigid)? Under what circumstances do
you get and not get erections? When did the problem start, and how has it
changed since then? How is your general health, and what medications are
you taking? What about alcohol, nicotine, and recreational drugs? Have
you ever had pelvic trauma (being kicked in the balls, falling on the top
tube of your bicycle)? These questions are the ones you should address
yourself before seeing the doctor or therapist.

Typically a physical examination is also done. This usually includes tests
to determine the state of your arteries and blood pressure, since blood
flow difficulties may well be responsible for your erection complaints. The
physician may conduct a rectal exam to check your prostate gland, since
an inflamed or painful prostate can disrupt blood flow or sensation in the
penis; a check for anatomical abnormalities of the penis, such as Peyronie's disease (a curved and sometimes painful erection), that can im-
pede blood flow; and a determination of whether the nerves in the penis
are functioning normally.

Blood tests are usually taken to determine your level of testosterone.
Your blood sugar may also be checked for diabetes, a frequent contributor
to erection problems.

Several other tests may be given. One of them is the RigiScan, a device
attached to your penis that records its activity while you sleep. Since men
usually have erections during rapid eye movement sleep, the stage of sleep
when we dream, this is a way of determining if the problem is physical or
not. The RigiScan is painless and typically done for two consecutive nights
either at home or at a sleep laboratory. Most other tests have the goal of
determining if enough blood is getting into and staying in the penis. These

require the doctor to inject your penis with a drug, usually prostaglandin, that causes the smooth muscles to relax and the arteries to open, thereby allowing increased blood flow into the penis. (Giving yourself such injections is also used as a treatment, which I cover later in this chapter.) By using X rays, blood pressure cuffs, and ultrasound, important information is collected about what might be getting in the way of you getting and keeping erections. If these tests don't reveal significant pathology, the problem clearly lies elsewhere.

WHAT MEDICAL OPTIONS CAN AND CANNOT DO

Each of the medical interventions that I describe below can do one thing and one thing only: give you a usable erection when you want it. That's it—nothing more. Compared to what was available twenty-five years ago, that's miraculous enough, but some people have let their expectations get out of control. The resources we have—Viagra, penile injections, penile implants, vacuum devices, and so on—will change only the stiffness of your penis, but not your personality, behavior, or lovemaking technique.

Some couples are doing fine even without an erection but would like to have intercourse. All they want from the medical tool is what it can offer. Simone and Paul were such a couple. Even though Paul had developed an erection problem, they still had a wonderful relationship and sex life. They had sex frequently and did all sorts of lovely things with their hands and mouths and a vibrator. Nonetheless, they both missed intercourse. After a few sessions with me and some medical tests, it seemed to be the case that Paul's problem with erections was caused by his long-standing diabetes. They tried a vacuum device for several weeks before deciding it wasn't for them. The penile injections they tried next worked very well for them. They tried Viagra as soon as it came on the market, but it was not as reliable as the shots, to which they returned. Because Simone and Paul only needed erections and found a medical tool that provided that for them, they are doing very well.

The situation for some other couples is different. Yes, there's an erection problem, but there are also other issues. Despite what many people think, these resources are not aphrodisiacs and in themselves will not make you desire sex more. (There is one exception. There are some men who have turned away from sex because of their erection problem. Because of the problem, sex was so full of tension and humiliation that they suppressed their desire. With the erection problem resolved, these men become more willing to have sex. But this is the only way in which it can be said that using any of the following tools creates more desire for sex.)

These tools will not help you to talk or listen to your partner or be more sensitive, will not make you a better lover, will not improve sensation or give you a better orgasm, will not resolve relationship tension, and most certainly will not save a failing relationship. All of these considerations may seem too obvious to be worth stating, but strange things happen. A client of mine in his fifties got Viagra, tried it by himself, and found that it worked. His wife was very angry that in the weeks after that discovery he didn't approach her. So he agreed that he would take a pill immediately after our session and make love with her that night. But he didn't. After he took the pill, they made out on the couch, but before things got too interesting he told her he wanted to watch "a few minutes" of the first game of the 1998 NBA playoffs. She went into the bedroom, and two hours later— when he had still not come to bed—she called me in a state of great distress. We interrupted his game watching and got him on the phone as well. He didn't have an explanation for what had happened, but it was clear that despite knowing that the Viagra he had taken would give him a good erection, despite knowing that his wife was expecting and wanting to make love with him, he chose Michael Jordan over his wife. Urologists and sex therapists, including myself, have talked with men who have gotten prescriptions for Viagra or vacuum devices which they never filled; others got the drug or pump and never used it. Some men have had surgery to have a penile prosthesis implanted and then never again had sex; some men have had sex only a few times in the years after surgery. Obviously, there is more to many men's "erection problems" than simply not having erections.

There is another issue to consider as well. In some relationships the woman likes not having sex and is actually grateful for the erection problem, perhaps because she didn't get much out of sex when they had it or because she feels estranged from her partner. So she isn't receptive, and may even be horrified, when he presents himself ready for action.

Unless your problem is a very simple one, like Simone and Paul's, consider a few sessions of sex therapy along with your new medical erection helper.

If you have refrained from sex for a long time because of your problem, it may be difficult to get started again after you have the pill, pump, or shot. Even though you know you can now get erect, there may be some shyness or hesitation on your part and perhaps your partner's as well. This is especially true if there were bad feelings and ugly words exchanged about not having sex. You may need professional help to get past the bad feelings and deal with the anxieties and hesitations still present.

Another reason to see a sex therapist is that most doctors today simply don't have the time to deal with all the concerns you may have. They may also lack the training or skill to deal with the relationship issues, anxiety, and other feelings that accompany erection difficulties. In addition, the partner may need to spend anywhere from a few minutes to several hours expressing how angry she is about all the rejections she endured before her man became willing to deal with the problem.

Don't kid yourself into thinking these are small matters. The partner is typically the key to whether any intervention will succeed. If your partner continually complains about the medical option the two of you have selected—it doesn't feel natural, it interferes with spontaneity, why can't you get erect without it, and so on—chances are good that there are still feelings of hurt and anger that need to be dealt with.

MEDICAL TREATMENTS

I start with the options available before the advent of Viagra that are still useful today, and then take a detailed look at the drug we've heard so much about. All of these therapies are FDA approved, but of course this discussion is not intended as a substitute for an in-depth conversation with your physician.

Yohimbine

A drug in pill form that comes from the bark of an African tree, yohimbine was, until recently, often the first intervention suggested by physicians for erection problems. It is being used less frequently now because its results have not been impressive: Only about 20 percent of patients received significant benefit. However, side effects—anxiety, headache, and a small increase in blood pressure—are infrequent and generally mild. Yohimbine may be worth a trial if your doctor suggests it. If it helps, fine; if not, look at other options.

Advantage:
▲ Yohimbine is safe, relatively inexpensive, and noninvasive.

Disadvantage:
▲ It is effective for only a small number of men.

Vacuum Devices

Vacuum pump devices and constriction rings are now available without prescription. The typical device consists of a plastic cylinder that fits over the penis. You then repeatedly press a lever that pumps the air out of the cylinder. This creates a vacuum, which draws blood into the penis, resulting in an erection. When you have a satisfactory erection, you remove the cylinder after placing a specially designed constrictor band at the base of your penis; this holds the blood in and keeps the penis erect during sex. The constrictor band should not be kept in place longer than thirty minutes. Vacuum devices work well almost regardless of the cause of the erection problems. A plus for some men is that they are entirely mechanical and noninvasive. Surveys indicate that the majority of men who've tried these devices like them and so do their partners, especially in established relationships. They are a bit cumbersome for the dating game.

Advantages:
▲ These devices, which can be used effectively by most men with erection difficulties, produce serviceable erections when you want them.
▲ Vacuum devices are inexpensive—a one-time fee of $150 to $450—and have few side effects.

Disadvantages:
▲ Some users complain that their erections are not as rigid as they want and somewhat wobbly at the base.
▲ Some men experience side effects because of the constrictor band: pain in the penis, numbness and bruising, and painful ejaculation.
▲ You can cause serious damage to the penis if you leave the band on for more than thirty minutes.

Injections of Prostaglandin and Other Drugs

Penile injections were introduced to American medicine in an unexpected and dramatic fashion. Because of his work with injections, British physiologist Giles Brindley was invited to present a paper at the meeting of the American Urological Association in Las Vegas in 1983. Knowing that many American doctors were skeptical, Brindley injected himself before his talk. He gave his lecture, announced that he had injected himself, then dropped his trousers and invited the astonished audience to view the results. (For some reason, Brindley was not again asked to address this group.)

The procedure consists of injecting one or more drugs into the shaft of your penis, just as in the diagnostic test mentioned earlier. These drugs relax the smooth muscles and arteries in the penis, thereby increasing blood flow. I realize putting a needle into your penis sounds painful, but it usually is not. A very fine needle is used. In some men, however, the medicine itself, not the shot, does cause pain. This method requires a prescription after your doctor determines the correct dose and teaches you how to inject yourself. Within five to thirty minutes after giving yourself a shot, you'll have a very stiff erection that will last from thirty minutes to an hour or longer. Injections have a very high success rate, higher even than Viagra, and often work for men for whom Viagra doesn't. They work with many cases of performance anxiety and also with problems based on physical causes that in the past would have required a penile implant.

The drugs used for the injections can vary. If pure prostaglandin doesn't work or causes pain, your doctor may try what's called a tri-mix, a combination of prostaglandin, papaverine, and phentolamine. This is the mixture that has worked best for my clients.

Squeamishness about needles, especially in the penis, has been a tremendous obstacle to the acceptance of this effective therapy. There are two kinds of help available. One is a powerful technique called eye movement desensitization and reprocessing (EMDR). I've used this method with numerous clients to overcome fears of all kinds. Unfortunately, there is no way to do EMDR on yourself; you need a trained therapist.

Other clients have used a little gizmo called a Pen-Inject or Auto-Injector. This is a small plastic case in which you insert the syringe after you've loaded it with the dose of medicine you need. You then put the tip of the Auto-Injector where you want the injection to go, press a button, and it does the rest. Of course, you're still getting a shot, but it's amazing how much it helps to hide the syringe and needle. One client was so fearful of needles that he started to sweat whenever the topic was broached and was certain that his girlfriend, a nurse, would have to do the injecting. But at the urology consultation the doctor introduced him to the Pen-Inject. My client was so excited, he called me as soon as he got home: "It's not a problem anymore. With this thing, it's not like actually taking a needle. I can do it myself."

Advantage:

▲ The ability to have good, long-lasting, natural-looking and -feeling erections when you want without incurring the cost, pain, and risks of surgery. Injection may work even when Viagra doesn't.

Disadvantages:

▲ Many men don't like to give themselves injections or even think about it. A very high percentage of men who start taking these shots soon discontinue them and seek other treatment. The Auto-Injector can help in this regard.

▲ A small percentage of men experience pain in the penis not from the injection but from the injected agent. This can often be remedied by changing the agent or the mixture of agents used.

▲ There is evidence that over time the injections form scar tissue in the penis in 5 to 10 percent of men, and sometimes cause Peyronie's disease (serious curvature of the penis).

▲ Most men continue to need these shots to get erections. It was once thought that many men would regain confidence after a few shots and be able to have erections without them. Unfortunately, this has proven to be true in less than 10 percent of cases.

▲ Although the risk is small, a few men who inject themselves get priapism, an erection that won't go down, almost always caused by injecting too much medicine. This can necessitate a trip to the doctor's office or a hospital emergency room for treatment. Priapism was more common when papaverine was the drug of choice. With prostaglandin and tri-mix, the incidence of priapism is less than 2 percent.

▲ Although the injections are effective with most cases of performance anxiety, they can be neutralized by massive anxiety.

Muse

This consists of a prostaglandin pellet inserted with an applicator into the urethra. It was developed for men who didn't want to take injections. Unfortunately, it also causes pain for some, and its effectiveness is somewhat less than that of the injections. However, because there are no injections, scar tissue is not formed in the penis. The maker of Muse has recently recommended that men use a constrictor ban around the base of the penis before inserting the pellet and during sexual activity; presumably this will raise the drug's effectiveness.

Advantage:
  ▲ A safe and modestly effective erection helper. Even though it uses the same agent as the injections, you don't have to inject yourself.

Disadvantages:
  ▲ Some men experience pain when using Muse.
  ▲ The drug is effective for only about 25 percent of men.
  ▲ As with injections, it can be neutralized by very strong anxiety.

Regarding vacuum devices, Muse, and injections, it's well to keep in mind that they can cause some difficulties in the beginning. Most couples, after all, are not accustomed to stopping love play in order to do something special to attain erection, and many couples are not accustomed to talking openly about sex. There can be embarrassment, anxiety, and hesitation. One client didn't have sex for weeks after he got his injection materials because he couldn't figure out how to tell his partner that he wanted to go to another room to inject himself—this despite the fact that she had been to the urologist with him and knew full well about the shots. Some men, even though they now have a way to get an erection, still feel like failures because they can't get "normal" erections. Such difficulties can usually be worked out easily if the partners are able to talk about them, but a few sessions with a sex therapist may be advisable.

Arterial and Venous Surgery

These are operations to repair or bypass clogged arteries and to seal leaky veins. Arterial surgery works very well for a very small group— young men whose blood flow problems are caused by accidents. Venous surgery, unfortunately, is not very effective in the long run. If your doctor recommends either type of surgery, find out what his or her results have been, especially on long-term follow-up, and insist on talking to several of the men who've had the operation. You might also want to ask for references in the medical literature regarding the effectiveness of these procedures.

Advantages:
  ▲ Arterial surgery, called revascularization, is very effective in select cases, and the men function as they did before the surgery.
  ▲ Both types of surgery are expensive but usually covered by insurance.

Disadvantage:

▲ Venous surgery has a very high relapse rate and is therefore not very effective.

Penile Implants

Since as far back as the 1930s, surgeons have been experimenting with ways to produce artificial erections. By now the art of penile implants is highly advanced. Though there are a great many implant models, they can be conveniently put in two groups.

Nonhydraulic (also called semirigid and malleable) implants consist of a pair of silicon rods placed inside the penis. With earlier models, the man always had an erection, and this obviously caused some embarrassment. Newer models are more flexible and can be bent down against the leg so the penis points toward the floor when the man is standing.

Hydraulic, or inflatable, implants come in a variety of styles. Their distinguishing characteristic is that they mimic the action of a normal erection process. A pair of hollow cylinders is placed inside the erectile tissue of the penis, and a fluid-filled reservoir is inserted in the belly; when you want to have sex, you activate a pumping mechanism, implanted in the scrotum, that inflates the cylinders with the fluid from the reservoir. Some newer models have the complete mechanism inside the cylinders; when you want an erection, you simply bend or squeeze the head of the penis and presto—as if by magic—you have an erection.

Hydraulic models have the advantages of seeming more natural since they mimic what the body would do under normal circumstances. The penis is truly soft when it's soft and only gets hard when you want it to. However, hydraulic models are also more complex than the nonhydraulic implants, and the chances of malfunction are greater. They are also more expensive and the surgery more involved.

These days, implant surgery is usually reserved for erection problems caused by severe vascular or neurological disease, pelvic trauma, and spinal cord injuries. Surveys show that a large majority of men with implants and their partners are satisfied with their devices, although many of them have various complaints. Nonetheless, the popularity of implant surgery has waned in recent years with the advent of less invasive tools such as penile injections and vacuum devices. Viagra will undoubtedly further reduce its popularity. But implant surgery remains an important last resort when other options do not work or lose their effectiveness over time.

Advantages:

▲ The ability to have a usable erection whenever you want one without having to give yourself shots and without having to go through sex therapy.

▲ Although implants are expensive (over several thousand dollars), they are covered by many insurance plans.

▲ These devices tend to be given high ratings by the men and their partners.

Disadvantages:

▲ Implants should be considered irreversible. They can injure or destroy the natural erection system. This will likely mean you can't decide to have an implant taken out and try another method.

▲ Erections produced by an implant may be smaller in length and circumference and also less rigid than those produced naturally. They are certainly rigid enough for vaginal insertion and enjoyable intercourse. However, what you get may not look like what you had before.

▲ Implant operations have the same risks as all surgery. Postoperative pain in the groin typically lasts for four to six weeks, and most patients require medication for pain control during some of that period. The risk of infection is small, but if it does occur, the implant will need to be removed temporarily.

▲ Mechanical failure is always a possibility in hydraulic devices. In such cases, further surgery is required to replace the offending component or the whole device.

With the addition of sex therapy, these were the main interventions that existed for men with erection problems before the spring of 1998. Then came the blue pill. And that's a story in itself.

Viagra

Humanity has been searching for an oral agent to cure erection problems since prehistoric times. By 2000 B.C.E. the Egyptians and others were experimenting with natural substances such as belladonna, henbane, jimsonweed, and the mandrake plant, not to mention oysters and ginseng. But while there were reports of success here and there, there was no convincing evidence that any of these substances was a reliable remedy.

And now—after four thousand years—it's here, the magic pill we wanted. We already have diet pills, birth control pills (and look what a revolution they caused), and happy pills (all sorts of antianxiety and antidepressant medicines), so why not a sex pill? No needles, no gadgets, no surgery—just pop a pill and you're ready to go. It's not surprising that more than six million prescriptions were written for Viagra in the first eight months it was on the market, making it the fastest-selling drug in history.

The researchers at Pfizer, Inc., were not looking for an erection pill. Rather, they hoped that the drug then called sidenafil citrate would alleviate angina, the chest pains caused by blockage of the blood vessels leading to the heart. They were disappointed and were ready to give up on the drug until some of the men in the study reported the side effect of having erections. The rest, as they say, is history. The name Viagra was chosen later. Pfizer knew it had a winner when, after it announced it was bringing its clinical trials of the drug to an end, the study subjects wrote in droves begging to be allowed to keep a supply of the pills.

To understand how Viagra works, we need to get into a little detail about how erections are created. When a man is aroused, the brain causes the penis to release the chemical cyclic GMP, which opens the blood vessels, allowing blood to rush in and create an erection. But another chemical, PDE5, is also released, and it works to degrade cyclic GMP. In a man without erection problems there is a balance between the release and degradation of cyclic GMP, and the erection remains as long as there is effective stimulation of some kind. Viagra blocks PDE5 and thereby boosts and prolongs the effects of cyclic GMP. This allows many men to have and keep erections who ordinarily would not be able to do so.

Several men have asked why other body parts don't stiffen when they take Viagra. Why, for instance, don't they get stiff necks, as Jay Leno has suggested a number of times in his monologues? One reason is that a stiff neck is caused by mechanisms very different from those that cause penile erection. The other reason is that PDE5 operates only in the penis.

Viagra produces good erections in about 70 percent of the men who take it. These erections are full and firm and feel—as clients never tire of telling me—"totally natural." The agent stays in the system for some time, although it gradually starts losing strength after four to five hours. Clients have reported erections from it seven or even ten hours later. Some have had sex in the evening after taking the pill, gone to sleep, and had sex again with a good erection in the morning.

As you might imagine, an agent this powerful must also have a downside. When Viagra was first introduced, the side effects seemed almost inconsequential, the main one being headaches, experienced by 16 percent of those participating in the clinical trials. Other side effects are flushing (10 percent of patients), indigestion (7 percent), nasal congestion (4 percent), and, in about 3 percent of patients, temporary vision problems, mainly a blue tinge but sometimes also blurred vision. Taking more than 100 mg of Viagra at a time increases the frequency of these side effects but does *not* increase the drug's benefits.

But a much more serious problem has come to light. In the year since Viagra's introduction, over 130 deaths have been attributed to its use. A few of these deaths were due to an interaction between Viagra and drugs containing nitrates (either prescription medicines used to control angina and high blood pressure or street drugs known as "poppers" used to enhance orgasm). The combination of Viagra and nitrates can cause a dangerous and sometimes fatal drop in blood pressure. Most of the reported deaths, however, resulted from "cardiovascular events"; that is, heart problems. For some older men taking Viagra, the exertion of sex is too much for their damaged hearts and blood vessels.

Because of the risk, the American College of Cardiology and the American Heart Association recently issued a caution on prescribing Viagra to men in the following categories:

▲ Those with angina
▲ Those who on an exercise stress test show evidence of blocked arteries
▲ Those taking multiple medications to control blood pressure
▲ Those with congestive heart failure with borderline low blood pressure
▲ Those taking other drugs that can prolong the effect of Viagra, including the common antibiotic erythromycin

Viagra can be wonderfully helpful to many men, but it has serious risks. You should get it only from a doctor who already knows your medical status or who is willing to ask the right questions and do tests to determine it.

As already noted, Viagra is effective, even at its highest allowable dose of 100 mg, for only about two-thirds of men. Because of this, penile injections and implant surgery will not disappear anytime soon. I know of several men who pinned their hopes on Viagra, and when it didn't work for them, they became open to considering injections for the first time. Viagra is less likely to work for men who have serious physiological problems—for example, those who have had radiation for prostate cancer and those with nerve and vascular damage due to diabetes.

Viagra also has the same drawback as injections: While it works very effectively in cases of typical performance anxiety, it can be neutralized by massive anxiety. Some consider it a drawback that Viagra takes thirty or more minutes to get into gear. Injections can produce erections in as little as five minutes. Viagra's effect can be speeded up a bit by taking it on an empty stomach.

A statement frequently heard about Viagra in the media is that "it doesn't work without stimulation," the implication being that the stimulation has to come from your partner. It is true that if you take Viagra and then spend the next three hours painting the house or watching the Super Bowl on the tube, you won't get erect during that time. With an injection, you get an erection no matter what you do (although stimulation from self or partner can speed up the process). But the stimulation needed to get Viagra going need not be from your partner and need not even be physical. Watching an erotic movie or having a sexy fantasy will do it.

As a practicing sex therapist, I'm very happy we now have Viagra. It is a revolutionary tool and has already been helpful to hundreds of thousands of men. It is also changing how we think about sexuality and sex therapy. While the penis may continue to have a mind of its own, its behavior can now be made to conform to its owner's wishes. And Viagra itself is just the beginning. There are other oral agents being developed, and some of these may work for men who don't benefit from Viagra.

Advantages:

▲ Take a pill and have a full, rigid, natural-feeling erection in thirty to sixty minutes. No messing with shots, pellets, or gizmos.

Disadvantages:

▲ Works only for about 70 percent of men.

▲ At about $8 to $9 a pill, it is expensive in the long run. Some health plans pay for Viagra, although perhaps not for as many pills as you would like, and others do not.

▲ Cannot be taken by men who are taking any kind of drugs containing nitrates (for example, nitroglycerine), and has to be used with caution and under strict medical supervision by those with heart and blood pressure problems.

▲ Reliance on Viagra may obscure other important underlying problems such as depression and diabetes.

QUESTIONABLE TREATMENTS

Given the huge number of men experiencing erectile difficulties, it's not surprising that all sorts of nostrums have been offered, many of which are unproven. This doesn't necessarily mean they don't work for some men, only that there's no convincing scientific evidence of their general effectiveness. If I lined up a hundred men with erection problems and had them all drink a cup of organic camel urine daily for a week, at least ten or twenty would probably report that their erection problems had vanished. While this is not sufficient to demonstrate that camel urine is a reliable cure for erection problems, those who benefited won't care.

I recently had a client who erection problem had been resolved by taking L-arginine (an amino acid available without prescription in health food stores). Then, after five years, the pills suddenly stopped working for him. He's now doing fine on Viagra. In the meantime, I'd suggested L-arginine to over twenty other clients, but it never did a thing for any of them. Other therapists report similar nonresults. However, since L-arginine is not expensive and has no known side effects, you might want to give it a try. Just don't be surprised if it doesn't do the job.

If you're wondering how a substance can help some people even though scientific studies can't demonstrate its effectiveness, you need to remember the placebo effect. In serious studies there is always a control group whose members receive a therapy (such as a pill or shot) that has no therapeutic properties. Yet in all these studies some of those receiving the inert medicines get better. In the clinical trials of Viagra, about 20 percent of men in the control groups reported better erections. If camel urine, sugar pills, or some other substance works for you, more power to you. But if it doesn't, or if it does but then stops working, try something with more scientific backing.

A number of clients have asked if acupuncture could help with their erections, and a surprisingly large number of my clients have already tried acupuncture without benefit. I know acupuncture has its uses; I have had it several times for back pain and found it to be helpful. But when I searched the literature, I found no credible evidence that acupuncture is a reliable treatment for erection problems.

Some hypnotherapists have made grandiose claims about their success with sex and other problems. I'm no stranger to this method. I've used hypnosis in my sex therapy, although not much anymore, and I even co-edited a book on the method. Unfortunately, the conclusion regarding hypnosis is the same as with acupuncture: There is no evidence that it is a reliable treatment for erection problems.

Here are some of the substances sometimes touted as potency aids, none of which have proven efficacy: cholestatin; deprenyl; ginkgo biloba; ginseng; melatonin; muira puama; oysters; saw palmetto; testosterone taken orally (not recommended because of the risk of inducing liver problems); trazodone (brand name Desyrel), an older antidepressant sometimes given in combination with yohimbine; vitamins B12, C, and E.

.   .   .

In considering your options, I think it's sound policy to try the least invasive, least risky, and least expensive alternatives first. For example, since you already have this book, doing the exercises in the next chapter will cost you only some time and energy; as far as I know, they have no negative side effects. If they don't seem to help, see a sex therapist or a physician. Even if you and your partner decide to try one of the methods discussed in this chapter, proceed with caution. Vacuum devices, yohimbine, and Viagra have few side effects. And while penile injections can have serious side effects, they are a much less invasive undertaking than surgery.

Of course, some men are in a hurry. They want the problem solved right now, even if they've had it for years and done nothing about it. I have no trouble understanding the impatience—I too want all my problems fixed this second. But with sex problems, as with many of life's difficulties, some degree of patience is a virtue, and often less is more. You can always escalate if the method you start with doesn't live up to your expectations.

WHAT IS COMING

Now that erection problems have come out of the closet, the pharmaceutical companies are busily at work. We are promised more effective injections, faster-working pills, tablets you put under your tongue, gels you smear on the penis, smaller pellets for another Muse-like system, and so on. How many of these will actually make it to market is another question entirely, but the man with an erection problem two, three, or five years from now will surely have far more choices than he does today.

Three drugs should be available sometime in 1999. One of them is a new injectable called Invicorp (made by Senetek). It contains two agents that promote arterial flow into the penis. This drug may be the answer for those men who have serious problems getting blood to stay in the penis. The two others are oral phentolamine, brand name Vasomax (made by Zonagen), and oral apomorphine, brand name Pentech (made by Tap). They work faster than Viagra and may be effective for some men for whom Viagra is not helpful. And side effects seem to be minimal, nasal congestion being the most common. By the year 2000, we may see on the market a pill still known only by its distinctly unsexy research label, IC351 (from Eli Lilly and Icos). From the clinical trials so far, it seems that IC351 works much like Viagra but with the advantage of fewer side effects.

Whatever the future, we have plenty to work with right now. If you are open to and willing to explore different treatments, there is almost certainly a satisfactory solution for you.

CHAPTER TWENTY - TWO

Resolving Erection Problems
with Sex Therapy

I don't think anyone who hasn't had the problem themselves can understand what it's like not feeling confident you'll have an erection during sex. This has taken over my whole life. I think about it at work and home, at night, during the day, constantly. As my son would say, this sucks.
—*Man, 52*

I know I was very reluctant at first, but I'll be the first to say that the therapy was very helpful. I've developed a very different relationship with my penis, which now usually works quite well, thank you, and have come to see sex as much more for pleasure and closeness than just for performance. My wife and I are much closer as a result and having a lot more fun.
—*Man, 40*

IF THERE'S NO physical reason for your erection problem, the main difficulty may well be in how you think your penis *should* function. A great many men uncritically accept the superhuman standards and myths about penises, then get upset when they discover they are merely human.

A married man of thirty-nine called early one morning and virtually demanded an immediate appointment. When he arrived, it was obvious he was in a panic. While still standing at the door to the building, he started talking with great emotion about his "impotence" and his need to know whether he needed a penile implant. I finally got him into my office, but couldn't get a word in for fifteen minutes. After he calmed down a bit and I was able to ask some questions, it turned out that the impotence consisted solely of a failure to have an erection with his wife the night before. Then, in response to my question of how last night had differed from other times he had sex with her, he began to sob. The previous day, with no warning at all, he had lost the job he had held for fourteen years and that meant the world to him. After wiping his eyes and making an obvious attempt to pull himself together, he smiled weakly and said without a trace of humor, "Other than that, everything was as usual. I just don't understand it." It hadn't occurred to him that his feelings about being fired might have affected his sexual functioning.

Nonmedical erection problems are almost always due to one or more of the following: unrealistic expectations, lack of arousal, absence of the proper conditions, and the anxiety generated by the need for an erection. For example:

▲ A sixty-year-old man getting upset because his penis doesn't jump to attention when he kisses his partner. He's not taking into account that a sixty-year-old penis differs from a twenty-year-old one and that he's not getting the direct penile stimulation he now requires.

▲ A man who expects an erection even though he isn't feeling aroused. He just expects his penis to function regardless of how he feels, as if his penis has nothing to do with the rest of him.

▲ A man who is very tense during sex. He's been criticized by his partner for his "failure to perform" in the past, and he's anticipating more criticism. Because of the way men have been trained, it doesn't occur to him to ask how anyone could get an erection in that situation.

If you are tense or anxious, if you are angry at your partner, if you aren't getting the physical and emotional stimulation you like, if you aren't turned on, if you are preoccupied with other matters—if any of these things is true, what makes you think you should have an erection? The answer, of course, is our sexual conditioning, the nonsense I discussed in Chapter 2.

Recall the example in Chapter 19 of Bud and Art, of how they think differently about sex. If you're having erection difficulties and there's nothing physically wrong, chances are good you're behaving like Art. That is, you're worried about sex even before it begins—you're focusing on how your penis is doing rather than on what you feel.

In order to resolve an erection problem, you need to start thinking and acting less like Art and more like Bud. I know this isn't easy—in fact, at this moment it may seem impossible—but it's necessary and can be done. You need to look forward to sex with positive anticipation, focus on the pleasurable sensations, and accurately judge the signs of increasing arousal.

To increase your sexual pleasure and improve your erections, stop stacking the deck against yourself and start stacking it on your side. This means getting your mind on your side, meeting your conditions for good sex, having sex only when you are aroused, and decreasing your anxiety.

USING A MEDICAL ASSIST IN ADDITION TO SELF-HELP

Some couples going through sex therapy or a self-help program can benefit from also using Viagra, injections, or Muse. Here are two examples.

Siri was ambivalent about going through sex therapy with her husband, Hector. On one hand, she was happy and relieved that he was finally, after years of nagging, willing to get help. On the other hand, she was angry that she hadn't had intercourse in five years and wouldn't be able to have it for at least another few months. I suggested Hector talk to his doctor about injections, which he did. This allowed him to get good erections and have intercourse with Siri several times while they went through therapy. Siri was impressed by his willingness to do this for her and by the actual intercourse. This made her much more cooperative and contributed significantly to the success of the therapy.

Using medical aids to get erections is more often than not, as in Siri and Hector's case, for the partner's benefit. But since nothing is more important than getting her cooperation, it is well worth it.

Winston and Emma were making progress in the beginning of their counseling for his erection problem when we ran into trouble. He still was not having reliable erections, and the thought that they probably couldn't have intercourse on their upcoming fortieth anniversary was causing sadness and anxiety, which in turn was negatively affecting therapy. They had celebrated all the previous "big" anniversaries by staying in a romantic resort and having intercourse several times. At my suggestion, Winston talked to his family doctor and got a prescription for Viagra. The sadness and anxiety quickly dissipated. On the anniversary weekend Winston was able to have intercourse one time without Viagra but needed the pill for the second intercourse. They were both pleased with the results. They had sex one more time that weekend, but it was their choice to do mutual oral stimulation instead of intercourse. This weekend was the only time during our four-month therapy that they took Viagra. That one time made them feel better and reduced the anxiety that was getting in the way of our therapy.

If using Viagra or one of the other medical resources sometimes during your therapy or self-help program will gain your spouse's cooperation, give you more confidence, or produce any other positive result, by all means speak to your physician.

MIND POWER FOR BETTER ERECTIONS

To derive maximum benefit from sexual activity, you need to get your mind working with you. Starting as soon as possible, you need to frequently imagine yourself as you'd like to be, and spend as little time as you can imagining how you've been. You are going to apply some of the information and suggestions contained in Chapter 19. If you haven't read that chapter and digested its contents, now would be a good time to do so.

Mind Power A: Whenever you're aware of telling yourself that you're impotent or inadequate, or having an image that embodies that idea, argue with it and change it. For example: "It's true, I've had troubles getting it up for the last few months. But I'm going to do this program and change that. I'm going to have good erections again."

Mind Power B: This is an image, really more like a movie, that you should spend thirty to ninety seconds on every day; doing it several times a day is even better. Imagine yourself having good erections with a partner, which includes several components. Imagine having a good erection, entering your partner, feeling relaxed and comfortable, and just being still inside her for a moment or two. You're not moving, just enjoying being in her. Then imagine slow movements, just taking it easy, still enjoying the feeling of being in her. Then gradually increase the pace of your thrusts. Now slow down again. Now again increase the pace gradually, until you're moving almost as much as you want, still feeling calm and easy. Now imagine slowing down and stopping all movement. Stop thrusting and just experience the pleasure. Then gradually increase the movements, slowly building up until you're moving with abandon, letting your body do what it wants. When you want, and only when you want, imagine a wonderful ejaculation. When you're done with the movie, be sure to end with a statement to yourself of this kind: "As it is in my mind, so it shall be in reality" or "This is how it's going to be."

Mind Power C: Before you do a physical exercise, spend a few seconds imagining yourself doing it perfectly, exactly as it is supposed to be done.

Be sure to imagine all the parts: for example, asking your partner to participate, attending to your arousal and physical sensations, asking her to stop if you get anxious, asking her to resume stimulation, and so on.

This mental rehearsal takes only a few seconds and can be very helpful. You can do it anyplace. For example, if you and your partner are getting ready to do an exercise, you can close your eyes and do your mental rehearsal right there or you can go into another room and take a few seconds to do it there.

Mind Power D: Every day, preferably just after awakening or just before retiring for the night, take a few seconds to imagine how good you're going to feel once your erections are back on track.

Mind Power E: Whenever the problem recurs, make every effort not to let it get you down. Instead of telling yourself that this is further proof you'll never get it together, ask yourself what you can learn from this experience. Maybe you were too anxious, too tired, too much in a hurry, too little aroused. Then tell yourself something like this: "No reason to get upset. I learned that it doesn't work to have sex when I'm this anxious and tired. Next time I'm this nervous, I'll stop and just talk to Jeannie about what's going on."

Mind Power F: This is the pep-talk exercise given in Chapter 19, on pages 273–274. Use it whenever you feel discouraged or think you failed in an exercise.

MEETING YOUR CONDITIONS

You should now turn to and reread Chapter 6 to determine the conditions you need to have met for having more or better erections. Consider your desire, arousal, anxiety, mental and physical stimulation, time of day, the state of your relationship, your partner's attitude and behavior, and anything else that seems relevant. Some men need for their partners to be more enthusiastic or aroused. Others need to be less preoccupied and more focused on matters at hand when they have sex.

There are only two important considerations about your conditions: finding out what they are and fulfilling them. You are who you are and you need what you need. Make sure you get it.

INCREASING AROUSAL

As I said in Chapter 15, arousal is basically what powers erections. If there's nothing seriously wrong with you physically, if you are relatively relaxed, if your conditions are met, and if you are aroused, you will get good erections. Since arousal is crucial, you should read or reread Chapter 15 before going on.

Pay particular attention to what I say about focusing on sensation in that chapter. One of the major ways of increasing arousal is to focus on physical sensation, to attend to and fully experience your partner's touching, kissing, caressing, and stroking you. Another way of increasing arousal is to ensure that you get the kinds of stimulation that are most arousing to you.

REDUCING ANXIETY ABOUT PERFORMANCE

Since worrying about how your penis will perform is perhaps the major obstacle to good functioning, anything that reduces this worry is helpful. All the methods discussed above play a role in this endeavor, but there are several other things that can help as well.

Since intercourse is the act that causes the greatest anxiety for men with erection problems, **it's best to agree not to have intercourse until you are confident of your erections.** Your partner needs to understand and accept this point. She also needs to agree that until that time she will satisfy you without intercourse and will allow you to do the same for her. Without agreement on these points, the chances of success after doing the exercises are drastically reduced.

If you have experience with any relaxation method—meditation, biofeedback, self-hypnosis, yoga, relaxation tapes—I suggest you resume that activity as soon as possible. If you've never done any of these things, you might want to invest in a good relaxation audiotape, many of which are available in bookstores, and listen for ten to fifteen minutes each day. Whatever method you use, your goal should be to be able to get relaxed quickly in almost any situation, without special equipment or postures.

JUST PLAY

One effective approach to resolving erection problems involves no exercises beyond those already given. To follow this approach, you do the steps above, and get together with your partner to play sexually as often as both of you desire. You can do whatever you want except have intercourse. When she's stimulating you, you should focus on sensation and try to build excitement as high as possible. Arousal and pleasure, not erection, are the only goals. And that's all there is to it.

This approach is so simple that some men have trouble with it. It seems too easy to them. It *is* simple and easy, but it's also effective.

It will help to keep a few things in mind. One is that the goal really is pleasure and arousal. You will of course note how your penis is doing, but try not to get concerned if it's not acting as you would like. It will in time. Be sure that all your conditions are met, that you have the best stimulation, and that you focus on the pleasurable physical stimulation.

If this approach doesn't work, you may want to do some of the exercises given below.

Which Exercises You Should Do

Everyone should do the mind-power exercises and the two masturbation exercises that follow. If you think you don't need to do the masturbation, it's a good idea to do each of them once just to make sure you can easily and comfortably handle them. If you don't want to masturbate, you can skip those exercises and start with the first partner exercise.

How Often to Do the Exercises

Good results can be achieved by doing the exercises anywhere from every other day to once or twice a week. Masters and Johnson noticed two things about penises that work against doing the exercises as often as you want. The first is what they called a refractory period, a time after ejaculation when your penis will not respond to stimulation no matter how skillfully done and no matter how long it lasts. For many teenagers the refractory period lasts only a few minutes. But it definitely increases with age. Some men in their fifties and sixties can't get another erection until days after their last ejaculation. Masters and Johnson also noticed that many older men can't regain an erection for a day or more after sex even if they don't ejaculate. Take account of these facts in deciding how often to do the exercises.

It is essential that you do the exercises only when you are relaxed and feeling sexy, or believe you can get into a sexy mood with a little time and stimulation. Doing the exercises when feeling under pressure or with gritted teeth will not help at all.

What About Ejaculating While Doing the Exercises?

In general, the less you ejaculate, the more easily you will become aroused and perhaps erect the next time you do an exercise. This does not mean you should never ejaculate, only that it is in your interest not to ejaculate unless you really want to.

What About Having Intercourse While Doing the Exercises?

Many men with erection problems develop an understandable but destructive habit. As soon as they notice they have an erection—whether they are engaged in love play or not, whether they are doing an exercise or not—they automatically try to stick it in their partners before it goes away. Although this sometimes results in a few thrusts or minutes of intercourse, it usually doesn't because the mind/body tends to interpret the frantic effort to stick it in as anxiety, which it is. This stick-it-in-before-you-lose-it practice causes all sorts of problems. It usually results in lost erections, which makes the man feel more hopeless, and it reinforces the idea that he has a serious problem. It does nothing to alleviate the anxiety that is a large part of the problem to begin with. And it often makes the man's partner upset or angry, because in entering her so frantically he may not notice that she's not ready or interested at the moment.

WHAT IF YOU DON'T HAVE A REGULAR SEX PARTNER?

If you don't have a partner with whom to do the couples exercises, you should attend to the steps given above and do the two masturbation exercises below. When you do get into a relationship, follow the advice about getting into sex very slowly, as per the discussion in Chapter 17. Also consider the discussion in that chapter about telling your partner about your problem. Then, as you desire it, just play as discussed on page 330. If it seems necessary, you can also do the partner exercises in this chapter with your new friend. An alternative is to go through surrogate partner therapy.

MASTURBATION EXERCISES FOR BETTER ERECTIONS

If you're willing to masturbate, I recommend doing these masturbation exercises before you begin working with your partner. If you're not willing to masturbate and have a partner, you can begin with the first partner exercise.

EXERCISE 22-1: PLEASURING YOUR SOFT PENIS

The goal is to get comfortable with touching your soft penis and learn what kinds of sensations that produces. Put some lubricant on one or both of your hands and touch your penis for about fifteen minutes in ways that feel arousing. Try different kinds of touches and strokes. You want to focus on the sensations and feel as sexy as possible, but you don't need an erection. In fact, an erection will only get in the way. Don't try not to get hard, just follow the instructions already given. If you find your penis getting hard, just pay attention to the sensations as it does so. But when it's reached what you consider to be about 50 to 80 percent of fullness and rigidity, stop touching it. Enjoy looking at it and let it go down. The session is over for you.

Repeat this exercise two or three times, until you feel comfortable touching your nonerect penis and feel that you've improved your ability to focus on the sensations in your penis.

EXERCISE 22-2: LOSING AND REGAINING ERECTIONS

Stroke your penis with a lubricated hand and focus either on the sensations produced or on an exciting fantasy. When you have an erection, enjoy it for a moment and then stop stimulation. Take your hand away from your penis and let your erection subside completely, which may take from a few seconds to a few minutes. When your penis is soft, resume stimulation and focus on sensation or fantasy. Most of the time your erection will return, in which case you should again stop and let it get soft. Two complete cycles of this sequence—stimulation, erection, stopping, losing erection, stimulation—are sufficient for one session.

If your erection does not return within a few minutes after resuming stimulation, ask if there is anything you can do to get into a more relaxed and more arousing frame of mind. Taking a few deep breaths or looking at some stimulating pictures may help. If the changes you make result in erection, just continue with the exercise. If not, call it quits for now and return to the exercise another time. Whatever you do, don't try to force an erection.

This exercise should be repeated as many times as necessary, with at least one day's rest between repetitions, until you are reasonably confident that an erection can often be regained by proper mental and physical stimulation.

PARTNER EXERCISES

Before starting on the partner exercises, it's a good idea to do Step A of Exercise 14-1 (nongenital body rubs) in Chapter 14. This will give you some useful experience before you get to genital stimulation in the following exercises.

Exercises 22-3 and 22-4 may surprise you, because in both of them you are asked not to have an erection. You may wonder why, after all the travail not having erections has caused you, I would be asking you to again not have an erection. My answer is simple. After working with hundreds of men with erection problems, I realized that two of their greatest fears are their partner's touching their soft penis ("She'll notice I'm still not hard") and losing an erection ("Here we go again"). As long as these fears are unaddressed, they remain in the background or foreground and get in the way of serious progress. Once they are addressed, on the other hand, the other exercises tend to be much easier and proceed more smoothly. Exercises 22-3 and 22-4 are ways of directly dealing with these fears and putting them to rest. Despite what I've said, after reading them you may be tempted to skip them. Do what's necessary to resist this temptation.

EXERCISE 22-3: NOT GETTING OR LOSING YOUR ERECTION

You are to do two things: reenact your old erection problem and handle it differently than you usually did. If your problem was that you did not get an erection while your partner stimulated you, then have her stimulate you and see to it that you don't get an erection. If your problem was getting soft during intercourse, then have intercourse and make your erection go away. Whatever the old problem, re-create it.

There are many ways to not get or to lose an erection. Distracting yourself from the pleasurable stimulation by worrying about a myriad of things can help—anything from whether you'll get or keep hard, to whether the kids are listening, to how much money the IRS will want from you this year—is probably the best way.

After you've managed not to get hard or to lose your erection, deal with the situation in ways that are enhancing to both you and your partner. Acknowledge what's happened but don't apologize. Instead, offer something that sounds good. Here is an example: "I don't think I can get hard again, but I'd love to love you. Anything interest you?" When the two of you agree on something, do it. It can be sexual or not. The only important thing is that you both feel good about yourselves, each other, and what you do.

Repeat this exercise as many times as necessary for you to feel comfortable about losing your erection and dealing with the situation after that. Some men find one or two repetitions sufficient; others can benefit from many more.

Exercise 22-4 is designed to help you feel more comfortable about having your partner touch your unerect penis. Many men are horrified at the prospect. They believe it should be hard before she touches it or, at the very least, should get hard as soon as she touches it. After all, that's the way a real man is. That's the fantasy. The realities are somewhat different. Being comfortable while your unerect penis is being touched is very important. It allows you to enjoy stimulation that might get you erect. Even if you don't get hard, it can still feel very good. The more comfortable you are with her touching your soft penis, the better all the following exercises will go.

EXERCISE 22-4: PARTNER PLAYING WITH YOUR SOFT PENIS

After making sure you are both in a comfortable position, let your partner play with your soft penis for ten to fifteen minutes. Try not to get an erection; you want the experience of being touched when soft. If you do get hard, stop for a while until your penis gets soft again, then have your partner resume.

She can explore, caress, stroke, and just generally play with your penis in any ways she wants. Don't let her do anything that's painful or uncomfortable, but, aside from that, keep your hands to yourself and your attention on the sensations produced. Be aware of what it feels like to be touched by her.

Do this exercise at least two or three times, until you are quite comfortable with her touching you when you're soft.

POSSIBLE PROBLEM

You find yourself trying to get an erection or feeling bad because you don't have one. Given what men are taught, this is natural. Use your mind-power techniques to turn negative thoughts and images into positive ones, and resist the temptation to try to get hard. Talking to your partner about the feelings you're having can be very helpful. And keep in mind that you have to keep your penis soft to derive benefit from the exercise. Having an erection interferes with this goal.

EXERCISE 22-5: PARTNER STIMULATION OF PENIS

This time your partner is to touch and stroke your genitals, with a lubricated hand, as you direct her, for ten to fifteen minutes. It's the same as the regular body rub but focused on genitals. Some men prefer to do some touching and kissing before getting to penile stimulation, while others prefer getting to genital stimulation right away. Do whatever feels right to you and your partner.

The goal is to get you as turned on as possible. Arousal, not erection, is what we're interested in. If you get an erection, that's fine, but no finer than if you don't. But if you do get one, don't try to stick it anyplace. Just continue with the exercise.

Give her feedback and directions, using words that turn you on. As you get excited, pay attention to the feelings and feel free to follow them through your body. A feeling may develop in your penis, and then you may notice differences in the way your chest and stomach feel. Go with these cues of arousal as long as you like. If sexual images or ideas appear, feel free to go with them.

As usual, deal with negative thoughts and images as per the discussion on pages 268–270.

You can touch your partner, *but only for your own pleasure.* You are not to try to turn her on during the exercise. If it would increase your own excitement to touch her breasts while she stimulates your genitals, it's fine, but touch her breasts only in ways that excite *you.* If you realize you're trying to excite her, change the kind of touching you're doing or stop it altogether.

If you do get aroused and do focus on your sensations, you will probably get an erection some of the time. You can ejaculate, but only if you really want to.

Men vary tremendously in how many times they need to do this exercise. It can be anywhere from three to twenty times, depending on how much time it takes to feel comfortable with it, to get good at focusing on sensation and refocusing when the mind wanders, to turn negative thoughts and images into positive ones, and to be able to give directions to get the best possible stimulation.

POSSIBLE PROBLEMS

You never get an erection in this exercise, or never keep it for long, even after a number of repetitions. Sometimes the problem is obvious. You can't get your partner to stimulate you the way you like, you can't focus on sensation, negative thoughts keep intruding, and so on. If one of these causes is manifest, you need to determine how to resolve it. Going back and redoing one or more of the earlier exercises may help.

If you usually get erections in masturbation but not with this exercise, there's something in the relationship that's getting in the way. Ask what it would take for you to be able to have an erection with your partner. What issues, attitudes, or behaviors would have to be resolved or changed? See if you can work them out. If not, you may need to seek professional help.

If you respond neither to masturbation nor this exercise, you should definitely see a competent urologist or sex therapist.

If you're like many of the men I've worked with, you are now convinced that things aren't as bad as you had imagined. You may, in fact, think that everything is fine and be in a hurry to get to intercourse. I hope you're willing to resist that temptation for now.

The next exercise, like Exercise 22-4, deals with the fear of losing an erection, but it also goes further in demonstrating that lost erections can often be regained, an important lesson for you to learn. Losing an erection is not a catastrophe. If you keep your cool, you can probably regain it. And if not, that's not a tragedy, either.

EXERCISE 22-6: LOSING AND REGAINING ERECTIONS

Have your partner stimulate your penis with her hand or mouth in ways that you like. Your goal, as always, is to attend to the sensations and get as aroused as possible. When you have an erection, enjoy it for a moment, then tell her to stop and allow your erection to go down. You can do anything you want to accomplish this—have a talk, give her a back rub or a sexual massage, or whatever. Take as much time as you need for your penis to get soft. Then have her resume stimulation. When it gets hard again, repeat the procedure given above. Two or three repetitions of the whole procedure—stimulation, erection, stop stimulation, erection fades, resume stimulation—constitute one session.

You will not always regain your erection and you will not always get one to begin with. When either of these things happens, let her know ("I guess it's not going to get hard today. I'd like you to stop"). Then talk with her about what the two of you want to do that would be enjoyable. Maybe she'd like you to sexually stimulate her. Maybe one of you wants a back rub. Whatever it is, do it.

It's crucial that you master this step. You can be sure your penis will not always respond the way you want. You need to feel comfortable letting your partner know that and talking with her about how to have a good time without an erection.

Do this exercise at least four times, until you are confident that your erection will usually return with proper stimulation and that when it doesn't, you can still have a good time.

POSSIBLE PROBLEMS

1. You never get an erection. This usually means you haven't yet mastered the previous exercises. Go back to the ones you skipped and do them.

2. Your erection doesn't go down in a reasonable length of time. This isn't a bad problem to have, but it does increase the amount of time it takes to do the exercise. Check to see if what you're doing while waiting for it to get soft is arousing. If it is, do something else. Getting up and walking around the room or the house will usually do the trick.

3. Your erection, once lost, doesn't return in a reasonable length of time. The problem often lies in anxiety about getting it back. In other words, you're forgetting some of the lessons you've learned in this chapter. You might want to reread it and mentally mark the important passages. Try to remember that you don't have to do anything to make your penis hard. It will take care of that itself as long as you focus on sensations or arousing thoughts or images and build arousal. It might also help to talk to your partner about any concerns you have about regaining the erection.

The exercises that follow require some kind of erection, so care must be taken not to create anxiety or pressure to perform. You can use spontaneous erections or those that occur in loveplay. Say you want to do an exercise and you ask your partner to stimulate you in ways you like. If you get a good erection (meaning one you feel good about, even though it's not 100 percent hard), feel free to go on to the exercise. If you don't get an erection in what seems a reasonable length of time, or if the erection you do get doesn't seem stable, don't try to force it. Do something enjoyable with your partner, sexual or not, and let it be.

These exercises also require that your partner's vagina be well lubricated. Talk with her about whether an artificial lubricant such as K-Y jelly or Astroglide would be helpful.

EXERCISE 22-7: GRADUAL INSERTION INTO VAGINA

Using a position that is comfortable for both of you, you are to gradually insert your penis, in stages, into her vagina. First place your erect penis just at the opening of her vagina. Take a few seconds to get used to having it there. When that feels comfortable, move it in a little bit, about an inch. Again, take a few seconds to get used to the feeling. Continue in this fashion until your whole penis is inside of her. Then stay that way for a few minutes and focus on the sensations in your penis. See how it feels to have your penis surrounded by her vagina. Be aware of the texture, temperature, and wetness of the vagina. Get used to being there; it's a nice place.

If at any time you feel your erection start to go down, stay focused and see if you can enjoy the sensations of your erection going down.

If you want to ejaculate after a few moments and it's okay with her, do so, but move slowly and be aware of what's happening to you.

You can proceed to the next exercise when you are comfortable being inside of your partner and can keep your erection for a minute or so without movement.

Now we're going to extend your ability to be inside her with movement. The position usually recommended for these exercises is you lying on your back and her sitting on top of you; this allows you to fully relax, letting the bed support your weight so you don't have to flex any muscles, and works well for many couples. But others prefer something else. So use any position that works best for you; just remember that it has to be sufficiently comfortable for both of you so that changes in it aren't necessary for five to ten minutes.

EXERCISE 22-8: PENIS IN VAGINA WITH MOVEMENT

Step A: This is similar to the previous exercise, except that now one of you thrusts slowly for ten to fifteen minutes. Which one moves largely depends on the position you're using. If she's on top, she'll do the moving. If you're on top, it will be you. Regardless of what position is used and who moves, you have to be in charge of how much movement and when to stop and resume thrusting. Your job is to focus on sensations and get as aroused as possible. It's important that your partner *not* start thrusting to satisfy herself. That will come later.

Start with a very slow pace. Make sure you're comfortable with it before increasing movement. Then go a little faster. When that feels fine, no anxiety or negative thoughts, increase the pace again.

Continue with this step until the active one is moving at a pretty good pace but not all out, say about 80 percent of abandoned movement. This will probably *not* be achieved in one fifteen-minute session. Use as many sessions as you need. Then do Step B.

Step B: The same as Step A, with the other one moving. This may well require a different position.

Step C: The same as the two previous steps, except both of you move. Start with very slow movements and only increase the pace as you feel comfortable. Use as many sessions as required until you are both moving as fast as you desire.

POSSIBLE PROBLEM WITH ANY OF THE STEPS

You lose your erection during intercourse. This happens occasionally to most men, but there are some things to try if you feel it's really a problem. Make sure you are relaxed; if you're not, take some deep breaths and have some positive thoughts and images. If your penis is still in her vagina, you can leave it there and try to get the stimulation you want; moving in certain ways or having your partner squeeze her pelvic muscles may do the trick. Or you can take your penis out and get the kind of stimulation you want, resuming intercourse when you are hard.

If you find that you usually lose your erection at a particular point—say, when your partner is thrusting very quickly—here's something you can do. When you are alone, take a few moments to get relaxed and imagine her moving slowly in intercourse. Continue to relax and imagine her moving a tad faster. Continue in this fashion, relaxing and then imagining her moving at increasingly faster speeds, until you can calmly imagine her moving at full speed. Then do the same thing for real with your partner. Relax and have her move slowly in intercourse. Check to see that you're still relaxed and, if so, have her increase the pace. If at some point you find you are getting tense, get her to slow down immediately to a speed you're comfortable with. Then, in very small steps, have her increase the pace. Always back away from speeds that make you tense and go back to those you are comfortable with. Done consistently, this procedure will allow you to tolerate and enjoy more and more movement.

By fulfilling your conditions, by having sex only when you desire it and are aroused, by making sure you are relaxed, and by getting the kinds of stimulation you like, you are ensuring that your penis will function most of the time you want it to. And when it doesn't meet your expectations or when an erection goes away at an inopportune moment, you no longer have to worry about it. You are prepared to have a good time no matter what your penis does.

As time goes on and your sexual confidence continues to develop, you will not need to be as careful about your conditions. Just don't forget about them altogether. If you should find yourself backsliding, if you notice you're tense in sex or find that sex isn't as satisfying as it is now, give more attention to conditions, arousal, relaxation, and stimulation, and it probably won't be too long before the situation improves again.

CHAPTER TWENTY-THREE

Surrogate Partner Therapy

FOR MEN WHO have any sex problem—shyness, lack of experience, lack of interest, erections, rapid ejaculation, or inability to ejaculate with a partner—and don't have a regular sex partner and aren't likely to get one until the problem is resolved, the most effective and certainly the most controversial treatment is what's called surrogate therapy. The word *surrogate* means "substitute" and was chosen by Masters and Johnson to refer to a woman associate who did the sexual exercises that ordinarily a man would do with his partner.

Despite lots of publicity about surrogate therapy in the media, there is still much confusion about it. Some people think that a surrogate is nothing more than a prostitute because she has sex for money. It's true that surrogates—just like therapists, lawyers, and physicians—like to get paid for their work. But the similarity ends there. A prostitute's job is to give her customers a good time and get them off, usually as quickly as possible.

A surrogate's role is different. Her job is to teach clients skills they need to be more effective socially and sexually. Reputable surrogates work with therapists—that is, the client has a session with the surrogate and then goes to see the therapist, with or without the surrogate—and function more as the therapist's associate rather than as a wife substitute. The surrogate's job is not getting the man off or giving him a good time. Rather, it is working with the therapist to diagnose and treat the client's problem.

A lot of the time the man spends with the surrogate is devoted to the development of social skills and talking, which in itself is different from what happens with a prostitute. Talking usually takes up most of the first session, followed by a relaxation exercise or two and perhaps some light touching with both surrogate and client fully dressed. In subsequent sessions, there is a progression to communication exercises, nudity, sensual touching, and finally more direct sexual activity. The physical/sexual activities they engage in, often called body work, are similar to the partner exercises given in this book. Depending on the surrogate, therapist, and the nature of the problem, there may or may not be much intercourse. In almost all cases, a large amount of time is spent by the surrogate helping the client to learn ways to reduce the anxiety he feels in sex and to increase his confidence.

Surrogate partner therapy is extremely beneficial to men of all ages who have little or no sexual experience and who are shy and fearful. I have worked with virgins or near-virgins as young as eighteen and as old as fifty-seven. Enrico is an example. He was forty-three when he came to see me. He had several experiences with prostitutes when in the army, and a number of hand jobs at massage parlors since then, but never sex that hadn't been paid for. He'd never had a date. Needless to say, he was painfully shy, fearful of both rejection and acceptance.

It took several sessions with me before he was even willing to meet the surrogate. For the first ten sessions with her, he kept his clothes on and the work focused on overcoming his social anxiety. I did a number of confidence-building and fear-reduction techniques with him, and he practiced talking to the surrogate and then role-playing meeting her in various places and initiating conversations. This progressed to getting her phone number and asking for a date.

He and the surrogate then went on simulated dates. They actually went for walks and to coffee shops. Then we got to initiating physical contact and, finally, to sexual contact. An essential element in every step was practicing talking with the surrogate; for example, in explaining why he wanted to proceed gradually in sex instead of rushing into bed on the second date.

The work with Enrico took a number of months because of his extreme shyness and fear. But in the end it was successful. He started dating and after a while met a woman he fell in love with. Now, some years later, he is happily married and a father.

You may be surprised by all the work we did with Enrico on social skills and communication, yet this is a common and crucial feature of surrogate partner therapy. We have had a number of clients who were taking penile injections for their erection problems, and now Viagra or antidepressants for their quick ejaculations, but who still wanted help to reduce their anxiety and to learn skills to become more confident and satisfying lovers. There is a lot more talking and relating in surrogate therapy than most clients and even referring therapists and physicians realize.

There is an exception to my earlier statement that surrogate work is only for men without partners. I have also worked with some men who had partners who absolutely refused to participate in any way in the treatment; they wouldn't even talk to me on the phone. Some of these women have themselves suggested a surrogate; they wanted their men to "get the problem fixed" or learn better lovemaking skills, but they didn't want to have anything to do with it. I have always had mixed feelings about doing surrogate work with these men, even when their partners are the ones pushing the idea. I haven't liked helping them have sex with a woman other than their mates. But given that the partners either wanted this solution or wouldn't cooperate in helping the men with their problems, there didn't seem to be much choice. Some of these cases have worked out, by which I mean the man overcame a problem by learning better skills with the surrogate and was able to transfer the learning to sex with his partner. But in a significant number of these cases the result was that the man left his partner. This isn't surprising, because her refusal to participate in treatment is a definite sign that the relationship was not in good shape. I don't exactly know how to categorize these cases—can a divorce ever be considered a success?—but without exception the men reported that the therapy was very helpful. Several of them even said that going into therapy with the surrogate and me was the smartest decision they had ever made.

Surrogate therapy at its best involves the therapist and surrogate working toward a common goal, with each contributing his or her own expertise. For example, the surrogate may tell me that our client is fine with sex play as long as there's no thought of intercourse. When intercourse is a possibility, he immediately tenses up and loses his erection. To help prepare him for intercourse, I may do some relaxation work with him followed by processes to reduce the specific fears. Then we have him imagine moving toward intercourse in a positive way. What I do with him in his imagination, she does in reality.

The main advantage of surrogate therapy is that it is highly effective. Other therapists I know who do this kind of work agree with me in thinking it is the most effective therapy for men without regular sex partners. It has been almost 100 percent effective with male virgins of all ages. Usually these men have failed with several women and been so humiliated that they refuse to try again until they feel their problem is resolved.

Some people make the assumption that while surrogate work will help the client function with the surrogate, it won't carry over to other partners. Fortunately, this assumption is incorrect. The surrogates I've worked with and I are very much aware of the issue and direct our efforts to resolving it. We would view it as an unmitigated failure if a man could function with the surrogate but not with real-life partners. So we are always focused on the partner(s) he doesn't yet have. Say a client is able to do something today with the surrogate that he's never been able to do before. When we ask him why, he usually gives credit to the surrogate: "She made me feel so relaxed (or confident) by saying X or doing Y." Then we ask the crucial question: Suppose you're with a woman who doesn't say X or do Y? What could *you* do to feel as relaxed (or confident)? And then we work on what he needs to be able to do, often involving role-playing with the surrogate and the therapist. In the many cases I've worked with, the ability to function as well with a real-life partner as with a surrogate is over 90 percent.

Surrogate therapy is hard work for the client. The work causes his problems to surface, and then he has to learn and perfect the skills necessary to resolve or handle them. In many ways the therapy is more difficult than real life. Many clients have told us long after the therapy, after they have dated one or more women and are involved in a relationship, "After what I went through with you, everything is easy."

Surrogate treatment also has disadvantages. First, it is applicable only for a small segment of the population: those men with sex problems who don't have a regular sex partner and who probably won't find one until their problem is resolved. Second, it is expensive, because two people are being paid. Surrogates generally charge less per hour than therapists but their sessions are longer, usually an hour and a half or two hours. Third, this kind of therapy is not widely available. As far as I know, the main places to find reputable surrogate therapy are in the large metropolitan centers on the East Coast and in California, especially Los Angeles and the San Francisco Bay area. In my practice, we have had clients from all over the country and abroad come to us for treatment because surrogate therapy wasn't available closer to home. This means that men living elsewhere may have to consider coming to one of these cities for two weeks or so of intensive therapy, which of course involves the additional expenses of travel and lodging.

An important question has to do with sexually transmitted diseases. After all, surrogates have sex with many partners and seem like prime candidates for contracting one or more of the many common diseases. The fear of spreading or getting AIDS, or of being sued for transmitting it, has caused some therapists to stop doing surrogate therapy.

The surrogates I have worked with are extremely careful about disease and were this way before the advent of AIDS. As far as I know, not one has ever had a sexually transmitted disease. The surrogate I now work with gets an HIV antibody test every six months and demands two negative test results from every new client. Safe sex is the name of the game, and it is played compulsively. Clients learn far more about safe sex than they want to know.

If you're interested in this kind of therapy, I have a few suggestions.

1. Work only with a surrogate-therapist team, not a surrogate alone. You see both of them and they keep in touch about you. In my own work, I call the surrogate after every session I have with the client to go over what came up and how that affects our work. She does the same after every session she has with the client. The therapist is a crucial element in the therapy. Surrogates are trained in sexuality and surrogate work, but they are not trained psychotherapists. Besides, as many surrogates will be the first to admit, it's often hard to be objective when you're doing body work with someone. Some therapists refer clients to surrogates and then have nothing further to do with the case. This is not a good idea and I caution against it. Both client and surrogate need support and assistance from an experienced therapist.

Speaking of which, it is important that your therapist be experienced in working with a surrogate. Most therapists, even most sex therapists, do not have this experience. If your therapist does not, ask for a referral to someone who does.

2. Before making any appointments, ask about safe-sex practices and proof that the surrogate has had a recent negative HIV antibody test. If the surrogate and therapist don't seem concerned about safe sex, if she won't provide the proof, or if she doesn't require similar proof from you, stay away.

3. Work only with a surrogate who respects who you are. Good surrogate work, like any good therapy, requires an understanding of and respect for you and your problem. It should begin where you are and gradually take you to where you want to go. It should not ask you to do what you can't do, and it should not humiliate or terrify you. I have heard a number of horror stories over the years about surrogates working alone. One of them asked a very anxious man with erection problems to undress and masturbate in front of her—after he had known her only half an hour! If he could have done that, he wouldn't have needed her help. The only effects were to further embarrass and humiliate him and to convince him that he would never get better.

4. Feel free to bring up any complaints or problems with the surrogate and the therapist. Years ago a man was telling me about a difficult session he had just had with the surrogate. In trying to determine what went wrong, we finally hit upon the temperature at her place. He said it was as hot as a sauna and he felt totally depleted. When I asked why he didn't ask her to turn down the heat or open a window, he answered, "I thought the heat was part of the program." Don't make the same mistake. Anything that bothers you or that makes you uncomfortable should be expressed as soon as possible. This is also good training for what you need to be able to do with your own partners: Express what's on your mind.

Since surrogate therapy is so expensive (you should figure on at least two thousand to three thousand dollars, unless your problem is quite specific and you don't need work on overcoming shyness or the development of social skills), you may want to try other treatment options first—for example, the exercises in this book relevant to your problem. If you make some progress but not as much as you want, you can still see a surrogate later; the work you've done on your own will probably decrease the number of sessions you'll need with her.

CHAPTER TWENTY-FOUR

Resolving Problems of Sexual Desire and Frequency

I don't know what to do about my girlfriend. I love her and we get along fine, but her idea of good sex is once, maybe twice, a week. I can't survive on such a meager quota.—*Man, 27*

I feel like shit. I just don't want to make love to my wife. She feels ugly and thinks I'm having an affair, which I'm not, and I feel guilty and awful. Why can't I get turned on to her anymore?—*Man, 44*

DESPITE ALL THE news on the media about erection and orgasm problems, the complaint that has brought the largest number of individuals and couples to sex therapy in the last fifteen years has to do with desire and frequency. Michael, for instance, is upset with his lover because "she rarely wants sex. I go around angry at her and horny all the time." Barney, on the other hand, is upset with his wife because "she's always hounding me for sex. It's gotten so I'm almost afraid to come home." Edward and Janet are upset because they rarely have sex even though they both miss and want it: "It's just that we're too busy and too tired; when one of us is in the mood the other either isn't or is already asleep."

When you first hear about such complaints, they sound easy to resolve. Surely Michael could just make do with less sex than he's used to and Barney could interest himself a little more often in order to make his wife happier. And certainly Edward and Janet could set aside a time each week when they'd both be awake and interested in making love. Of course, some people do come up with these solutions on their own and make them work. Yet many other couples cannot resolve these problems on their own. Their egos are involved, their feelings are hurt, and they find it difficult even to discuss the issues constructively with their partners, let alone make any changes. Yet assuming goodwill on both sides and a reasonably functional relationship, most of these complaints can be worked out.

DESIRE PROBLEMS

Problems of sexual appetite and activity usually come up as a discrepancy in a relationship: One partner wants more or less sex than the other, and they are unable to work out a compromise. It may always have been this way—A wanted more sex than B from the first days of their relationship—or it may be a more recent development. The problem may be or at least seem absolute; that is, A "always" wants sex or B "never" wants it.

A woman I saw in therapy complained that absolutely nothing dented her husband's sex drive. When she was angry with him, he still wanted sex, as he did when he was angry with her. One night, she recalled, she was suffering from the flu, had a temperature of 103 degrees, "was coughing and sneezing every minute and, as I noticed later, even had snot running down my face," but was awakened to find her husband rubbing her breasts, trying to turn her on.

On the other side of the continuum, a male client complained that ever since they had moved to California four years earlier, his wife has never, "not once," wanted sex. She did not initiate nor did she respond positively to any of his initiations.

The problem may also be less extreme, with B being interested some of the time but not nearly enough to satisfy A. A man in his early forties complained, "It's not that Marge never wants sex. Occasionally she does, but that requires that the kids be out of the house or sound asleep, that we've been lovey-dovey for at least a week, and that she isn't engaged in an important project at work. What this comes down to is sex once or twice a month, and I just can't deal with that."

WHAT ARE WE TALKING ABOUT, ANYWAY?

Since much more is often entailed in desire problems than that term implies, let's try to define exactly what is involved. There are three key concepts: desire itself, the object or purpose of the desire, and the willingness to act on the feeling of desire.

I take the first concept, *erotic desire*, to mean a physical/emotional interest in engaging in sexual activity. While desire often has cognitive elements (thoughts or images of sex), it is more than a vague intellectual itch. For example, the idea "I should want to make it with such a beautiful woman," if unaccompanied by any feeling or physical sensation, is not desire as I define it. Neither is the idea "Gee, we haven't made love in several weeks, so I guess it's time." As I use the term *desire,* it is similar to the messages we get from our bodies signifying a desire for food. But just as we don't always eat when we get a message saying, "*Beep, beep,* hungry," so too we don't always engage in sex when we get a "*Beep, beep,* horny" message. And just as we sometimes eat without having received a "*Beep, beep,* hungry," message, so too we sometimes have sex without a "*Beep, beep,* horny" message.

In some people interest itself is low; that is, they don't have many sexual thoughts, feelings, or fantasies. Seeing or talking to an attractive person doesn't evoke any surges of sexual energy or any thoughts or images of what they might want to do sexually with these people. This total or relative lack of interest in sex can be either long-term—and for a few men it's always been like this—or of recent origin.

Although there are some women who want more sex than the average man and some men who want less sex than the average woman, in general men seem to have a greater libido than women. The observation of sex therapists and researchers Sandra Leiblum and Raymond Rosen fits my own impressions:

> Overall, it does appear that men have a more insistent and constant sexual appetite, which is readily accessed through a large variety of internal and environmental prompts. Women, on the other hand, have less intense and more sporadic sexual desires, which they are more likely to suppress or to ignore if a host of conditions are not met.

An example of men's more constant appetite is that they think about and want sex regardless of whether they are in a relationship, while many women seem to automatically turn off their erotic interest when they're not connected to someone. As one woman reported: "When I don't have a partner, I don't think about sex. And to tell the truth, I don't miss it much. As soon as I'm in a new relationship, though, and sexually active again, I think about it all the time!"

Women's desire also fluctuates with their menstrual cycles. Very few women, for instance, have much sexual interest just before and during the first two or three days of their periods. And most women do not have much sexual appetite in the last trimester of pregnancy or for a while after giving birth.

Despite what I've said about men generally being more interested in sex than women, there are many exceptions. In my own practice, in the vast majority of couples consulting me about desire complaints it's the woman who wants more and the man who always has a headache.

For both men and women, sexual desire does decrease gradually with age. The height of sexual interest for both males and females comes fairly early—in adolescence and the twenties. It's like everything reminds you of sex and everything makes you feel sexy. This feeling tends to diminish over the years, although there can be resurgences at various times.

There is no physical reason for sexual desire to entirely disappear with age. The production of testosterone, which largely controls sexual appetite in men and women, does decline over time, but it never ceases altogether in healthy individuals. There are many men in their sixties, seventies, eighties, and beyond who remain interested in sex and have it when they can, although factors like lack of a partner or medical problems may get in the way. But interest remains, and not only for men. A friend of mine is a doctor who routinely asks her patients about safe sex. One day, without thinking, she asked a ninety-year-old single woman patient if she was practicing safe sex. The woman smiled sweetly and said, "No, but I'd like to."

Despite what I've said about the constancy of male libido, it can ebb and flow, depending on a number of variables. Some men, for instance, can lose interest when they're deeply involved in their education, work, or athletics. This can be for days, weeks, or longer. Various stresses can also deflate desire. One man with a usually ravenous sexual appetite reported that he didn't think about sex or engage in any form of it for four months—the period beginning when he was first contacted by the IRS until the day after the audit was completed.

The same things affect different men in different ways. Although some men forget about sex when involved in their work, other men get turned on while working and use sex as a relief from work and as a way of recharging their batteries. Certainly the stressful job of being president of the United States didn't dampen John F. Kennedy's enormous sexual appetite.

Many men's desire, or willingness to act on desire, is heavily dependent on the physical characteristics of their partners. These men report that their sexual appetites decreased after their partners gained weight or developed stretch marks as a result of pregnancy. Some men's sexual desire is severely affected by relationship problems. If they feel angry at or rejected by their partners, their libido disappears. Other men barely seem to notice. It's as if their sexual urges are in a separate compartment and are unaffected by other considerations. And for a great many men, almost regardless of their age and situation, the appearance of a new partner, especially if she's young and attractive, can greatly increase erotic desire, at least for a short time.

The second crucial concept is the *object of desire,* which really comes down to the question of, desire for what? There are men who desire and engage in sex frequently, but only with themselves. While this can be the result of a block to sex with the partner—for instance, feeling that sex with her isn't fun or worthwhile—it can also be a preference. There are men who get all their erotic needs met in masturbation and, left to their own devices, would almost never have sex with a partner. It's as if they believe intercourse is a poor substitute for masturbation. While there is nothing specifically wrong with such an attitude, it can wreak havoc in relationships where the partner wants more sex with the man and realizes that although he's unwilling to have sex with her, he's doing it regularly with himself.

Even when we're thinking about sex with a partner, the question of desire for what remains. People don't have sex only to satisfy sexual urges. Many men, for example, sometimes or often have sex in the absence of any specific sexual desire; what they do feel, however, is a wish not to disappoint their partners or a desire to live up to their ideas of masculinity. And there are certainly women who have sex in the absence of any specific sexual interest in order to please their partners, to avoid hassle or argument, to avoid feeling guilty, and so on. One woman whose appetite for sex was so ravenous that her husband was fearful of coming home from work said the following when I asked why she wanted so much sex: "It's the only time I have his full attention." Another woman in a similar situation said, "Sex is the only time I get the touching I crave." What these women wanted, strictly speaking, was more attention and more touching, not more sex. But they believed sex was the only way to get what they really wanted.

There are many men who don't know how to get a hug, to express love or feel loved, or to feel strong and masculine except by having sex. Such individuals are often experienced by their partners as oversexed. The way out of this situation is for them to learn to express nonsexual feelings in nonsexual ways.

Just as the purpose or object of the sex that is wanted is an important question, so too is the kind of sex. Couples often have arguments about sexual frequency that could be easily resolved if only they could state precisely what it is that they want more or less of. Those wanting less sex usually believe that they are being asked to get aroused and go through a lengthy process, when in fact the partner who wants more may simply want, or be willing to settle for, a helping hand or a quickie. And even if this isn't the case at first, a discussion of the possibilities can often bring about a compromise on what at first seemed like an insurmountable problem.

Our third important concept is *willingness,* going along with the desire for sex by engaging in it or even initiating and having sex in the absence of a specific desire for it. Without this willingness, the motor just idles. Willingness is putting the car in gear and stepping on the accelerator.

A pattern of unwillingness in the presence of interest often signifies personal or relationship problems. If you feel desire but are unwilling to do anything about it with your partner, this could mean that you're angry or upset with her or don't find her attractive. Despite her many overtures, one man with a healthy sexual appetite didn't make love to his wife for two years after the birth of their child because he was so upset about what he perceived as her exclusive relationship with the child, which caused him to feel "totally left out." Or it could mean that something you believe and may not even be aware of is getting in the way; for example, that sex is too dirty an activity to have with someone you love. This might explain the behavior of a man who feels desire but instead of approaching his wife either masturbates or goes to prostitutes.

Willingness in the absence of desire could be a problem if it means that you're feeling pressured by your ideas of what a real man should do or by fear of your partner's reaction if you don't have sex. Yet willingness without much desire doesn't have to be a problem, as in Gunther's case:

Dee wants sex three or four times a week no matter what. I would be happy with less, but there's no way I'm going to let this sour our relationship. So I accommodate her as best I can. Sometimes I don't have much interest, but she gets my penis up anyway and we make love. If we don't get it up, I service her with my tongue and hand. I usually don't get highly aroused with that, but I feel good giving her pleasure. It's a fair trade-off.

CAUSES OF DESIRE PROBLEMS

Problems of sexual desire and frequency usually stem from one of two factors: different preferences, or obstacles to desire or willingness.

Difference in Sexual Preferences

Difference in preference for sexual frequency has barely been mentioned in the professional literature, yet I consider it to be crucial to an understanding of desire discrepancies. We assume that couples are or should be well matched sexually; in the words of another era, they should be sexually compatible. Both partners should want sex about, say, twice a week. If that's not the case, there must be some block or problem. But why should they agree on sexual frequency? Couples disagree on many things: how often to go out or have company in, how to raise children or even whether to have them, whether to squeeze the toothpaste tube from the top or the bottom, and so forth. Why should sex be different?

My idea is that by the time people reach the age of twenty-five or thirty, they have arrived at some natural or preferred level of sexual frequency. Some people, for example, really like sex. Almost everything turns them on and makes them desire sex. Most of us can easily think of a man who fits this pattern, but so do some women. Witness the heroine in Peter Benchley's novel *The Deep:*

> To Gail, sex was a vehicle for expressing everything—delight, anger, hunger, love, frustration, annoyance, even outrage. As an alcoholic can find any excuse for a drink, so Gail could make anything, from the first fallen leaf of autumn to the anniversary of Richard Nixon's resignation, a reason for making love.

There are also lots of women and men for whom very few stimuli evoke sexual interest or response.

Kurt is such a man. Even as a teenager, he noticed that his interest in sex seemed much less than that of his friends. He didn't think or fantasize about sex much and used masturbation only occasionally as a sleeping aid. The pattern continued in adulthood. A problem developed in his relationships because his partners all "wanted more sex than I did and would get upset when I rejected their overtures." Kurt was evaluated by several doctors and therapists, none of whom could find anything wrong with him. If left to his own preferences, he would have sex with a partner maybe once a month and masturbate two or three times a month when he had trouble getting to sleep. Although he said sex was "enjoyable" and he had no trouble functioning, sex didn't do a lot for him, and having it didn't make him want to have it again anytime soon.

You can get a sense of a person's natural or preferred level of sexual interest and activity by looking at his history. How much sex did he want and have over the years in different relationships? And how much does he desire and have now? People vary considerably in their answers.

Unfortunately, just as people who squeeze the toothpaste tube from the bottom often marry people who squeeze from the top, so people who want sex once a month often marry people who want it five times a week. And that's a real problem. There may be no blocks, no barriers, nothing neurotic, and nothing weird, just different preferences. This is no different from a couple in which one person needs physical activity almost every day—jogging, swimming, or what have you—and the other is quite sedentary. Neither one is crazy; they just have different patterns.

It's important in cases like this to look at both ends and not just focus on bringing up the desire of the one who wants less sex. It may be just as necessary to decrease the desire of the one who wants more sex; maybe Gail can find other satisfying ways of celebrating the first day of spring than by having sex.

Obstacles to Desire or Willingness

Below I discuss some of the most common inhibitors of desire or the willingness to act on it. I start with obstacles having to do with medical and drug issues.

▲ **Low hormone levels.** Testosterone is the desire hormone in both women and men. If there's little or no desire—no sexual thoughts or fantasies, no appetite for sex alone or with a partner—you should definitely talk to a physician and get your hormones checked.

▲ **Medical conditions.** Any acute or chronic medical problem will tend to decrease sexual interest. If someone is chronically ill, there is a host of variables that may affect sexual interest and functioning. Among these are the effects of the disease itself, the effects of the patient role and the meaning the patient attaches to the illness, fears of rejection by the partner, and so on. Then, of course, there are the treatments—not only drugs, but also surgery, radiation, and so forth, any of which can affect one's desire and ability to function.

▲ **Drugs.** Modern medicine has been quite successful in producing a number of drugs with the unintended side effect of decreasing sexual desire. Many recreational drugs have the same effect. See the Appendix for a list of the drugs that can cause problems.

▲ **Depression.** Millions of Americans suffer from it, and a great many of them experience decreased interest in sex. If someone has lost interest in sex because of depression, the chances that sex therapy will work aren't very good unless the depression is treated first. If it's successfully treated, whether by brief psychotherapy, drugs, or both, the chances are good that no other treatment will be necessary. One problem to be aware of is that certain antidepressant drugs themselves cause decreased desire in some people.

There is an interesting exception to depression decreasing sexual desire. There are some folks in whom it produces the opposite effect: They want more sex. It's as if sex is the only way they have of gaining relief from the depression, so the more depressed they get, the more sex they want. This can cause huge relationship problems. There he or she is, very morose and hardly an appealing partner, yet wanting lots of sex. And it's hard to turn them down, even though they're not very attractive in this state, because you can see this is the only medicine that works for them. Obviously they need to see a doctor or therapist for help with the depression.

▲ **Dissatisfaction with partner sex.** This category encompasses a number of issues. Perhaps the sex you have with your partner isn't all that great. It seems like too much work for what you get out of it. Perhaps your partner isn't that attractive to you sexually; there are things about her looks, attitude, or behavior that make sex with her not appealing. Another possibility is that you're having difficulties functioning as you like; per-haps you have trouble keeping erections or delaying ejaculations. Not having sex is a way of not confronting these problems.

▲ **Dissatisfaction with the relationship.** If either partner feels unap-preciated, unloved, taken for granted, or in any other way discontented with or angry at the partner or the relationship, he or she may lose their desire to have sex with their partner. What is needed in such cases is recti-fying the cause of the discontent; in other words, work on the relationship.

▲ **Scheduling issues.** Some couples are so overscheduled with work, children, visitors, meetings, hobbies, and so on that they have neither the time nor the energy for sex. These couples often staunchly maintain their desire for a sex life, yet strongly resist any suggestion they change their schedules. Of course, being busy with busyness is a good way to avoid hav-ing to deal with deeper issues such as a fear of sex or closeness.

▲ **Fear of too much closeness.** Some men and women I have worked with seemed to believe that more sex or better sex would make them too vulnerable. They would end up feeling too close and too dependent on their partners and this would lead to huge problems. This fear caused them to avoid sex with their partner even when they were horny. They would find a reason not to have sex at all or to masturbate.

▲ **Sexual fears.** Millions of Americans, not all of them women, were abused as children, both sexually and otherwise. Some of these people have developed fearful reactions to sex. Although they may feel turned on, these feelings come into conflict with the fears, and a struggle ensues.

▲ **Tension about sex.** In many couples a tremendous amount of anxiety has grown up around making love. There has been criticism, hostility, or distance, often because of a problem such as not having much sex or an erection or orgasm difficulty. Even after the original problem is resolved, the strain remains. Instead of looking forward to sex as a joy, there is foreboding. As one man put it, "Although I love my wife and find her sexy, there's been so many arguments about how we make love, and how often, that when I think of approaching her, I get this terrible knotted-up feeling in my stomach. I have to take Alka-Seltzer to get rid of it—and that's hardly a turn-on." This couple needs to find ways to reduce their stress about making love and to increase their comfort and arousal with one another.

In many couples, more than one of the above reasons is operating. One woman was very unhappy about the lack of sex in her marriage and sought counseling. Her husband maintained he enjoyed sex with her, but even he couldn't remember the last time they had actually done it. At first he tried to brush off the problem by suggesting they were just going through a phase because of how busy they both were. When I asked what he was busy with, I got a clue as to what was going on. He absolutely glowed when he talked about his passion for old records—searching for them on the Internet and in newspapers, going to hear them, buying them, cataloging them, and listening to them and playing them for others. His wife started crying and said, "That's it—I want him to feel that way about me." The energy, enthusiasm, and excitement he manifested toward records certainly seemed similar to what other men feel for their wives. It turned out that this man had been raised in a violent family and had learned not to trust people; for him, it was far safer to put one's trust in the solidity of things. Getting close to his wife, on the other hand, was terrifying for him. Not having sex was for him a great way not to get too close. We worked in therapy for a number of months on reducing this fear, and as it diminished he approached his wife more often. While his interest in records continued, it did so at a much less intense level, and he spent less time with them.

The point isn't to have more sex or less sex. Rather, the only point is to arrive at an arrangement that satisfies the two of you, that makes each of you feel good about yourself, about your partner, and about sex and the relationship. The one who is more desirous should not automatically conclude that he is okay while his partner is deficient and needs to be changed. Both partners need to be willing to be open and consider solutions that will work for both of them.

TOWARD RESOLUTION

I devote the rest of this chapter to suggestions for trying to resolve the desire/frequency difficulties you are having. These are the kinds of things I do with clients in my office. I have arbitrarily divided them into six steps: enhancing the relationship; starting to talk about the problem; defining the goal; determining if there has been a change; determining if medical or drug issues are involved; and deciding what needs to be done. In reality, the steps often merge into one another and in some cases can be dealt with in one conversation. For other couples, one or more steps are sticking points and need lots of time and energy, even professional help. You should at least read over what I say about each step and not cavalierly dismiss any of them.

1. **Enhancing the Relationship.** Since resolving most desire problems requires a functional relationship and lots of talk, this is a crucial step. When couples can't agree on how much sex to have, things can quickly turn ugly. Both people end up feeling bad. The person wanting more sex (let's say it's you) feels unloved, undesirable, and cheated. All you're asking for is some loving. Why can't she just go along with that? Is it because she finds you unattractive, undesirable? Maybe, you think, it's because you're not a good lover. So you alternate between feeling angry and frustrated, on one hand, and doubting yourself, on the other.

The one wanting less sex doesn't feel any better. She feels always under attack; you're always after her for sex, and that makes her angry. She's afraid to be close to you in any way—holding hands, hugging, kissing, or snuggling—because you might interpret it as a desire for sex. At the same time, she feels guilty. After all, you're not asking for much. Why can't she just go along?

When it's the man who wants less sex, things can get even worse. After all, who ever heard of a man rejecting, even running away from, a willing partner? As one man in this situation put it: "The only word I have for it is *crazy*. I can't imagine any other man turning down sex, and if I could, I would say he's flat-out nuts. And that's what I think of myself."

Obviously, there are more than enough bad feelings to go around. As long as the bad feelings exist, they make resolution of the problem difficult. You should do what you can about any bad feelings between you and your partner. Get the relationship on as sound a footing as possible. The material in Chapters 7 through 14 can help in this respect.

You are going to need a lot of empathy for your partner. It is likely that you have been seeing her as willfully withholding sex and not caring about your needs and feelings, or as someone who's deliberately demanding far more sex than you can offer, constantly badgering you and making you feel guilty, and not caring about your needs and feelings. You need to try to understand her position. Can you see her as a person who is as hurt and frustrated by the situation as you are and who is doing her best to deal with it even though her best, like your best, so far hasn't had the desired results? The more you can truly understand her situation and the more you can truly understand that the two of you are stuck, the better things will go. It's extremely rare to find a villain in these situations. Don't create one; doing so is easy but only makes the situation worse.

You will also need empathy for yourself. You may well have been blaming yourself for being too demanding or not giving enough. Such thoughts, even if based on some truth, don't help. What we have is a problem: You aren't getting what you want and neither is she, but the problem can usually be worked out if both of you can keep cool, remember that you're in this together, and have some tolerance for each other and yourselves as fallible but lovable human beings. Do what you need to get to this place.

And try to keep in mind what I said earlier: The only reasonable goal is a situation that works for both of you and makes both of you feel good about yourselves and the relationship. With this perspective, chances are excellent the problem can be resolved.

2. Start talking with your partner about the problem. Whether or not you have talked before, what's needed is a relatively calm discussion where each of you gets to say what you want to say and where each of you listens to the other. This discussion could take only a few minutes, although that is rare, or it could consist of several sessions, taking several hours in all.

If you have already read Chapters 10 through 14, you have a good idea of what's required. Later in this chapter I give examples of how to open communication with your partner about the problem and negotiate for change.

3. Precisely define the goal. Try to define as clearly as possible what you want more or less of. On the more side, is it the feeling that your partner sees you as attractive and desirable, the feeling that your partner loves you, a sense of closeness or love, a sense of being important to your partner, a feeling of passion or excitement, more physical affection, more sexual contact (which could mean a number of things), more intercourse, more orgasms, or what? The more differentiated and specific you and your partner can be, the greater the chance that a solution can be found.

In some cases this part is easy. For example, Thelma and Chris had a good sex life until the birth of their son four years ago. Since then, the few times they tried to be sexual had been fraught with tension, with each blaming the other for their lack of a sex life. Their goal was simple: to return to the quality and quantity of sex they had previously enjoyed. What would be more difficult for them was determining how to get there.

Lenny and Marilyn's situation was more complicated. Marilyn had always wanted more sex than Lenny, and so much distance and hostility had built up around the issue that they were barely on speaking terms. Lenny felt that Marilyn was hounding him, asking for sex when she herself wasn't interested, just to make him feel bad. Although there was no evidence she was trying to make him feel bad, there was some truth to what he believed, because Marilyn is the woman I mentioned earlier who was going after sex in order to get her husband's attention. It turned out that, attention aside, Marilyn usually did have a greater interest in sex than Lenny. But she also wanted more of his attention and presence than he was giving. For his part, Lenny did want to make love with his wife, but he didn't want to feel hounded.

He was greatly relieved when he heard that Marilyn would want less sex if he would attend more to her in nonsexual ways: for instance, by listening to her talk about her day and her troubles with her family, and by going out with her more to events and activities they both enjoyed. He was also relieved when she said that sex didn't always have to include intercourse. This had been his big fear, that he would have to get aroused and hard every time she wanted sex. She realized she could often be happy if he would just give her a helping hand or hold her while she used her vibrator—assuming, of course, that he was present and did not drift off.

4. Determine if there has been a change over time. If someone's desire or willingness has significantly increased or decreased during the relationship, that change needs attention. The following exercise can help.

EXERCISE 24-1: WHEN DID THE CHANGE OCCUR AND WHAT LED TO IT?

This exercise can be done alone or with your partner. What you want to do is focus on the time just prior to the changed desire or activity. What happened during that time that may have contributed to the alteration of desire? Consider all of the following: changes in physical health or medications; changes in the relationship (engagements, weddings, trying to have or having children, affairs, big arguments, and so on) and in other important relationships (such as with your parents); changes in job (hers and yours); changes in living arrangements (moving in together, moving out, moving to another city); changes in finances; changes in how you feel about yourself; changes in friendships. If the answer isn't obvious, pull out old calendars, appointment books, and anything else that might jog your memory. If your sexual desire seriously changed in November 1998, it's probable that something else that happened in October or November had a lot to do with it. Knowing what that something is can help.

I did a version of this exercise with Jennifer and Chip, who had come to see me after almost a year of tension and bickering because of Jennifer's "loss of interest," which turned out to be more a case of loss of willingness. Although at first she said she didn't have any idea why her feelings had changed, she was able to pinpoint the time when they had; it was the week after she realized that they would have to move once again because Chip had taken a new job. This had been the pattern in their thirteen-year marriage. Chip was a professor and would take a post at a different college every two years or so. Jennifer felt that just as soon as she started making friends and feeling comfortable in a new city, they'd have to move. As we talked about this, she realized that the most recent time was simply the last straw. She felt that her feelings weren't even considered and that Chip just did whatever he wanted to further his career.

Chip was shocked. He hadn't even known she was unhappy about the moves. It's easy to jump to the conclusion that he was an insensitive lout, but Jennifer had never directly voiced her complaints until this therapy session; it's not even clear she had fully recognized how upset she was about them. Chip was deeply concerned about her unhappiness, and the two of them had a series of constructive conversations about what to do. As a result, Chip offered to make no more moves without Jennifer's consultation and agreement.

Although very little was said about sex, Jennifer's willingness to make love steadily increased as she became convinced that her wishes were being given fair consideration.

5. Determine if drugs, medical factors, or depression is involved. If your desire, or your partner's, is zero or close to it, or has sharply decreased, or if you are taking drugs of any kind or have a serious medical condition, or think one of you is depressed, it's a good idea to have a talk with your family doctor or a doctor who specializes in sexual medicine. Any of these factors can lead to desire problems.

6. Decide what changes can be made. After you have done the preceding steps, you are ready to negotiate for change, what you can do differently, what she can do differently. Sometimes these talks are relatively easy, at other times very difficult. Just remember that you're dealing with someone you love and keep your cool as best you can. As always, time-outs are encouraged when needed; name-calling, spacing out, and walking out are not acceptable. Here are some examples of how these conversations can go.

If there are already bad feelings between you and your partner about the desire conflict, you may want to write her a note like this:

I feel terrible about the conflicts and bad feelings we're having about sex. It hurts me to see you in pain, and I don't like feeling it myself. I love you and want to make things better.

I'd like us to have a different kind of talk than we've had. I'd like for each of us to get as much time as we want to say exactly where we're at. I'd be happy to go first, but I'd also be happy for you to start. When you talk, I'll just listen to what you have to say. When you're done, I'll summarize what you said to make sure I understand. I'd like you to do the same for me when I talk. At least we'll know we're hearing what the other is saying.

It's not easy being nondefensive about sex, especially after what we've been through, but I promise to do my best not to attack or criticize you, to listen as openly as I can, and to say exactly where I'm at. I hope you'll be willing to do the same.

I'd like to do this as soon as possible. This Saturday morning would be good for me. Does that work for you?

Now we turn to several examples of what to say when your partner wants more sex than you do. The reason for including all these examples is that the men in this situation I've worked with have had a great deal of trouble expressing themselves.

> YOU: I guess I need to be more open than I've been. The reason I turn you down so often when you initiate is that I'm scared I won't be able to get hard and give you what you want. See, when I initiate, that means I'm already turned on and either have an erection or know I can get one. When you initiate, I don't know that. I'm concerned that we'll start and I won't be able to deliver.

Here's another way:

> YOU: After thinking about it, I realize the reason I'm not more interested in lovemaking is that I haven't been enjoying it very much. I love you but I feel pressured and burdened in our lovemaking. I'm not sure this is how it really is, but it feels to me that I've got to do a lot of work. Even when you initiate, it seems like I have to spend a lot of time getting you ready and then a lot more time stimulating you to orgasm. Only then can I take my pleasure, and it doesn't feel to me that you do a lot about that. Maybe the way I'm seeing this is unfair and not how it is, but this is my perception and it's affecting my behavior.

Another kind of situation might call for something like this:

> YOU: I don't really know why I'm less interested in sex. All I do know is that I don't look forward to making love and don't take advantage of many opportunities. And I know this is making you miserable, which bothers me a lot. I wish I knew more, but I don't. I'd like to get to the bottom of this, but I'm not sure what to do next.

In this example, it would help if you could make a distinction between desire and action. That is, is it the case that you don't feel much desire (don't have many sexual thoughts, fantasies, or feelings), or you do but are not allowing yourself to fulfill those thoughts and fantasies with your partner? This is a crucial distinction.

If you're not having much desire for sex at all, that could indicate a physical or drug-related problem, or maybe high stress. Whatever the reason, your partner may feel a bit better knowing that the lack of feeling is general and not just about her. On the other hand, if your desire is greater than your willingness to have sex with her, you're making a statement about the relationship or how you feel about sex with her. This may not make her feel very good, but it clearly indicates where to look for solutions.

Here's another kind of situation:

YOU: I have less interest in sex than before because I'm exhausted and overwhelmed most of the time, especially in the evenings. I feel totally strung out. It may be different for the two of us. It seems to me that even when you're tired, you're still up for sex. But for me, when I'm tired and overwhelmed, sex just seems like one more burden. I realize that sounds terrible, but that's how it feels. I would like to change. I miss our lovemaking. But to make a change, something has got to give. If you're up to discussing it, I can go over some of the things I'd like to stop doing or do less often.

YOUR PARTNER: Go ahead.

YOU: The first thing is the meals. When you proposed that I cook half the meals, I thought it was a great idea. But now I don't. I'm not good at it, and it's a tremendous strain. After picking up food on the way home and cooking and serving it, I'm a wreck and not up for sex or anything. I want to stop cooking. I'm willing to pick up something already cooked and serve it, but that's all I can do. Or maybe we can eat out more.

And one more possibility:

YOU: I never thought I'd be saying this, but I think it's true. As you've pointed out many times, our lovemaking is good when we have it. We both enjoy it. So why don't I want more? The fact is that I'm scared. Often when we have sex, I feel incredibly close to you. All the barriers are down; I'm just fully open. I know that sounds good, but it's also scary. I don't know exactly why, but it's like I have to draw back from it. There's something threatening there. As long as we don't have sex too often, I can keep the scary part under control. But my fear is that if we have sex more often, I'll lose control of it. That's as far as my thinking has gone so far, but I wanted you to know where I am.

After having a discussion like one of these, the door is open for some kind of action. The man in the last example may want to talk more with his partner. Maybe together they can find out what's frightening him. Or maybe he'll want to spend more time alone trying to figure it out. Another alternative is for him to get professional therapy. And sometimes it happens that just giving voice to the fear will resolve the problem.

METHODS TO INCREASE SEXUAL DESIRE OR WILLINGNESS

Most of the following methods, with the exception of the first, can be helpful whether your concern is to increase or decrease sexual desire or activity. But since they're easier to explain if I take a consistent point of view, I'll focus on increasing desire or activity. By changing a few words in the exercises, they are equally applicable to decreasing desire.

Simmering

If the reason you're not having much sex is because you are not feeling much desire, and if this lack of interest is *not* the result of depression, drugs, relationship difficulties, or work stress, it will help to get your sexual juices flowing again. The simmering exercise on page 209 is an excellent way of doing this, and you should turn to it now.

Conditions for Greater Desire or Activity

There must be certain things that, if they were present or absent, would make you be more willing to have sex. These things are what I call conditions. You should do the conditions exercise in Chapter 6, substituting desire for arousal. That is, compare times when you felt greater desire with times when you felt less desire, or imagine what it would take for you to want more frequent sex. Another possibility is to just think about what changes in your life, broadly considered, would make you want more sex.

In looking for answers, consider all of these issues that can negatively affect sexual desire: fatigue, stress from any source, drugs and alcohol, the quality of the sex you have and any concerns you may have about your functioning, problems with children, negative beliefs about sex, and fear of too much closeness.

If your situation is such that you want to determine what would help you want less sex, adjust the wording of the exercise in that direction. The question in the exercise then becomes something like, "What would have to happen for me to want less sex?" What kinds of nonsexual activities might satisfy your desire for sex some of the time? Men I've worked with have often gasped in disbelief, "Only sex can satisfy my desire for sex!" But almost all found that's too hasty a judgment. Although it may be true that you desire sex three times a night, or five times a week, that does not mean that only sex can satisfy you. Many people who once thought that certain of their desires could be satisfied only by a cigarette, food, or alcohol have found that other things will do as well, or almost as well.

Improving the Quality of Sex

One reason some people don't want much sex is because the sex they have isn't all that hot. I'm not talking about a dysfunction here; they function fine, but it doesn't seem to be worth the effort. In working with a number of men like this, the problem has usually come down to a lack of assertiveness—they aren't going after what they want.

It took some time and effort before Daniel was able to locate the problem. The best sex he'd had in his life had been with women he didn't have a lot of feelings for. He was very forceful with them and went directly after what he wanted, which resulted in very high arousal. But now he was married and very much in love with his wife. He was much more focused on her feelings and pleasure than his own, which kept his arousal low.

One thing that helped was the idea of paying dues. By having lovemaking sessions where he focused totally on her pleasure, he felt he had paid his dues and earned the right to do the same for himself. So in the subsequent "Daniel-focused" sessions, he could focus more on himself and let himself go. Interestingly—and this almost invariably happens in such cases—his wife loved these sessions and didn't think he was being too self-centered. She too had been missing his excitement and passion. If being assertive with your partner is a problem, reading Chapter 11 will help.

Improving the quality of sex covers a lot of ground. Perhaps there's something about your partner's behavior that you'd like to be different. A conversation with her will probably help. Remember to focus on what you want her to do and not on what she is doing that you don't like. I recall one man who had lost much of his interest in sex and had developed sporadic erection difficulties, which further decreased his willingness to engage in sex. As we talked about how he felt about sex with his partner, he kept mentioning how "enthusiastic and active" she had been when they were dating. When I asked if she was still the same, he thought for a moment and then yelled, "That's it, she isn't. She doesn't fuck me back. I do all the work, and she's like a dead person." In the following week, he had several conversations with her about this, and also about her complaints, which had caused her to be less active. He was able to hear her and change his behavior accordingly. Not surprisingly, her behavior then changed. I got a big charge out of the message he left me one day: "Don't need another appointment. She's fucking back. Feels great."

Resolving Erection and Ejaculation Problems

A major reason some men lose interest in sex is because of an erection or ejaculation problem or the fear of one of them. Because the men aren't sure they can have erections when required or last as long as their partners want, it seems easier just not to have sex at all. If you think this might be your situation, the appropriate action would be to resolve the erection or ejaculation problem. You should turn to the relevant chapters for information and decide, with your partner, whether you want to use the appropriate exercises in this book to work on your problem or to see a sex therapist. Whatever the two of you decide, do it!

Scheduling and Having Time Together

See the discussion in Chapter 9 and follow the suggestions for making time to have fun together.

Having Sex in the Absence of Strong Desire

The model of sex we all hold is that desire motivates us to act; that is, we feel an inner urge and this makes us move toward our partner. Although there is nothing wrong with this model and it often reflects reality, it isn't the only possibility. Take, for example, Gunther, who I quoted earlier.

Although his wife wanted more sex than he did, he often went along in order not to "sour our relationship." And it's clear he invariably felt good about having sex with her even though he initially lacked desire.

Many of us have experienced something similar with physical exercise. Although I've been an exercise buff since I was a child, there are days when I just don't feel like working out. But I usually do anyway—unless I'm physically ill—because I know it's good for me and also because I generally enjoy it once I get started. And I am always glad I did it afterward.

I'm not suggesting you have sex when doing so would make you feel coerced or feel bad about yourself. But if there's anything positive about the idea of sex on a particular occasion—knowing you might get into it as the action proceeds, knowing it's important for your relationship, wanting to satisfy your partner—why not go along and see what happens?

Men and women who make it a practice to have sex in the absence of strong desire often find that in the long run their desire increases. (Be sure, however, to resist the temptation to try to force erections or orgasms.) If you discover having sex without desire brings up strong feelings of fear or anger, that in itself may be beneficial by putting you in touch with what's getting in your way. You should discuss these obstacles with your partner and, if necessary, with a therapist.

WHEN SHE'S LESS INTERESTED THAN YOU ARE

The best thing you can do in this situation is to help your partner talk to you about what's going on with her. In order for that to happen, she needs to feel that she can trust you not to judge her responses or to use them against her. If you've been critical of her comments in the past, you need to apologize and assure her that it won't happen again. You want to hear what's going on with her, and you want the two of you to be able to resolve the issue in a way that honors both of you.

You may well hear things you don't like. That may not seem like an enticing prospect, but I assure you it's a good one. I say this in all seriousness because if it's true that her relative lack of interest or willingness has to do with your behavior (you're not romantic enough, you don't do things she likes, and so on), you're in a great position to change your behavior and therefore to change hers.

What follows is an edited transcript of a conversation between a couple I saw.

HIM: I feel sad that you so often don't want to make love. I'd like to make this better for us. Could you tell me what's going on with you and our lovemaking?

HER: Every time we've tried to talk about this, you get defensive and we have a fight.

HIM: I know that's the way it's been. But we've got to talk, so I'm ready to listen. I promise I won't get defensive. I want to understand.

HER: Well . . . okay. But I don't want you to attack me. Promise?

HIM: Yes.

HER: When we were first together, you wanted to please me. You were very romantic. You told me how beautiful I was, how I turned you on. And you used to enjoy satisfying me. You'd take your time and do what I liked and make sure I had an orgasm before or after intercourse. But it's changed. I feel like you don't care anymore. You rarely tell me nice things, and you don't take time to turn me on. You give me a quick kiss and a touch or two, then you stick it in me and have your orgasm and that's it. I don't feel included or needed. So I've just turned off. And that's it.

HIM: Boy, that's really hard to hear. . . . Let's see if I understand. You're saying that I've become selfish. Instead of acting romantically, like I used to, and instead of making sure both of us are turned on and satisfied, I just do what's necessary to get my rocks off. Because of this, you've lost interest. Is that it?

HER: It sure is.

HIM: I can't say it's good to hear, but I'm glad I heard it instead of not hearing it. Tell you what. I need some time to let this sink in. Could we break this off for now and meet again tonight to continue? [In effect, he's asking for a time-out.]

HER: Fine. How about after dinner?

HIM: That's good.

HIM (LATER): What you said earlier was hard to hear. But I thought about it and have to admit you're right. I don't know how or why it happened, but it did. And I can see why you're not enjoying sex and not even wanting it.

HER: I'm glad you understand.

HIM: I want to change things. I miss the sex we used to have. Are you up for that?

HER: Sure, that's what I've always wanted. But you're going to have to put more time and energy into lovemaking.

It is also possible that what is bothering your mate has nothing to do with you. One client couldn't figure out what was going on with his wife. Although she had always seemed more hesitant about sex than other women he had been with, she had usually been a willing participant. Until, that is, they moved to California several years before, to the very city she had grown up in. As a child, she had been sexually molested by a neighbor for several years. This experience ended only when her family moved to another state. Coming back to the city of her molestation brought up all her old feelings of powerlessness and shame. She knew what was going on but was too ashamed to tell her husband until they were in therapy.

But it may also be true that nothing is bothering your partner and she just naturally has a lower sexual appetite than you. It's a mistake to assume that everyone else has or should have the same level of interest in sex that you do. If your partner enjoys sex, isn't hung up, yet doesn't want it as often as you do, you're going to have to work out some compromises.

It will not work to make her feel guilty. Many men do this. When their partners turn them down, they sulk for days until the partner gives in because she feels so guilty. This giving in is usually not a joyous event. It's clear she's doing it out of guilt, and with resentment for being coerced. The result is hardly ecstatic sex.

Far better, I think, to go over the list of sexual options with her and see what she's willing to do for you when you're in the mood and she isn't.

Here's a way one of these conversations might go.

YOU: I guess I have to accept the fact that you're not as interested in sex as I am.

HER: I think that's true. I enjoy our lovemaking and have no complaints about it, but I don't want it five times a week. That was true before I met you. Twice a week or so is about right for me.

YOU: I'm not sure where to go from here. You know me, I always want intercourse. But I read about the other options in the book and I think I could be satisfied with them sometimes. Do you have any interest in that?

HER: I've said many times that I'll be happy to get you off when I'm not in the mood.

YOU: I know. It's just a little hard for me to accept. I'm getting all the pleasure.

HER: I'm not excited the way you are, but why can't you understand it makes me happy to give you pleasure?

YOU: I'm trying, but it's a new idea. Okay, next time I'm in the mood and you're not, I'm going to ask you for something else. How about we agree to two things? One is that you accept only if you really want to. I need to know you're not doing anything you don't want to do. And the second is that I'll try to accept and appreciate what you can do. Is that a deal?

Now let's try a variation in which the partner isn't as agreeable as the one above. The man has just asked her if she'd be willing to get him off when she's not up for intercourse.

HER: I know the right answer would be yes, I'll get you off whenever you want. But I don't feel that. Sure, I'd be willing to do that sometimes, as I already have. But I'm not going to want to do that every time you want something. We have intercourse once or twice a week, and that's plenty for me. I'm afraid you're going to want something else every day, and I can't honestly say I'd be up for that. I'd rather do something else.

HIM: Like what?

HER: Lots of things. I think it could be very romantic to take a short walk with you before going to sleep. Or just cuddle. I love it when we lie in bed or on the sofa and just hold each other for a few minutes. Or a short body rub. You know how much I like them.

HIM: So there are a number of things you'd like to do sometimes instead of sex, like walking, cuddling, and body rubs. Right?

HER: Sure.

HIM: You'd also be willing to get me off when you're not in the mood for sex, but not every night. Right?

HER: Yes.

HIM: What about this? I'll ask for what I want, and you feel free to answer as you want. If I ask for sex and you don't want that, you say no and also suggest what you want to do. One more thing: You feel free to request a body rub or a walk when that's what you feel like doing. How's that?

HER: Sounds perfect, but I'm worried you'll sulk when I refuse you sex. That's happened so many times. That doesn't make me want to suggest a walk.

HIM: I'm going to have to learn not to do that, to just accept your refusal without taking it personally. You know what would help? If you could make the rejection a little easier. Instead of just saying you're not in the mood, maybe you could say, "I'm not up for sex now, but I'd love to be with you. What about some cuddling?" That would soften the blow.

HER: You're asking me to show I care even though I don't want sex. That's very reasonable, and I'll do that.

MIND POWER FOR DESIRE PROBLEMS

Getting your mind on your side is an important part of resolving desire and frequency complaints. Since these complaints often involve a feeling of discouragement for one or both partners ("We'll never find a solution"), it's important to combat these discouraging thoughts with positive statements. I've given a number of examples of using positive self-statements in Chapter 19 and will not repeat them here. You should reread that chapter at your convenience and develop a number of positive statements to use. The more hopeful you feel about finding a solution, the better the chances of finding one.

The partner who wants less sex often feels inadequate or guilty ("I should want to make love more often" or "It's not fair to deny her the love-making she wants"). When you're aware of telling yourself things like this, argue with the statement and change it. For example: "I'm not a bad person and I'm not denying her. We just have different appetites. But we're working on it and will come up with something better."

Since monstrification of partners frequently happens in couples with desire/frequency differences, it's important to remind yourself as often as possible that your partner is not a demanding or withholding bitch. She's not a bad person, and neither are you. You just have some differences that need to be worked out.

Another helpful technique is mental rehearsal. In a number of the examples above, people promised to do certain things—for example, to ask for sex or something else, or to react in a certain way when they are turned down. Since these promises may be easier made than kept, rehearsing in your mind how you will do what you promised can help. The more often you imagine asking for sex when you want it, for example, the better the chances you will actually do it. The same is true for reacting in a given way when you get rebuffed. If you have said that you will respond to a rejection by asking for something else, you can make a mental movie that goes something like this: You make a sexual advance; she says she's not interested; you tell yourself, "It's no big deal"; you suggest something else to do or are open and interested as she suggests something else. Run through this mental movie as many times as possible.

When the typical frequency problem recurs, and you can be sure it will, make every effort not to let it get you down. Instead of telling yourself that this is further proof that you'll never resolve the problem, ask yourself what you can learn from the experience. Maybe you need to do more mental rehearsing of how you want to react when she turns you down, or maybe you need more practice with new ways of initiating sex. Then tell yourself something like this: "No reason to get upset. We tried, but were both tired and just got back into old habits again. I have to be careful about initiating when I'm tired, and I need a lot more rehearsing on not getting upset when she says no."

And last, don't forget the self–pep talk exercise in Chapter 19. Use it whenever you feel discouraged or think you failed in something you said you would do.

The suggestions in this chapter have been helpful to many couples with complaints about sexual frequency. If you find you can't put them into practice or that they don't work for you and your partner, make an appointment with a competent sex therapist. The sooner you do this, the better the chances you'll achieve the results you want.

Appendix:
The Effects of Drugs
on Male Sexuality

The issue of drug effects on sexuality is complex, and the following discussion and charts are intended to be suggestive rather than exhaustive. The charts comprise three major categories: prescription drugs that may cause adverse sexual side effects, street drugs including tobacco and alcohol, and prescription drugs that have beneficial effects on sex.

In dealing with drugs, prescribed or not, it is crucial to understand that they are not innocuous substances. Any drug you take can have serious side effects. Even aspirin, probably the most widely used over-the-counter drug in the world, causes distressing side effects for many people.

If you consult a physician or sex therapist about a sexual difficulty, it is crucial that you inform them of all chemicals you are putting into your body.

PRESCRIPTION DRUGS WITH ADVERSE EFFECTS

The main thing that needs to be said about these drugs is that **under no circumstances should you fiddle with dosages or stop taking them without the consultation of a physician who is knowledgeable about drugs and your medical and sexual situation**. If you think a prescribed drug you are taking may have something to do with a sex problem you are having, talk to the physician who prescribed it or with a physician who specializes in sexual problems.

It is also important to understand that hardly any drug has the same effects on all the people who take it. A drug that is known to have adverse effects, for instance, may have these effects on only 10 to 15 percent of the men who take it. So even if you have an erection problem and are taking a medicine known to produce this result in some people, this does not mean the drug is the cause of your erection problem. It may be, and then again it may not be.

Some detective work is needed to determine what is going on. **Such work should always be done in conjunction with a physician.** Perhaps a different dose of the same drug will help, or a different drug in the same category. Or perhaps the drug is having the adverse sexual effect only in conjunction with other drugs you are taking. There is also the possibility that the drug has nothing to do with your erection problem. If, for instance, you are having trouble keeping an erection with your partner but not with masturbation, it's doubtful that the drug is what needs changing. Sex therapy, either with a qualified professional or by using the appropriate exercises in this book, may help.

We have not differentiated between drugs that cause negative sexual effects on large numbers of users and those that cause these effects in a small percentage of users. If there are any reports of negative effects, the drug has been marked. Whether or not it is having a negative effect on your sexuality is something you and your doctor need to determine.

STREET DRUGS

These drugs, including alcohol, can have both positive and negative effects, depending on the amount. Many men, for example, find that small amounts of alcohol make them feel more relaxed and sexier. But alcohol is a central nervous system depressant, and too much can lead to difficulty with erections in both the short and long run. Marijuana and cocaine have been used by some to enhance sex, and there are reports that they increase desire and confer the ability to delay ejaculation longer than usual. But at higher doses and over the long haul they cause erection and ejaculation problems. MDMA, or Ecstasy, can make people who take it feel closer to their partner and allow them to delay ejaculation. We don't have information about its effects with high doses and over time. The vast majority of street drugs can cause sexual enhancement in low doses and sexual dysfunctions of various kinds with increased doses or prolonged use. And virtually every single one of these drugs causes dependency or addiction.

PRESCRIPTION DRUGS WITH BENEFICIAL EFFECTS

This chart, unfortunately the shortest one, lists prescription drugs that have positive sexual side effects for some users. All of them are discussed in detail in appropriate places in the text of the book. If you would like to consider trying one of them, talk with a knowledgeable physician.

The following charts were prepared by John Buffum, D. Pharm., a leading expert on the effects of drugs on sexual functioning. Dr. Buffum is Psychiatric Clinical Pharmacist Specialist and Associate Clinical Professor of Pharmacy, University of California, San Francisco.

PRESCRIPTION DRUGS WITH ADVERSE EFFECTS
ON MALE SEXUAL FUNCTION

Cardiovascular Drugs	Decreased desire	Erectile problems	Ejaculation problems	Priapism/ painful ejaculation
Diuretics				
Bendroflumethiazide (Naturetin®)		X		
Benzthiazide (Exna®)				
Bumetanide (Bumex®)				
Chlorothiazide (Diuril®)		X	X	
Chlorthalidone (Hygroton®)		X		
Cyclothiazide (Anhydron®)				
Furosemide (Lasix®)		X		
Hydrochlorothiazide (Hydrodiuril®)	X	X		
Hydroflumethiazide (Diucardin®, Saluron®)				
Indapamide (Lozol®)				
Methyclothiazide (Enduron®)				
Metolazone (Diulo®, Zaroxolyn®)				
Polythiazide (Renese®)				
Quinethazone (Hydromox®)				
Spironolactone (Aldactone®)	X	X		
Torsemide (Demadex®)				
Trichlormethiazide (Metahydrin®, Naqua®)				
Beta-adrenergic blockers				
Acebutolol (Sectral®)		X		
Atenolol (Tenormin®)		X		
Betaxolol (Kerlone®, Betoptic®)				
Bisoprolol (Zebeta®)		X		
Carteolol (Cartrol™)		X		
Carvedilol (Coreg®)	X	X		
Labetalol (Normodyne®, Trandate®)		X	X	
Metoprolol (Lopressor®, Toprol XL®)		X		
Nadolol (Corgard®)		X		
Penbutolol (Levatol™)		X		
Pindolol (Visken®)		X		
Propranolol (Inderal®)	X	X		
Sotalol (Betapace®)		X		
Timolol (Blocadren®)	X	X	X	

P = Priapism/Painful erection   E = Painful ejaculation

PRESCRIPTION DRUGS WITH ADVERSE EFFECTS (CONTINUED)

Cardiovascular Drugs (cont'd)	Decreased desire	Erectile problems	Ejaculation problems	Priapism/ painful ejaculation
Central-acting alpha-2 adrenergic inhibitors				
Clonidine (Catapres®)		X		
Guanabenz (Wytensin®)		X		
Methyldopa (Aldomet®)	X	X	X	
Peripheral-acting adrenergic inhibitors				
Guanadrel (Hylorel®)		X	X	
Guanethidine (Ismelin®)	X	X	X	X(P)
Reserpine (Serpasil®)	X	X	X	
Alpha-1-adrenergic blockers				
Prazocin (Minipress®)		X		X(P)
Phenoxybenzamine (Dibenzyline®)			X	
Terazosin (Hytrin®)	X	X		X(P)
Vasodilators				
Hydralazine (Apresoline®)				X(P)
Minoxidil (Loniten®)				
ACE inhibitors				
Captopril (Capoten®)		X		
Enalapril (Vasotec®)		X		
Fosinopril (Monopril®)		X		
Lisinopril (Prinivil®, Zestril®)		X		
Quinapril (Accupril®)		X		
Ramipril (Altace®)		X		
Angiotensin II antagonists				
Losartan (Cozaar®)	X	X		
Valsartan (Diovan®)	X			
Calcium channel blockers				
Amlodipine (Norvasc®)		X		

P = Priapism/Painful erection   E = Painful ejaculation

PRESCRIPTION DRUGS WITH ADVERSE EFFECTS (CONTINUED)

Cardiovascular Drugs (cont'd)	Decreased desire	Erectile problems	Ejaculation problems	Priapism/ painful ejaculation
Bepridil (Vascor®)		X		
Diltiazem (Cardizem®)		X		
Calcium channel blockers (cont'd)				
Felodipine (Plendil®)		X		
Isradipine (DynaCirc®)				
Nicardipine (Cardene®)				
Nifedipine (Procardia®)		X		
Nimodipine (Nimotop®)				
Nisoldipine (Sular™)				
Verapamil (Calan®, Isoptin®)		X		
Lipid-lowering agents				
Clofibrate (Atromid-S®)		X		
Colestipol (Colestid®)				
Cholestyramine (Questran®)				
Gemfibrozil (Lopid®)	X	X		
HMG-CoA reductase inhibitors				
Atorvastatin (Lipitor®)				
Cerivastatin (Baycol®)				
Fluvastatin (Lescol®)				
Lovastatin (Mevacor®)				
Pravastatin (Pravachol®)				
Simvastatin (Zocor®)		X		
Antiarrhythmic drugs				
Amiodarone (Cordarone®)	X	X		
Digoxin (Lanoxin®)	X	X		
Disopyramide (Norpace®)		X		
Mexiletine (Mexitil®)				
Procainamide (Procan®)				
Quinidine (Quinaglute®)				
Tocainide (Tonocard®)				

P = Priapism/Painful erection   E = Painful ejaculation

PRESCRIPTION DRUGS WITH ADVERSE EFFECTS (CONTINUED)

Psychiatric Drugs	Decreased desire	Erectile problems	Ejaculation problems	Priapism/painful ejaculation
Antidepressants				
Amitriptyline (Elavil®)	X	X	X	
Amoxapine (Asendin®)	X	X	X	X(E)
Bupropion (Wellbutrin®)	X	X		X(P)
Citalopram (Celexa®)	X	X	X	
Clomipramine (Anafranil®)	X	X	X	X(E)
Desipramine (Norpramin®)	X	X	X	X(E)
Doxepin (Sinequan®)	X	X	X	
Fluoxetine (Prozac®)	X	X	X	X(P)
Fluvoxamine (Luvox®)	X	X	X	
Imipramine (Tofranil®)	X	X	X	X(E)
Maprotiline (Ludiomil®)	X	X	X	
Mirtazepine (Remeron®)	X		X	
Nefazodone (Serzone®)	X	X	X	
Nortriptyline (Aventyl®)	X	X	X	
Paroxetine (Paxil®)	X	X	X	X(P)
Phenelzine (Nardil®)		X	X	
Protriptyline (Vivactil®)	X	X	X	X(E)
Sertraline (Zoloft®)	X	X	X	X(P)
Tranylcypromine (Parnate®)		X	X	
Trazodone (Desyrel®)			X	X(P)
Trimipramine (Surmontil®)			X	
Venlafaxine (Effexor®)		X	X	
Mood stabilizers				
Lithium (Lithobid®)	X	X		
Divalproex (Depakote®)				
Antipsychotics				
Chlorpromazine (Thorazine®)	X	X	X	X(P)
Clozapine (Clozaril®)		X	X	X(P)
Fluphenazine (Prolixin®)	X	X	X	X(P)
Haloperidol (Haldol®)	X	X	X	X(P,E)
Mesoridazine (Serentil®)	X	X	X	X(P)
Molindone (Moban®)	X	X	X	X(P)

P = Priapism/Painful erection   E = Painful ejaculation

PRESCRIPTION DRUGS WITH ADVERSE EFFECTS (CONTINUED)

Psychiatric Drugs (cont'd)	Decreased desire	Erectile problems	Ejaculation problems	Priapism/ painful ejaculation
<u>Antipsychotics (cont'd)</u>				
Olanzapine (Zyprexa®)				
Perphenazine (Trilafon®)	X	X	X	
Pimozide (Orap®)		X	X	
Quetiapine (Seroquel®)				
Risperidone (Risperdal®)	X	X	X	X(P)
Thioridazine (Mellaril®)	X	X	X	X(P,E)
Thiothixene (Navane®)	X	X	X	X(P)
Trifluoperazine (Stelazine®)	X	X	X	X(P,E)
<u>Sleep/antianxiety agents</u>				
Alprazolam (Xanax®)	X	X	X	
Buspirone (Buspar®)				
Clonazepam (Klonopin®)	X	X		
Chlordiazepoxide (Librium®)	X			
Clorazepate (Tranxene®)	X			
Diazepam (Valium®)	X	X	X	
Estazolam (ProSom®)	X			
Flurazepam (Dalmane®)	X			
Lorazepam (Ativan®)	X		X	
Oxazepam (Serax®)	X			
Quazepam (Doral®)	X			
Temazepam (Restoril®)	X			
Triazolam (Halcion®)	X			
Miscellaneous Drugs				
<u>Gastrointestinal drugs</u>				
Cimetidine (Tagamet®)		X		
Famotidine (Pepcid®)		X		
Lansoprazole (Prevacid®)				
Metoclopramide (Reglan®)	X	X		
Omeprazole (Prilosec®)	X	X		
Ranitidine (Zantac®)		X		
Corticosteroids				

P = Priapism/Painful erection   E = Painful ejaculation

PRESCRIPTION DRUGS WITH ADVERSE EFFECTS (CONTINUED)

Miscellaneous Drugs (cont'd)	Decreased desire	Erectile problems	Ejaculation problems	Priapism/ painful ejaculation
Antiandrogens				
Cyproterone (Androcur®)	X	X		
Ketoconazole (Nizoral®)	X	X		
Medroxyprogesterone (Provera®)	X	X		
Carbonic anhydrase inhibitors				
Acetazolamide (Diamox®)	X			
Methazolamide (Neptazane®)	X			
Antiepileptic drugs				
Carbamazepine (Tegretol®)	X	X	X	
Gabapentin (Neurontin®)		X		
Lamotrigine (Lamictal®)				
Phenobarbital (Luminal®)	X	X		
Phenytoin (Dilantin®)	X	X		
Primidone (Mysoline®)	X	X		
Valproic Acid (Depakene®)				
Other drugs				
Cancer chemotherapy agents	X	X		
Etretinate (Tegison®)		X		
Flutamide (Eulexin®)	X	X		
Hydroxyzine (Atarax®, Vistaril®)				X(P)
Indomethacin (Indocin®)	X	X		
Naproxen (Naprosyn®)			X	
Narcotic analgesics (morphine, codeine, etc.)	X	X	X	
Tamoxifen (Nolvadex®)		X		
Thiabendazole (Mintezol®)		X		

P = Priapism/Painful erection   E = Painful ejaculation

EFFECTS OF STREET DRUGS ON MALE SEXUAL FUNCTION

	Acute, Low-dose	Acute, High-dose	Chronic	Withdrawal	Recovery
Alcohol	Increased desire Delayed ejaculation Decreased tumescence	Erection problems Delayed ejaculation Decreased orgasmic intensity	Decreased drive Erection problems Ejaculation problems	Decreased desire Erection problems; fewer nocturnal erections	Return of normal sexual desire and erections for most, but damage to erections and sex drive may be permanent in some cases of severe alcoholism
Dissociative anesthetics (PCP)	Sexual enhancement	Erection problems Ejaculation problems Decreased orgasm intensity	Erection problems Ejaculation problems Decreased orgasm intensity	Depression Decreased desire	No information
Opiates and opioids (e.g., heroin, morphine, methadone)	Orgasmlike subjective effects	Erection problems Ejaculation problems Pharmacogenic orgasm	Decreased desire Erection problems Ejaculation problems	Increased nocturnal emissions, morning erections, and sex dreams	Return to normal sexual functioning

EFFECTS OF STREET DRUGS ON MALE SEXUAL FUNCTION (CONTINUED)

	Acute, Low-dose	Acute, High-dose	Chronic	Withdrawal	Recovery
Stimulants (e.g., cocaine, amphetamine, methamphetamine)					
	Increased desire	Increased desire	Dose-driven desire	Decreased desire	Return to normal sexual
	Delayed ejaculation	Delayed or total	Erection problems	Increased erectile ability	functioning
		ejaculatory inhibition	Ejaculation problems		
		Erection problems			
Psychedelics (LSD, MDMA, MDA)					
	Increased intimacy	Ejaculation problems	No information	No information	No information
	Heightened genital				
	responsiveness				
	Delayed ejaculation				
Nitrous oxide					
	Increased arousal	No information	Erection problems due	No immediate	Erection problems slowly
	Increased orgasm	Probable decreased	to myeloneuropathy	improvement in	reversed
	intensity	sexual function due		erectile function	
		to anesthesia			

EFFECTS OF STREET DRUGS ON MALE SEXUAL FUNCTION (CONTINUED)

	Acute, Low-dose	Acute, High-dose	Chronic	Withdrawal	Recovery
Tobacco	Possible decreased erection (greater with increased age and diabetes)	Erection problems	Dose-driven erection problems	Possible return to baseline function, but erection problems may be irreversible with long-term use	Possible return to baseline function, but erection problems may be irreversible with long-term use
Volatile nitrites	Increased desire Enhanced perception of orgasm Facilitated anal sex Erection problems	Increased desire Erection problems	No reported chronic negative effects	None reported	None reported
Marijuana	Increased desire Increased sensuality Delayed ejaculation	Decreased desire Erection problems Anorgasmia	Dose-dependent increased/decreased desire Delayed ejaculation Erection problems Anorgasmia	Return to preexisting function (may include sexual boredom and premature ejaculation)	Return to normal sexual functioning

EFFECTS OF STREET DRUGS ON MALE SEXUAL FUNCTION (CONTINUED)

Acute, Low-dose	Acute, High-dose	Chronic	Withdrawal	Recovery
Sedative hypnotics (e.g., benzodiazepines, methaqualone, barbiturates)				
Enhanced arousal	Enhanced arousal	Decreased desire	Return to preexisting function	Return to normal sexual functioning
Decreased anxiety	Erection problems	Erection problems		
Delayed ejaculation	Anorgasmia	Ejaculation problems		

PRESCRIPTION DRUGS WITH BENEFICIAL EFFECTS ON MALE SEXUAL FUNCTION

Drug	Increased Desire	Increased Erection	Comments
Drugs Used for Reversal of Sexual Dysfunction			
Due to Illness			
Zinc salts	X	X	Reverses zinc deficiency
Bromocriptine (Parlodel®)	X	X	Reverses hyperprolactinemia
Testosterone	X	X	Reverses low testosterone
L-dopa (in Sinemet®)	X	X	Reverses Parkinsonian sexual dysfunction
Selegiline (Eldepryl®)	X		Treatment for Parkinsonism
Pergolide (Permax®)	X		Treatment for Parkinsonism
Injectable Drugs Used for Erectile Dysfunction			
Alprostadil (Caverject®)		X	Injected into penis, usually with papaverine and phentolamine
Papaverine (Pavabid®)		X	Injected into penis, usually with alprostadil and phentolamine
Phentolamine (Regitine®)		X	Injected into penis, usually with alprostadil and papaverine
Vasoactive intestinal polypeptide (VIP)		X	Injected into penis in combination product with phentolamine (Invicorp™)

PRESCRIPTION DRUGS WITH BENEFICIAL EFFECTS ON MALE SEXUAL FUNCTION

Drug	Increased Desire	Increased Erection	Comments
Oral Drugs Used for Erectile Dysfunction			
IC351		X	Investigational
Phentolamine (Vasomax®)		X	Investigational
Quinelorane (LY163502)		X	Investigational
Sildenafil (Viagra®)		X	Prescription drug
Trazodone (Desyrel®)		X	Prescription drug
Yohimbine (Yocon®)		X	Prescription drug
Yohimbe bark extract		X	Available in health food stores
Topical Drugs Used for Erectile Dysfunction			
Alprostadil (Muse®)		X	Urethral suppository
Alprostadil (Topiglan®)		X	Topical gel applied to glans
Nitroglycerine 2% Topical (Nitropaste®)		X	Applied to penis
Minoxidil 2% topical (Rogaine®)		X	Applied to penis for neurogenic erectile problems

References

Although space considerations preclude listing all the materials that have been helpful in working with men and writing this book, I list those works that are of particular interest for further reading, and also document quotations and information taken directly from other sources.

Introduction

ix. "Challenging because masculinity itself. . . ." A survey conducted in the 1990s demonstrates that while images of women have improved since the 1970s, those of men have "soured." Men are now seen as jealous, moody, fussy, temperamental, deceptive, narrow-minded, and heedless of consequences. One of the researchers called the phenomenon "negative masculinity." "Stereotypes: From the '70s to the '90s," *Psychology Today*, November/December, 1998, p. 8.

xi. "New solutions have also emerged . . ." R. Rosen et al., "The Effects of SSRIs on Sexual Function," *Journal of Clinical Psychopharmacology*, forthcoming, 1999.
"Nondrug sex therapy has also become . . ." Numerous examples of the increased sophistication and flexibility of sex therapy can be found in R. Rosen & S. Leiblum, *Case Studies in Sex Therapy* (Guilford, 1995).

xii. "In this new edition, I draw on . . ." J. Gottman, *What Predicts Divorce* (Lawrence Erlbaum, 1994) and *Why Marriages Succeed or Fail* (Simon & Schuster, 1994). Gottman's actual therapy interventions are in *The Seven Principles That Make Marriage Work* (Crown, forthcoming, 1999) and *The Marriage Clinic* (Norton, forthcoming, 1999).

xv. "I suggest that it's not easy being a woman or a man . . ." Among the helpful works in recent years on how men get to be how they are and the price they pay are: J. Balswick, *The Inexpressive Male* (Lexington, 1988); W. Farrell, *Why Men Are the Way They Are* (McGraw-Hill, 1986); M. Kimmel & M. Messner (eds.), *Men's Lives* (Macmillan, 1989); A. Kipnis, *Knights Without Armor* (Tarcher, 1991); R. Levant & G. Brooks, *Men and Sex* (Wiley, 1997); M. Miedzian, *Boys Will Be Boys* (Doubleday, 1991).

Chapter 1

1. On manly characteristics, see D. S. David & R. Brannon (eds.), *The Forty-nine Percent Majority* (Addison Wesley, 1976), and J. Doyle, *The Male Experience*, 2nd ed. (Wm. C. Brown, 1989).

3. H. Robbins, *The Adventurers* (Pocket, 1966), 8; S. Sheldon, *The Sands of Time* (Warner, 1989), 353; C. Schuler, *Sophisticated Lady* (Harlequin, 1989) 8–9.

   "Nature had different purposes . . ." Sociobiologists are the people who most strongly, and in my mind most cogently, make the case for genetic differences between males and females. A good place to start is the outstanding book by D. Symons, *The Evolution of Human Sexuality* (Oxford, 1979).

4. "little girl burst into tears . . ." J. Kellerman, *Time Bomb* (Bantam, 1990), 1.

5. On the differences between girl-girl and boy-boy friendships, see M. Caldwell & L. Peplau, "Sex Differences in Same-Sex Friendships," *Sex Roles*, 1982, 8, 721–731; P. Erwin, "Similarity of Attitudes and Constructs in Children's Friendships," *Journal of Experimental Child Psychology*, 1985, 40, 470–485; L. Kraft & C. Vraa, "Sex Composition of Groups and Pattern of Self-disclosure by High School Females," *Psychological Reports*, 1975, 37, 733–734.

   The terms "face-to-face intimacy" and "side-by-side intimacy" were coined by P. Wright, "Men's Friendships, Women's Friendships, and the Alleged Inferiority of the Latter," *Sex Roles*, 1982, 5, 1–20.

   N. Mailer, *The Armies of the Night* (Signet, 1968), 16.

   D. Gilmore, *Manhood in the Making* (Yale, 1990), 11.

6. "Western societies long ago got rid of these rituals. . . ." To those who might argue that the Jewish bar mitzvah remains, let me suggest that it is

no longer a rite of passage. The thirteen-year-old boy still can't work in the adult world, still can't support himself, still can't vote, drink, or drive. There is no substantive way in which his life changes. Despite the ceremony, he remains a boy. On the relationships between fathers and sons, of over seven thousand men respondents to Shere Hite's questionnaire, "almost no men said they had been or were close to their fathers"; *The Hite Report on Male Sexuality* (Knopf, 1981), 17. As extreme as this finding seems, it doesn't differ that much from those in other surveys: S. Osherson, *Finding Our Fathers* (Fawcett, 1986), 6–8.

R. Heckler, *In Search of the Warrior Spirit* (North Atlantic, 1990), 38–39.

6. T. O'Connor, "A Day for Men," *Family Therapy Networker* (May/June 1990), 36.

8. J. Lester, "Being a Boy," *Ms.* (July 1973), 112.

A. Pines, personal communication.

Because of the emphasis on competition, strength, and self-reliance, men have a difficult time forming close friendships. On the basis of his research, D. Levinson states, "close friendship with a man or woman is rarely experienced by American men." *The Seasons of a Man's Life* (Knopf, 1978), 335.

9. D. Tannen, *You Just Don't Understand* (Morrow, 1990).

"They are slow to admit to illness . . ." A. Kipnis, *Knights Without Armor*, (Tarcher, 1991), 38–41.

10. J. Lester, "Being a Boy."

11. "He was after all . . ." C. Schuler, *Sophisticated Lady*, 87.

12. B. Cosby "The Regular Way," *Playboy* (December 1968), 288–289.

13. "Her hands left my neck . . ." Kellerman, *Time Bomb*, 121.

I. Wallace, *The Guest of Honor* (Dell, 1989), 223.

14. L. Barbach and L. Levine, *Shared Intimacies* (Bantam, 1981), *33*.

"For women, sex is intertwined . . ." J. Carroll et al., "Differences Between Males and Females in Motives for Engaging in Sexual Intercourse," *Archives of Sexual Behavior*, 1985, *14*, 131–139; M. Brown & A. Auerback, "Communication Patterns in Initiation of Marital Sex," *Medical Aspects of Human Sexuality*, 1981, *15*, 107–117.

Chapter 2

16. "magical instruments . . ." S. Marcus, *The Other Victorians* (Basic, 1966), 212.

17. "She was a month away . . ." J. Higgins, *Season in Hell* (Pocket, 1990), 52. J. Gardner, *The Secret Houses* (Jove, 1990), 58.

"That's right, honey, . . ." H. Robbins, *The Adventurers* (Pocket, 1966), 251.

18. H. Robbins, *The Betsy* (Pocket, 1972), 101–103.

21. L. Rubin, *Erotic Wars* (Farrar, Straus, Giroux, 1990), 9.
    "A man in a research study . . ." M. E. McGill, *The McGill Report on Male Intimacy* (Perennial, 1985), 194.
    "A woman in the same study . . ." *McGill Report*, 190.

22. The classic study of touching is A. Montagu, *Touching* (Perennial, 1971).

24. "Ike Vesper . . ." R. Gorton, *The Hucksters of Holiness* (Bart, 1989), 128.
    "Now all Alexis wanted . . ." R. Latow, *Three Rivers* (Ballantine, 1981), 113.
    On the difficulty men have saying no to sex, research indicates that men actually have more unwanted sex than women. Unlike women, however, most men who have unwanted sex aren't forced into it. Rather, they go along largely because of the fear of being thought less than men if they refuse. C. Muehlenhard & S. Cook, "Men's Self-reports of Unwanted Sexual Activity," *Journal of Sex Research*, 1988, *24*, 58–72.

25. E. Jong, *Parachutes and Kisses* (Signet, 1985), 340–341.

26. "She reached inside . . ." B. Sassoon, *Fantasies* (Pocket, 1991), 461.
    "She swears . . ." S. Sheldon, *If Tomorrow Comes* (Warner, 1986), 202.
    M. Puzo, *The Godfather* (Fawcett, 1969), 28.
    H. Robbins, *Dreams Die First* (Pocket, 1978).
    "She wailed . . ." D. Morrell, *The Covenant of the Flame* (Warner, 1991), 406.

27. "She captured . . ." H. Robbins, *The Adventurers*, 475.
    "The lingering kiss . . ." I. Wallace, *The Guest of Honor* (Dell, 1989), 226.
    "With Dax it's like having . . ." and "She looked at him . . ." H. Robbins, *The Adventurers*, 427, 386.

30. The original description of orgasm experienced as the earth moving is in Hemingway's *For Whom the Bell Tolls* (Scribner's, 1940), 160.

31. "Then Jeff rolled . . ." S. Sheldon, *If Tomorrow Comes*, 369.
    S. Filson, *Nightwalker* (New American Library, 1989), 176–177.
    "Alix felt as if . . ." E. Lustbader, *French Kiss* (Fawcett, 1989), 119.
    "You're good, Ezra . . ." I. Wallace, *The Guest of Honor*, 226.
    "Deeper, harder . . ." C. Schuler, *Sophisticated Lady* (Harlequin, 1989), 82.
    "With three violent thrusts . . ." and "Within seconds . . ." B. Sassoon, *Fantasies*, 428, 411.

32. "No wonder that faking orgasms. . . ." C. Darling & J. Davidson, "Understanding the Feminine Mystique of Pretending Orgasm," *Journal of Sex & Marital Therapy*, 1986, *12*, 182–196. See also S. Carter & J. Sokol, *What Really Happens in Bed* (Evans, 1989), 315, who claim that "almost every women has faked orgasm."

33. J. Collins, *Lucky* (Pocket, 1986), 344, 352.

Chapter 3

37. W. Brinkley, *The Last Ship* (Ballantine, 1988), 452–453.
39. Carol Ellison, "Intimacy-based Sex Therapy," in W. Eicher & G. Kockott (eds.), *Sexology* (Springer-Verlag, 1988), 234–238.
41. "women were given permission and encouragement . . ." See, for example, L. Barbach, *For Yourself* (Doubleday, 1975).
47. M. Brenton, *Sex Talk* (Stein & Day, 1972), 61–62.

Chapter 4

52. "The producers of these films . . ." Not only do they use the largest penises they can find, they also give them some help. E. McCormack, "Maximum Tumescence in Repose," *Rolling Stone* (Oct. 9, 1975), 56–71.
56. "The parts and how they work . . ." A useful book is J. Gilbaugh, *A Doctor's Guide to Men's Private Parts* (Crown, 1989).
60. W. Masters & V. Johnson, *Human Sexual Response* (Little, Brown, 1966). Much of our current understanding of sexual anatomy and physiology stems from this important work. The sexual response cycle is another matter entirely. See L. Tiefer's devastating critique, "Historical, Scientific, Clinical and Feminist Criticisms of 'The Human Sexual Response Cycle Model,' in J. Bancroft (ed.), *Annual Review of Sex Research*, vol. 2 (Society for the Scientific Study of Sex, 1991), 1–23.
60. A. Kinsey et al., *Sexual Behavior in the Human Female* (W. B. Saunders, 1953), 594.
61. Masters and Johnson discuss the sense of ejaculatory inevitability in various places in *Human Sexual Response*.
63. For men raped by women, see P. Sarrel & W. Masters, "Sexual Molestation of Men by Women," *Archives of Sexual Behavior*, 1982, *11*, 117–132.
64. Two good books for laypeople on the medical aspects of erection problems, as well as medical treatment options, are R. Berger & D. Berger, *BioPotency* (Rodale, 1987), and I. Goldstein & L. Rothstein, *The Patient Male* (The Body Press, 1990). R. Berger and Goldstein are prominent urologists.
65. Performance anxiety, now almost a household term, is a relatively new concept in sexology. It was first used by the founder of behavior therapy, J. Wolpe, in *Psychotherapy by Reciprocal Inhibition* (Stanford, 1958), and later popularized by Masters & Johnson, *Human Sexual Inadequacy* (Little, Brown, 1970).
68. L. Schover, personal communication.

Chapter 5

71. "Similar nonsense was promoted . . ." I have relied heavily on two excellent sources, from which come all the quotes. R. Deutsch, *The New Nuts Among the Berries* (Bull, 1977), and J. Money, *The Destroying Angel* (Pantheon, 1985).

    On the efforts to prevent masturbation, see A. Comfort, *The Anxiety Makers* (Delta, 1967), an excellent historical survey.

72. "one-third of births in colonial America . . ." J. D'Emilio & E. Freedman, *Intimate Matters* (Harper, 1988), 22–23. This work is probably the best history of sex in America.

    "A majority of boys . . ." "Sexual Behavior Among High School Students" CDC, *MMWR*, Jan. 1, 1992, 885–888.

    On the incidence of oral and anal sex, see M. Hunt, *Sexual Behavior in the 1970s* (*Playboy*, 1974), 198–200.

73. J. Brown, *Out of Bounds* (Zebra, 1990), 205.

    S. Carter & J. Sokol, *What Really Happens in Bed* (Evans, 1989), 310.

    S. Hite, *The Hite Report on Male Sexuality* (Macmillan, 1976), 340–358.

74. I. Spector & M. Casey, "Incidence and Prevalence of Sexual Dysfunctions," *Archives of Sexual Behavior*, 1990, *19*, 389–408.

    S. Carter & J. Sokol, *What Really Happens in Bed*, 311.

    S. Hite, *The Hite Report on Male Sexuality*, 1097–1098.

75. "Estimates are that about 70 percent . . ." M. Hunt, *Sexual Behavior in the 1970s*, and R. Levin & A. Levin, "Sexual Pleasure," *Redbook* (Sept. 1975), 51–58.

77. Kinsey's definition of a nymphomaniac is given in W. Pomeroy, *Dr. Kinsey and the Institute for Sex Research* (Signet, 1972), 317.

78. "A controversy has raged . . ." Feminist viewpoints are given in L. Lederer (ed.), *Take Back the Night* (Morrow, 1980), and a wide range of men's opinions are in M. Kimmel, *Men Confront Pornography* (Crown, 1990).

82. "Studies of sexual fantasies . . ." C. Crepault & M. Couture, "Men's Erotic Fantasies," *Archives of Sexual Behavior*, 1980, *9*, 565–581; M. Hunt, *Sexual Behavior in the 1970s*; D. Sue, "Erotic Fantasies of College Students During Coitus," *Journal of Sex Research*, 1979, *15*, 299–305; D. Zimmer et al., "Sexual Fantasies of Sexually Distressed and Nondistressed Men and Women," *Journal of Sex & Marital Therapy*, 1983, *9*, 38–50.

Chapter 6

87.   J. Brown, *Out of Bounds* (Zebra, 1990), 205.

Chapter 7

102.   "Having the kind of relationship . . ." The finding of an intensive study of couples says it all: "When the nonsexual parts of couples' lives are going badly, their sex life suffers." P. Blumstein & P. Schwartz, *American Couples* (Morrow, 1983), 203.

On the importance of communication, see S. Metts & W. Cupach, "The Role of Communication in Human Sexuality," in K. McKinney & S. Sprecher (eds.), *Human Sexuality* (Ablex, 1989), 150–161, and A. Pines, *Keeping the Spark Alive* (St. Martin's, 1988), 171.

107.   On the reactions of boys and girls to the first experience of intercourse, see J. DeLamater, "Gender Differences in Sexual Scenarios," in K. Kelley (ed.), *Females, Males, and Sexuality* (SUNY, 1987), 127–140. The best survey I know of girls' first sexual experiences is S. Thompson, "Putting a Big Thing into a Little Hole," *Journal of Sex Research*, 1990, *27*, 341–361. Many of the girls describe the experience as painful, boring, or disappointing, and many of them talk about it as just sort of happening without any intention on their part.

Chapter 8

I have relied on a number of sources for the discussion in this chapter on sex differences. One of them is a series of interviews I conducted with women at three different times: 1977, 1991, and 1998. There was only one question: "What makes a man a good lover?" The responses at the three times were remarkably consistent. Most of the quotes and examples in the chapter are from these interviews. Aside from the books and articles noted below, I also made heavy use of the work of sociobiologist D. Symonds, especially *The Evolution of Human Sexuality*, (Oxford, 1979), J. Daniluk, *Women's Sexuality Across the Life Span* (Guilford, 1998), and A. Moir & D. Jessel, *Brain Sex* (Lyle Stuart, 1991).

109.   "If the first space visitor . . ." Quoted in F. Pittman, "The Masculine Mystique," *Family Therapy Networker*, May/June 1990, 42.

111.   On men's style of loving, see F. Cancian, *Love in America* (Cambridge, 1987). Cancian is one of the few writers I found who treats men's style as something of value, rather than as an inadequacy.

The story of the man who washed his wife's car is in T. Wills et al., "A Behavioral Analysis of the Determinants of Marital Satisfaction," *Journal of Consulting and Clinical Psychology,* 1974, *42,* 802–811.

114. "In one study . . ." J. Carroll et al., "Differences Between Males and Females in Motives for Engaging in Sexual Intercourse," *Archives of Sexual Behavior,* 1985, *14,* 131–139.

117. "Male fantasies, for example, include more visual content . . ." B. Ellis & D. Symons, "Sex Differences in Sexual Fantasy," *Journal of Sex Research,* 1990, *27,* 527–555. This is probably the best study yet done on the subject.
     On the differences between the sexual thoughts, fantasies, and activity of women and men, see R. Coles & G. Stokes, *Sex and the American Teenager* (Harper, 1985); J. Jones & D. Barlow, "Self-reported Frequency of Sexual Urges, Fantasies, and Masturbatory Fantasies in Heterosexual Males and Females," *Archives of Sexual Behavior,* 1990, *19,* 269–279; R. Knoth et al., "Empirical Tests of Sexual Selection Theory," *Journal of Sex Research,* 1988, *24,* 73–89; and S. Hite, *The Hite Report on Male Sexuality* (Macmillan, 1976), 599–615.

119. Regarding the importance of touching to women, perhaps the most dramatic evidence comes from the answers of 100,000 women to a question asked by advice columnist Ann Landers. The question was: "Would you be content to be held close and treated tenderly and forget about 'the act'?" Seventy-two percent of the respondents said yes, and 40 percent of them were *under* forty years old. "What 100,000 Women Told Ann Landers," *Reader's Digest,* Aug. 1985, 44–46.
     "In a study of sexual fantasies . . ." B. Ellis & D. Symons, 1990.

121. "Only a small number of men have problems . . ." These men are called "retarded ejaculators" by sex therapists, and they certainly do exist. But theirs is by far the least common of the male sexual problems.

122. "Some men are uncomfortable . . ." N. Denny et al. found that women wanted to spend more time in foreplay and afterplay than did men. "Sex Differences in Sexual Needs and Desires," *Archives of Sexual Behavior,* 1984, *13,* 233–245. J. Halpern and M. Sherman also found that women wanted more physical affection after sex than did men; *Afterplay* (Pocket, 1979).

Chapter 9

126. Regarding the physical and emotional consequences of not expressing emotion, see S. Jourard, *The Transparent Self* (Van Nostrand, 1964), and J. Balswick, *The Inexpressive Male* (Lexington, 1988). Also see the fascinating work by J. Pennebaker, *Opening Up* (Morrow, 1990). His research indicates that the prolonged inhibition of important thoughts and feel-

ings is unhealthy and, further, that expressing these feelings—confessing,
as he puts it—promotes physical and emotional well-being.
S. Hite, *Women and Love* (Knopf, 1987), 5.

127. "25 percent of husbands were surprised . . ." E. Hetherington & A. Tryon,
      "His and Her Divorces," *Family Therapy Networker,* Nov./Dec. 1989, 58.
      My requirements for happy relationships are similar to the characteristics
      John Gottman found in his research on happily married couples.

Chapter 10

135. The research indicating that our emotions are generated and maintained
      by our thoughts has been conducted by cognitive psychologists and thera-
      pists. A good introduction, and a useful self-help book as well, is D. Burns,
      Feeling Good (Signet, 1980).
139. A. Pines, *Keeping the Spark Alive* (St. Martin's. 1988).

Chapter 11

148. On what assertiveness is and is not, the best source is R. Alberti & M. Em-
      mons, *Your Perfect Right* (Impact), any edition. This is the book that
      started that whole assertiveness movement.
151. Yeses and Nos: L. Barbach, *For Yourself* (Signet, 1976), 50–51.
154. C. Tavris, *Anger* (Touchstone, 1989).

Chapter 12

My ideas about listening, talking, and dealing with conflict have been significantly
influenced by informal conversations over the years with psychologist Dan Wile.
His book *After the Honeymoon* (Wiley, 1988) is not easy but can be very helpful to
couples willing to put out some effort. Two other useful works are J. Gottman,
Why Marriages Succeed or Fail (Simon & Schuster, 1994) and *The Seven Principles
That Make Marriage Work* (Crown, forthcoming, 1999).

166. On nagging, a study of divorced men and women had some interesting
      findings. Half of the women complained that lack of communication
      and affection was the main problem in their marriages. But the most
      common complaint of the men "was their wives' nagging, whining, and
      faultfinding." Hetherington & Tryon, "His and Her Divorces," *Family
      Therapy Networker,* Nov./Dec. 1989, 58.

Chapter 13

182. D. Wile, personal communication.
184. On forgiveness, a useful work is S. Simon & S. Simon, *Forgiveness* (Warner, 1990).
     "it has been estimated . . ." N. Jacobson, personal communication.
187. "it tends on the average to be six years . . ." J. Buongiorno, "Wait Time Until Marital Therapy," unpublished master's thesis, Catholic University of America, 1992.

Chapter 14

189. "Touching is a vital . . ." A. Montagu, *Touching* (Perennial), 1971.
191. A. Montagu, *Touching*, 192.
193. R. Heinlein, *Stranger in a Strange Land* (Berkley, 1961), 175.
196. These body rubs are similar in some ways to the sensate focus exercise Masters and Johnson give in *Human Sexual Inadequacy* (Little, Brown, 1970), 71–75.

Chapter 15

200. Many people, including some sex therapists, use *arousal* as a synonym for *erection*. But then they are faced with the problem of what to call the feeling or experience of excitement. Confusion is the inevitable result when they use the same term to refer to both. Clarity seems best served if we use separate terms for separate phenomena.
206. B. Apfelbaum, personal communication.
208. "Simmering . . ." B. Zilbergeld & C. Ellison, "Desire Discrepancies and Arousal Problems," in S. Leiblum & L. Pervin (eds.), *Principles and Practice of Sex Therapy* (Guilford, 1980), 79.
210. "collections of erotica written by women . . ." Two good ones are L. Barbach (ed.), *Erotic Interludes* (Doubleday, 1986), and *The Erotic Edge* (Plume, 1996).
214. Dr. Arnold Kegel started using this exercise with women who were incontinent after childbirth, and they told him their sex lives had improved. "Sexual Function of the Pubococcygeus Muscle," *Western Journal of Surgery*, 1952, *60*, 521–534.

Chapter 16

216. On the role of the clitoris in women's sexual pleasure, see S. Hite, *The Hite Report* (Macmillan, 1976), and W. Masters & V. Johnson, *Human Sexual Response* (Little, Brown, 1966), Chapter 5.

219. On women who can orgasm solely via fantasy, see B. Whipple, et al., "Physiological Correlates of Imagery-Induced Orgasm in Women," *Archives of Sexual Behavior*, 1992, *21*, 121–133.

"Three researchers . . ." A. Ladis, B. Whipple, & J. Perry, *The G-spot and Other Recent Discoveries About Human Sexuality* (Holt, 1982).

"the evidence for an anatomical structure is shaky . . ." W. Schultz et al., "Vaginal Sensitivity to Electric Stimuli," *Archives of Sexual Behavior*, 1989, *18*, 87–95.

221. On the physical similarities between male and female orgasm, see Masters & Johnson, *Human Sexual Response*. Regarding emotional similarities, the classic study is by E. Vance and N. Wagner: "Written Descriptions of Orgasm," *Archives of Sexual Behavior*, 1976, *5*, 87–98.

222. Masters & Johnson, *Human Sexual Response*, 1966, 76–78.

On the basis of her interviews and research, Susan Bakos concludes that "physiologically, all women are capable of having multiple orgasms, though probably less than 50 percent do." *Sexational Secrets* (St. Martin's Press, 1996), 192.

223. My sources for how women like to be sexually stimulated are, aside from my personal experiences, the following: conversations over the years with Linda Banner, Lonnie Barbach, Mary Buxton, Sandy Caron, Carol Ellison, Susan Hennings, Joyce Polish, Vivian Resnick, and Anne Weiwel; interviews I did with women in 1977, 1991, and 1998; and various books, including all of Lonnie Barbach's; S. Bakos, *Sexational Secrets;* and S. Kitzinger, *A Woman's Experience of Sex* (Penguin, 1988).

Chapter 17

237. "Surveys show that many men . . ." "Sex Partners Can't Be Trusted for AIDS Protection, Study Says," *San Francisco Chronicle*, Aug. 12, 1989, A-5; S. Cochran & V. Mays, "Sex, Lies and HIV," *New England Journal of Medicine*, 1990, *322*, 774–775.

238. The tragic story of Magic Johnson shows why using condoms is necessary for sexually active singles. The woman he got the HIV virus from didn't tell him she had the disease either because she feared the consequences of sharing this information or because she didn't know she was

infected. And he in turn didn't tell subsequent partners because he didn't know he was infected.

239. "A recent survey . . ." S. Cochran & V. Mays, "Sex, Lies and HIV."

Chapter 18

253. J. LoPiccolo's discussion of "good prognostic indicators" for sex therapy is similar in several ways to my list of ideal partner characteristics. He places particular emphasis on both partners holding realistic views of sexual functioning, on the woman being able to accept nonintercourse sex during treatment, and on the man believing that he can fully satisfy her without an erection. "Post-Modern Sex Therapy for Erectile Failure," in R. Rosen & S. Leiblum (eds.), *Erectile Failure: Assessment and Treatment* (Guilford, 1992).

Chapter 19

264. A. Ellis has published so many works it's difficult to know which to cite. Two of the most important are *How to Stubbornly Refuse to Make Yourself Miserable About Anything—Yes, Anything!* (Lyle Stuart, 1988) and *A New Guide to Rational Living* (Wilshire, 1975), coauthored by R. Harper.

265. On getting your mind on your side, there are a number of useful books. Among those I like are D. Burns, *Feeling Good* and *The Feeling Good Handbook* (Morrow, 1989); almost anything by A. Ellis; M. Seligman, *Learned Optimism* (Knopf, 1991); and one I wrote with A. Lazarus, *Mind Power* (Ballantine, 1988).

My summary of Greg LeMond's victory in the Tour de France is taken from two articles in *Sports Illustrated:* F. Lidz, "Vive LeMond!," July 31, 1989, 13–17; and E. Swift, "Le Grand LeMond," Jan. 1, 1990, 55–72.

Chapter 20

275. "It has been estimated . . ." I. Spector & M. Carey, *Archives of Sexual Behavior*, 1990, *19*, 389–408.

277. "According to a number of studies . . ." A few years ago P. Kilmann and I estimated that 75 to 85 percent of men develop better ejaculatory control in therapy: "The Scope and Effectiveness of Sex Therapy," *Psychotherapy*, 1984, *21*, 319–326. My current estimate—based on my own results, on

reading the therapy literature, and on discussions with colleagues—is a bit higher, but it applies only to men who stay in therapy for at least eight sessions and who are willing and able to do the homework exercises, including exercises with a partner.

278.   "rapid ejaculation is almost always due to . . ." In fairness, I should say that there may be a physical component for a small number of men. Some clients seem to be extremely sensitive to penile stimulation—that is, the same amount of stimulation that another man might describe as simply nice takes them very close to orgasm. One man like this who had the problem for many years and had given much thought to it said, "It's as if my arousal system is always in hyperdrive." My experience with such men is that although they need to spend more time than other men on the beginning exercises, they often do develop very good control.

Regarding the issue of how women have orgasms, S. Hite, *The Hite Report on Male Sexuality* (Macmillan 1976), and L. Wolfe, *The Cosmo Report* (Arbor, 1981), come up with almost identical figures: Only about a third of women reliably orgasm in intercourse and the rest, the large majority, require direct clitoral stimulation.

For information on antidepressants used to treat quick ejaculation, I have relied on the comprehensive review by Ray Rosen et al., "The Effects of SSRI's on Sexual Function," *Journal of Clinical Psychopharmacology*, in press.

282.   J. Semans, "Premature Ejaculation," *Southern Medical Journal*, 1956, *49*, 353–358.

287.   M. Perelman, personal communication.

Chapter 21

I could not have put this chapter together without the generous assistance of two psychologist/sex therapists, Joe LoPiccolo and Ray Rosen, and three of the most knowledgeable urologists in the country: Ken Goldberg, Irwin Goldstein, and Ira Sharlip. Aside from the specific references given below, I have also relied on R. Rosen, "Erectile Dysfunction: The Medicalization of Male Sexuality," *Clinical Psychology Review,* 1996, *16,* 497–519; R. Rosen et al., *A Process of Care Model: Evaluation and Treatment of Erectile Dysfunction* (The University of Medicine and Dentistry of New Jersey, 1998); and the proceedings of two conferences on the pharmacologic treatment of male sexual dysfunction, the first given in September, 1997, in Universal City, CA, the second at the American Urological Association, June, 1998, in San Diego.

302.   "It is estimated . . ." The estimate is formed by extrapolating from the results of the study that found that 52 percent of men between 40 and 70 have erection problems. H. Feldman et al., "Impotence and Its Medical

and Psychosocial Correlates: Results of the Massachusetts Male Aging Study," *Journal of Urology*, 1994, *151*, 54–61.

312. L. Sonda et al., "The Role of Yohimbine for the Treatment of Erectile Impotence," *Journal of Sex and Marital Therapy*, 1990, *16*, 15–21.

313. On vacuum devices, there are three important articles in *Journal of Sex and Marital Therapy*, 1991, *17*: R. Witherington, "Vacuum Devices for the Impotent," 69–80; L. Turner et al., "External Vacuum Devices in the Treatment of Erectile Dysfunction," 81–93; R. Villeneuve et al., "Assisted Erection Follow-up with Couples," 94–100.

     S. Althof et al., "Sexual, Psychological, and Marital Impact of Self-Injection of Papaverine and Phentolamine," *Journal of Sex and Marital Therapy*, 1991, *17*, 101–112; S. Althof et al., "Why Do So Many People Drop Out from Auto-Injection Therapy for Impotence?" *Journal of Sex and Marital Therapy*, 1989, *15*, 121–129; B. Fallon, "Intracavernous Injection Therapy for Male Erectile Dysfunction," *Urologic Clinics of North America*, 1995, *22*, 833–845.

317. J. McCarthy & S. McMillan, "Patient/Partner Satisfaction with Penile Implant Surgery," *Journal of Sex Education and Therapy*, 1990, *16*, 25–37; R. Lewis, "Long-term Results of Penile Prosthetic Implants," *Urologic Clinics of North America*, 1995, *22*, 847–855.

318. I. Goldstein et al., "Oral Sildenafil in the Treatment of Erectile Dysfunction," *New England Journal of Medicine,*1998, *338*, 1397–1404. A. Morales et al., "Clinical Safety of Oral Sildenafil Citrate (Viagra) in the Treatment of Erectile Dysfunction," *International Journal of Impotence Research*, 1998, *10*, 69–74.

320. "But a more serious problem . . ." M.D. Cheitlin et al. "ACC/AHA Expert Consensus Document: Use of Sildenafil (Viagra) in Patients with Cardiovascular Disease," *Journal of the American College of Cardiology*, 1999, *33*, 273–82. "Dying for Sex," *U.S. News & World Report*, January 11, 1999, 62–66.

Chapter 22

330. W. Masters & V. Johnson, *Human Sexual Response* (Little, Brown, 1966), 7, 252.

Chapter 23

341. W. Masters & V. Johnson describe their work with surrogates in *Human Sexual Inadequacy* (Little, Brown, 1970), 146–154.

343. "Other therapists I know . . ." One report of a very large number of cases

seen by a therapist-surrogate team is B. Apfelbaum, "The Ego-Analytic Approach to Individual Body-Work Sex Therapy," *Journal of Sex Research,* 1984, *20,* 44–70. Apfelbaum estimates that 90 percent of the cases were successful.

344. "this kind of therapy is not widely available . . ." One indication is that in a survey of the kinds of methods used by almost three hundred sex therapists, surrogate therapy was employed in less than 2 percent of the cases treated and was therefore the *least* used method. P. Kilmann et al., "Perspectives of Sex Therapy Outcome," *Journal of Sex and Marital Therapy,* 1986, *12,* 116–138. My impression is that this is simply because the vast majority of sex therapists don't work with surrogates.

Chapter 24

347. In 1977, Helen Kaplan criticized Masters and Johnson's sexual response cycle for not including a desire phase ("Hypoactive Sexual Desire," *Journal of Sex and Marital Therapy, 3,* 3–9), and Harold Lief reported that desire problems had become the most common presenting complaint in sex therapy clinics ("Inhibited Sexual Desire," *Medical Aspects of Human Sexuality, 7,* 94–95).

349. S. Leiblum & R. Rosen, "Introduction," in Leiblum & Rosen (eds.), *Sexual Desire Disorders* (Guilford, 1988), 12–13.

352. The willingness or motivation to act on sexual desire with one's partner is also part of the thinking of therapist Stephen Levine. His work is complex, subtle, and important. "An Essay on the Nature of Sexual Desire," *Journal of Sex and Marital Therapy,* 1984, *10,* 83–96; "Intrapsychic and Individual Aspects of Sexual Desire," in S. Leiblem & R. Rosen (eds.), *Sexual Desire Disorders,* 21–44.

353. P. Benchley, *The Deep* (Bantam, 1977), 63.

355. Relationship dissatisfaction and conflict—whether about things erotic or not—seems to be one of the most important reasons for desire problems. H. Lief, "Foreword," in S. Leiblum & R. Rosen (eds.), *Sexual Desire Disorders,* xii.

356. On sexually abused males, a subject one doesn't hear much about, see two books by M. Hunter: *The Sexually Abused Male* (Lexington, 1990) and *Abused Boys* (Lexington, 1990).

Acknowledgments

My heartfelt gratitude to the many people who made this book possible:

▲ The clients and workshop participants I've worked with over the last twenty-eight years, with special thanks to those who read and made comments on earlier drafts of the chapters.

▲ The many people who've called, written, and e-mailed me about the earlier editions of this book. By sharing their questions and concerns, these people and my clients provided the raw material on which the book is based. Many of their stories are recounted here, although their names and other identifying information have been changed.

▲ The friends and colleagues who read and commented on the changes made for this edition. Because of the very tight deadline under which they worked, their contributions were truly above and beyond the call of duty: Linda Banner, Mary Buxton, Ken Goldberg, Irwin Goldstein, Meg Keller, Joe LoPiccolo, Marilyn Mansfield, Lou Paget, Joyce Polish, Ray Rosen, Ira Sharlip, and Anne Weiwel.

▲ The friends and colleagues who read and commented on various chapters in earlier editions of the book or discussed the ideas in them with me: Bernard Apfelbaum, Robert Badame, Lonnie Barbach, Victor Barbieri, Dawn Block, David Bullard, Jill Caire, Sandy Caron, Isabella Conti, Gerald Edelstien, Albert Ellis, Carol Ellison, Suzanne Frayser, Joshua

Golden, Marsha and Allen Goodman, Jackie Hackel, Susan Hanks, Harriet Jacobs, Jo Kessler, Michael Kimmel, Arnold Lazarus, Sandra Leiblum, Joe LoPiccolo, Sumner Marshall, Diane Morrissette, Michael Perelman, James Peterson, Jackie Persons, Ayala Pines, Rebecca Plante, Richard Reznichek, Ray Rosen, Howard and Barbara Ruppel, Carolyn Saarni, Leslie Schover, Ira Sharlip, Deborah Tannen, Carol Tavris, Steve Taylor, Leonore Tiefer, Carol Wade, Anne Weiwel, Dan Wile, Robyn Young, and George Zilbergeld.

▲ John Buffum for preparing the charts in the Appendix and providing ongoing consultation about the effects of drugs on male sexuality.

▲ Marsha Goodman for helping with the illustrations.

▲ My agent of many years, Rhoda Weyr, always there with a sympathetic ear and good advice, and my wonderful and tireless editor, Toni Burbank.

Index

ABOUT THE AUTHOR

BERNIE ZILBERGELD received his Ph.D. in clinical psychology from the University of California, Berkeley, and is the former head of the Men's Program and co-director of clinical training at the Human Sexuality Program, University of California, San Francisco. He is in private practice in Oakland and is currently working on *Better Than Ever: Sexuality at Mid-Life and Beyond*, to be published by Bantam in 2001.